Birkhäuser Advances in Infectious Diseases

BAID

Coronaviruses with Special Emphasis on First Insights Concerning SARS

Edited by A. Schmidt, M. H. Wolff and O. Weber

Birkhäuser Verlag
Basel · Boston · Berlin

Editors
Axel Schmidt
University Witten/Herdecke
Faculty of Medicine
Alfred-Herrhausen-Str. 50
58448 Witten
Germany

Manfred H. Wolff
University Witten/Herdecke
Faculty of Biosciences
Stockumer Str. 10
58448 Witten
Germany

Olaf Weber
Institut für Molekulare Medizin und
Experimentelle Immunologie
Universitätsklinikum Bonn
Rheinische Friedrich-Wilhelms-Universität
Sigmund-Freud-Str. 25
53105 Bonn
Germany

A CIP catalogue record for this book is available from the Library of Congress, Washington, D.C., USA

Bibliographic information published by Die Deutsche Bibliothek
Die Deutsche Bibliothek lists this publication in the Deutsche Nationalbibliografie; detailed bibliographic data is available in the internet at http://dnb.ddb.de

ISBN 3-7643-6462-9 Birkhäuser Verlag, Basel - Boston - Berlin

Part of Springer Science+Business Media
Printed on acid-free paper produced from chlorine-free pulp. TFC ∞
Cover design: Micha Lotrovsky, CH-4106 Therwil, Switzerland
Cover illustration: With the friendly permission of Luis Enjuanes and SpringerWienNewYork (from: *Archives of Virology*, 2003, volume 148, pages 2207–2235, González et al.)
Printed in Germany
ISBN-10: 3-7643-6462-9
ISBN-13: 978-3-7643-6462-5
9 8 7 6 5 4 3 2 1

www. birkhauser.ch

In remembrance of

Friedrich August Johannes Loeffler

(1852, Frankfurt/Oder, Germany – 1915, Berlin, Germany)

Friedrich A.J. Loeffler was, with the discovery of foot and mouth disease (Maul- und Klauenseuche) in 1882, the first physician and scientist together with Paul Frosch to recognize a virus as a causative agent of an infectious disease within mammals.

He furthermore discovered *Erysipelothrix rhusiopathiae*, the cause of swine erysipela (Schweinerotlauf; 1885) and *Salmonella typhimurium* as the causative agent of typhus in mice (Mäusetyphus; 1891). Other outstanding scientific achievements were the discovery of *Corynebacterium diphtheriae*, the causative agent of diphtheria, in 1884 and the corresponding specific diphtheria toxin in 1889. This major finding was fundamental for the emerging research on antitoxic serum therapy of Emil von Behring (1854–1917) who was awarded with the Nobel Prize for Medicine in 1901. Friedrich A.J. Loeffler also found *Pfeifferella mallei* (*Pseudomonas mallei*) which causes malleus (Rotz) in horses.

Friedrich A.J. Loeffler accepted a professorship for Hygiene and Microbiology at Greifswald University, Germany in 1888. In 1910 he founded the first virus research institute in the world at the "Insel Riems". He became the President of the "Institut für Infektionskrankheiten" in Berlin in 1913.

He is one of the most outstanding researchers in history of in medical microbiology, virology and infectiology.

A. Schmidt, M.H. Wolff, O. Weber

Contents

List of contributors

Olusola Adegbunrin, Centre for Research on Environmental Microbiology (CREM), Faculty of Medicine, University of Ottawa, Ottawa, Ontario, Canada K1H 8M5

Andrea Ammon, Department for Infectious Disease Epidemiology, Robert Koch-Institut, Seestr. 10, 13353 Berlin, Germany; e-mail: AmmonA@rki.de

Kanchan Anand, Institute of Biochemistry, University of Lübeck, Ratzeburger Allee 160, 23538 Lübeck, Germany

Caroline R. Astell, Genome Sciences Centre, British Columbia Cancer Agency, Suite 100-570 West 7th Ave., Vancouver, B.C., Canada V5Z 4S6; e-mail: castell@bcgsc.ca

Mark Bartlam, Laboratory of Structural Biology, Tsinghua University, Beijing, China

Charlene E. Bush-Donovan, Bayer HealthCare LLC, 725 Potter Street, Berkeley, CA 94710, USA; e-mail: charlene.bush-donovan.b@ bayer.com

Dave Cavanagh, Institute for Animal Health, Compton Laboratory, High Street, Compton, Newbury RG20 7NN, UK; e-mail: dave.cavanagh@bbsrc.ac.uk

Jill J. Detmer, Bayer HealthCare LLC, 725 Potter Street, Berkeley, CA 94710, USA

Hans Wilhelm Doerr, Institute for Medical Virology, Johann Wolfgang Goethe University Hospital, Paul Ehrlich-Str. 40, 60596 Frankfurt/Main, Germany

Christian Drosten, Bernhard Nocht Institute for Tropical Medicine, Virology/Molecular Diagnostics, Bernhard-Nocht-Str. 74, 20359 Hamburg, Germany

Cynthia S. Goldsmith, Infectious Disease Pathology Activity, Division of Viral and Rickettsial Diseases, National Center for Infectious Diseases, Centers for Disease Control and Prevention (CDC), Atlanta, GA 30333, USA; e-mail: Cynthia.Goldsmith@cdc.hhs.gov

Rolf Hilgenfeld, Institute of Biochemistry, University of Lübeck, Ratzeburger Allee 160, 23538 Lübeck, Germany; e-mail: hilgenfeld@biochem.uni-luebeck.de

Robert A. Holt, Genome Sciences Centre, British Columbia Cancer Agency, Suite 100-570 West 7th Ave., Vancouver, B.C., Canada V5Z 4S6

Steven J. Jones, Genome Sciences Centre, British Columbia Cancer Agency, Suite 100-570 West 7th Ave., Vancouver, B.C., Canada V5Z 4S6

Arthur Chun-Wing Lau, Division of Respiratory and Critical Care Medicine, Department of Medicine, Pamela Youde Nethersole Eastern Hospital, 3 Lok Man Road, Hong Kong SAR, PR China

Marco A. Marra, Genome Sciences Centre, British Columbia Cancer Agency, Suite 100-570 West 7th Ave., Vancouver, B.C., Canada V5Z 4S6

Tony Mazzulli, Department of Microbiology, Mount Sinai Hospital, 600 University Avenue, Toronto, Ontario, Canada M5G 1X5

Wolfgang Preiser, Institute for Medical Virology, Johann Wolfgang Goethe University Hospital, Paul Ehrlich-Str. 40, 60596 Frankfurt/Main, Germany; e-mail: w.preiser@em.uni-frankfurt.de

Princess Margaret Hospital SARS Study Group: Po Oi Lee, Ping Tim Tsui(tsuipt@netvigator.com), Tak Yin Tsang, Tai Nin Chau, Chi Pong Kwan, Wai Cho Yu and Sik To Lai), Department of Medicine and Geriatrics, 2-10 Princess Margaret Hospital Road, Hong Kong Special Administrative Region, China

Zihe Rao, Laboratory of Structural Biology, Tsinghua University and Institute of Biophysics, Chinese Academy of Science, Beijing, China

Syed A. Sattar, Centre for Research on Environmental Microbiology (CREM), Faculty of Medicine, University of Ottawa, Ottawa, Ontario, Canada K1H 8M5

Axel Schmidt, Institute of Microbiology and Virology, University Witten/Herdecke, Stockumer Str. 10, 58448 Witten, Germany; e-mail: axel780961@aol.com

Loletta Kit-Ying So, Division of Respiratory and Critical Care Medicine, Department of Medicine, Pamela Youde Nethersole Eastern Hospital, 3 Lok Man Road, Hong Kong SAR, PR China

Johan Surtihadi, Bayer HealthCare LLC, 725 Potter Street, Berkeley, CA 94710, USA

Jason Tetro, Centre for Research on Environmental Microbiology (CREM), Faculty of Medicine, University of Ottawa, Ottawa, Ontario, Canada K1H 8M5

Olaf Weber, Institute of Molecular Medicine and Experimental Immunology, Rheinische Friedrich-Wilhelms-University Bonn, Sigmund-Freud-Str. 25, 53105 Bonn, Germany; e-mail: weberao@t-online.de

Manfred H. Wolff, Faculty of Bioscience, Institute of Microbiology and Virology, Stockumer Str. 10, 58453 Witten, Germany; e-mail: mhwolff@uni-wh.de

Loretta Yin-Chun Yam, Division of Respiratory and Critical Care Medicine, Department of Medicine, Pamela Youde Nethersole Eastern Hospital, 3 Lok Man Road, Hong Kong SAR, PR China; e-mail: lycyam@ha.org.hk

Haitao Yang, Laboratory of Structural Biology, Tsinghua University, Beijing, China

Sherif R. Zaki, Infectious Disease Pathology Activity, Division of Viral and Rickettsial Diseases, National Center for Infectious Diseases, Centers for Disease Control and Prevention (CDC), Atlanta, GA 30333, USA; e-mail: sherif.zaki@cdc.hhs.gov

Glossary

aa	amino acid
ACE	angiotensin-converting enzyme
AEI	antibody-enhanced infection
ARDS	acute respiratory distress syndrome
ARDS	adult respiratory distress syndrome
ATCC	American Type Culture Collection
BAL	bronchoalveolar lavage
BC CDC	British Columbia Center for Disease Control
BCoV	bovine coronavirus
BHK	baby hamster kidney (cell line)
BOOP	bronchiolitis obliterans organizing pneumonia
BToV	bovine torovirus
CAP	community-acquired pneumonia
CCoV	canine coronavirus
CCV	canine coronavirus
CDC	Center for Disease Control
CEA	carcinoembryonic antigen
CECoV	canine enteric coronavirus
CMK	chloromethyl ketone
CNS	central nervous system
CPAP	continuous positive airway pressure
CT	threshold cycle
CV	coefficient of variation
EPAP	expiratory positive airway pressure
ERGIC	endoplasmic reticulum-Golgi intermediate compartment
EToV	equine torovirus
FCoV	feline coronavirus
FIPV	feline infectious peritonitis virus
GI	gastrointestinal
GSC	Genome Sciences Center
HAART	highly active antiretroviral therapy
HAV	hepatitis A virus
HCoV	human coronavirus
HE	hemagglutinin esterase
HE	hemorrhaging enteritis
HEF	hemagglutintin esterase fusion (protein)
HEV	hemagglutinating encephalomyelitis virus

HRCT	high resolution computed tomography
HRV	human rhinovirus
IBV	infectious bronchitis (corona)virus
IC	internal control
ICU	intensive care unit
IEM	immunogold labeling electron microscopy
IHC	immunohistochemical (studies)
ILT	infectious laryngotracheitis
IPAP	inspiratory positive airway pressure
ISH	*in situ* hybridization
LoD	limit of detection
MBP	maltose binding protein
MHV	murine hepatitis virus
MPD	2-methyl-2.4-pentadiol
NCBI	National Center for Biotechnology Information
ND	Newcastle disease
NIV	non-invasive ventilation
NML	National Microbiology Laboratory
NP	nasopharyngeal
nt	nucleotide
NVRI	nosocomial viral respiratory infection
OIE	Office International des Epizooties
ORF	open reading frame
PDB	protein data bank
PEDV	porcine epidemic diarrhea virus
PEDV	porcine epizootic diarrhea virus
PLP	papain-like protease
PRCoV	porcine respiratory coronavirus
PToV	porcine torovirus
r.m.s.d.	root mean square deviation
RACE	rapid amplification of cDNA ends
RdRp	RNA-dependent RNA polymerase
RH	relative humidity
RLM-RACE	5'-RNA ligase-mediated rapid amplification of cDNA ends
Rt CoV	rat coronavirus
RT-PCR	reverse transcription-polymerase chain reaction
SD	standard deviation
SDAV	sialodacryadenitis virus
TAS	transcription-associated sequence
TCoV	turkey coronavirus
TGEV	transmissible gastroenteritis virus
TRS	transcription regulatory sequence
VLP	virus-like particle
WHO	World Health Organization

Preface

It is with great pleasure that we introduce the first volume of *Birkhäuser Advances in Infectious Diseases*. This book series will focus on relevant topics of microbiology and infectious diseases with emphasis (as much as possible) on emerging pathogens and related diseases. The series will also stress the inter-disciplinarity of the field and include "modern" aspects such as progress and new approaches in molecular biology, clinical aspects and modern insights relevant to human and veterinary medicine. In addition, questions of epidemiology, disease management, hygiene and prevention of infectious diseases will be discussed.

Emerging or recently classified pathogens are a great challenge in medicine. Therefore we focused the first volume of this series on the outbreak of SARS. The advent of SARS is a threat for people around the globe. Our modern technologies have figuratively transformed the world into a village. It is not a problem anymore for someone or something to travel to or trade with remote parts of the world. This traffic, however, reprensents a new opportunity to spread diseases, particularly such of infectious nature from tiny villages throughout the entire world.

The outbreak of a novel severe respiratory disease was first recognized in 2002 in Guangdong, China. It soon became clear that this apparent contagious disease was caused by a virus. The World Health Organization estimated an outbreak of 8,098 cases, with 774 resulting in lethality. Although each case is one too many, it is not the number that alarmed the authorities and people, but the uncertainties that prevailed. However, in an unprecedented effort, multidisciplinary teams identified the cause of SARS, the SARS-coronavirus (SARS-CoV) within weeks and suggested measures to control this novel threatening disease. Although of paramount importance in veterinary medicine, until the emergence of SARS coronaviruses had only been recognized as a cause of common cold in humans.

The challenge SARS mirrors the dynamic of viral diseases and reminds us of the ever-present threat of infectious diseases. The success in handling this challenge so far, however, underscores the importance of the progress that has been made in basic and applied research. We have been dedicated to develop novel anti-infective therapies and diagnostic systems. With respect to the plasticity of many infectious agents, this aspect remains a challenge.

The first volume of *Birkhäuser Advances in Infectious Diseases* reviews some of the current knowledge about coronaviruses with a special emphasis on SARS. The multidicplinary efforts that were made to identify the cause of SARS are described and diagnostic, clinical, pathological and therapeutic aspects of SARS are discussed.

All chapters are written by international experts and scientists in their respective field and we wish to thank all authors for their excellent and efficient collaboration despite their other duties and responsibilities. We especially would like to thank Dr. Beatrice Menz from Birkhäuser Publishing for the excellent collaboration, exchange of information and assistance within this ambitious book project. Finally, we wish to emphasize that the series editors are looking forward to suggestions, criticism and remarks from the reader, with the aim that this "young" book series may provide a benefit to its readership.

Wuppertal, Germany, August 2004

Axel Schmidt
Manfred H. Wolff
Olaf Weber

Coronaviruses with Special Emphasis on First Insights Concerning SARS
ed. by A. Schmidt, M.H. Wolff and O. Weber

Coronaviridae: a review of coronaviruses and toroviruses

Dave Cavanagh

Institute for Animal Health, Compton Laboratory, High Street, Compton, Newbury RG20 7NN, UK

Introductory remarks

From rags to riches, pauper to princess. Thus did Cinderella progress, literally overnight (well, three nights; Grimm & Grimm http://www.nationalgeographic.com/grimm/index2.html). Coronaviruses were described as being a "virology backwater", the SARS coronavirus (SARS-CoV; severe acute respiratory syndrome) likened to Cinderella, thrusting coronaviruses from the shadows to the spotlight in early 2003. Understandably, this is the view from a human disease standpoint; coronaviruses in humans are usually considered to be the cause of nothing more serious than the common cold. However, this group of viruses has long had a higher profile in the veterinary science field, most of our knowledge of coronaviruses being based on viruses of domesticated species – plus the mouse (Tab. 1). Most of the 40 000 000 000 chickens in the world annually succumb to infection by avian infectious bronchitis coronavirus (IBV), resulting in reduced production, including mortality. The death toll amongst newborn swine can be 90% when infected with porcine transmissible gastroenteritis coronavirus (TGEV). The names porcine haemagglutinating encephalomyelitis coronavirus (HEV) and porcine epidemic diarrhoea coronavirus (PEDV) tell their own story. Most of the coronaviruses replicate, at least initially, in either or both of the respiratory or enteric tracts (Tab. 1). Within a coronavirus species some variants may have a tropism for the respiratory tract, others for the enteric region, though usually causing pathology in only one of these regions. SARS-CoV might be an exception to this, it appearing to cause pathology in both tracts, although that might be strain dependent.

The advent of SARS-CoV served as a reminder of an important aspect that we already knew about coronaviruses, namely that their host range is greater than was often supposed. One of the human coronaviruses, human coronavirus-*OC43*, is extremely similar genetically to bovine coronavirus (BCoV), suggesting that these viruses might be capable of infecting each other's recognised host. BCoV, under experimental conditions at least, infects and causes disease in turkeys. Canine enteric coronavirus (CECoV)

Table 1. Species within the genera *Coronavirus* and *Torovirus*

Major host	Virus species	Acronym	Dominant pathology	Additional hosts
Coronavirus genus				
	Group 1			
Swine	• Porcine transmissible gastro-enteritis virus	TGEV	Enteric[a]	
Cat[c]	Feline coronavirus	FCoV	Enteric; peritonitis	Dog[b] Swine[b]
Dog	□ Canine enteric coronavirus	CECoV	Enteric	Cat[b] Swine[b]
Swine	• Porcine epidemic diarrhoea coronavirus	PEDV	Enteric	
Human	☼ Human coronavirus 229E	HCoV-229E	Respiratory; Enteric[d]	
	Group 2			
Swine	• Porcine haemagglutinating encephalomyelitis coronavirus	HEV	Central nervous system	
Cattle	Bovine coronavirus	BCoV	Enteric or respiratorye	Turkey[b] Humans?
Dog	□ Canine respiratory coronavirus	CRCoV	Respiratory	
Mouse	Murine hepatitis coronavirus	MHV	Enteric, Liver, CNS[f]	Rat[b]
Rat	Rat coronavirus	RtCoV	Sialodacryoadenitis	
Puffin	Puffinosis coronavirus	PuCoV	puffinosis	
Human	☼ Human coronavirus OC43	HCoV-OC43	Respiratory[d]	
	Group 3			
Chicken	Infectious bronchitis coronavirus	IBV	Respiratory (kidney)[g]	
Turkey	Turkey coronavirus	TCoV	Enteric	Chicken[b]
Pheasant	Pheasant coronavirus	PhCoV	Respiratory (kidney)[h]	
	Group 4[i]			
Human	☼ SARS-coronavirus	SARS-CoV	Respiratory, Enteric	Civet cat[j] Raccoon dog[j] Other?[k] Macaque[l] Cat[l,m]
Torovirus genus				
Swine	Porcine torovirus	PoToV	Enteric	
Cattle	Bovine torovirus (Breda virus)	BToV	Enteric	
Horse	Equine torovirus (Berne virus)	EqToV	Enteric	
Human	Human torovirus	HToV	Enteric	

[a]Some variants (often referred to as porcine respiratory coronavirus) of TGEV do not cause enteritis. They replicate largely asymptomatically in the respiratory tract
[b]Deductions from experimental infections.
[c]Apart from the domestic cat a similar virus has been isolated from a cheetah (*Acinonyx jubatus*) [261], in which it is widely detected [262].

(continued on next page)

[d]Although human coronaviruses have been shown to be associated with enteritis, their relatedness with the HCoV 229E and HCoV OC43 species has not been thoroughly investigated.
[e]The classical BCoVs are associated with enteritis, though there are respiratory forms.
[f]Central nervous system.
[g]Nephritis is not uncommon, though not all chickens are observed to be affected in this way. Notwithstanding, some strains of IBV are highly nephropathogenic.
[h]Nephritis has commonly been reported.
[i]SARS CoV has not been officially assigned to a group. It is placed here unofficially in a new group 4, on the basis that its structural proteins have very low amino acid identity with those of groups 1, 2 and 3, as is the case between viruses of groups 1, 2 and 3.
[j]Virus with ~99.9% genome sequence identity with the human SARS-CoV was detected in these species. Also, there was serological evidence.
[k]There may be one or more other species of wild animal that is the natural host of SARS-CoV.
[l]Infected experimentally.
[m]Cats might have been involved in the spread of SARS in some episodes of the disease e.g. the Amoy Gardens incident, Hong Kong.
The symbols ■□✲ draw attention to hosts that are known to be infected by more than one species of coronavirus, including species from more than one coronavirus group.

---

can cause disease in swine and cats. Indeed, a subset of feline coronavirus (FCoV) has been demonstrated to be a chimaera arising from recombination between an FCoV and CECoV. "Recombinant" was one of the spectres feared in the early weeks of the epidemic in Hong Kong. Subsequent sequencing of the genome has shown that SARS-CoV has not arisen by any recent recombination event. Notwithstanding, an appreciation of what has been learned from over half a century of studying coronaviruses helps to put SARS and SARS-CoV into perspective.

Delineating the roles of the various coronavirus proteins in pathogenesis and host range has been greatly facilitated by the development of procedures to make precise modifications to the coronavirus genome: targeted recombination for murine hepatitis virus (MHV) [1–4] and FCoV [1] and various "infectious clone" systems for HCoV-229E [5], TGEV [6, 7], IBV [73], MHV [8] and SARS-CoV [9]. Targeted recombination has been used to show that the gene order of MHV can be altered dramatically without reducing infectivity *in vitro* [10], demonstrating the plasticity of the coronavirus genome.

The family *Coronaviridae* comprises not only the genus *Coronavirus* but also *Torovirus*. Species in these two genera are morphologically very similar (Fig. 1), a prime reason for them being in the same family. Underlying this, they have similar structural proteins and overall genome organisation (Tab. 2). The *Coronaviridae* together with *Arteriviridae* and *Okaviridae* form the order *Nidovirales*, the members having some common features with respect to genome organisation, replication and transcription. The name *Nidovirales* is derived from the Latin *nidus* for nest, reflecting the large nested-set arrangement of the subgenomic mRNAs.

The first torovirus, Berne virus, now referred to as equine torovirus (EToV), was isolated in 1972, though no disease has been associated with it.

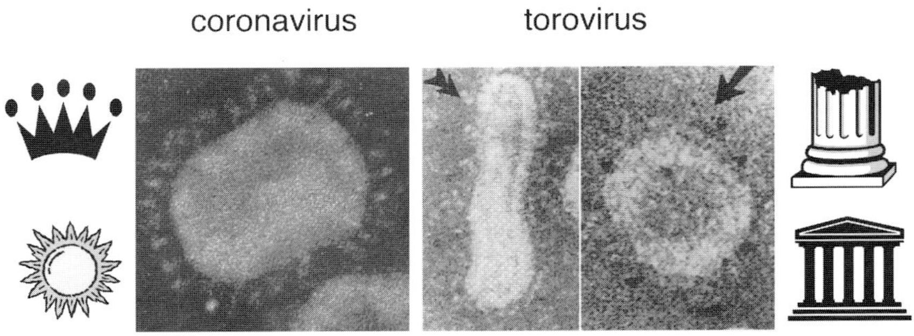

Figure 1. Appearance of a coronavirus (IBV) and torovirus (a human enteric ToV) by electron microscopy after negative staining. The appearance of coronaviruses was likened to that of some ornate crowns, the Latin for which is *corona*, and the corona of the sun, that also being derived from the Latin for crown, so *corona* was adopted for the name of this virus group. Toroviruses also derived their name from a Latin root, this time from *torus*, a semi-circular moulding such as is found at the base of a column. This name was chosen to reflect the appearance of the internal component of the virus which is torus- or doughnut-shaped (arrow). Some torovirus particles may appear rod-shaped (double arrowhead). Coronaviruses have a surface spike layer (20 nm) that may be more prominent than that of toroviruses. The shorter, 10 nm, projections on the torovirus particles in these pictures may be the haemagglutinin esterase protein rather than the spike protein which may be largely absent. (Reprinted by Duckmanton et al., 1997, by permission from Elsevier.) [265]

Similar viruses may infect a number of ungulate species, as serology has indicated infections with EToV-like viruses in cattle, sheep, goats and pigs. About 10 years after the discovery of EToV, a torovirus was shown to be the cause of gastroenteritis in humans, with antigenic relationship to bovine torovirus (BToV).

Superficially toroviruses and coronaviruses resemble each other; one could be mistaken for the other during electron microscope analysis (Fig. 1).

The key dimension of this review is breadth rather than depth, its purpose being to set the stage for the proceeding chapters. References to more in-depth reviews are given throughout this chapter. As the remainder of this book is about SARS-CoV, the major part of this chapter is on the coronaviruses, much less on toroviruses. Indeed, much more is known about coronaviruses than toroviruses.

Diseases in humans associated with coronaviruses and toroviruses

Whilst there is insufficient space within this chapter for a thorough description of all coronavirus- and torovirus-induced diseases, the advent of SARS in humans makes it appropriate to summarise what we know about other diseases in humans caused by coronaviruses and toroviruses.

Table 2. Features of coronaviruses and toroviruses

Feature	Coronavirus	Torovirus
Enveloped	+	+
Linear positive-sense ssRNA genome with poly(A) tail	+	+
5' polymerase gene-structural protein genes 3'	+	+
3' co-terminal nested set of ≥4 subgenomic mRNAs	+	+
Only the 5' unique region of an mRNA is translated	+	+
Polymerase gene has two ORFs, 1a and 1b	+	+
The 1b ORF is translated after ribosomal frameshifting	+	+
M protein has three membrane-spanning sequences	+	+
Virion formation at internal membranes	+	+
Genome size (kb)	27–31	~25
5' leader sequence	+	
Core shell	+	
Nucleocapsid (RNA plus N protein)	Helical	Tubular
Prominent S glycoprotein.	+	+
Coiled-coil structure in S protein	+	+

Adapted from [263] and [264].
The reader is referred to [59] and [32] for more detail of torovirus proteins.

HCoVs are generally thought of in the context of the common cold, some 25% of which are believed to be caused by HCoVs [11, 12]. Subclinical or very mild infections are common and can occur throughout the year. In a study of children with otitis media with effusion, HCoVs were associated with 10% of them, respiratory syncytial virus being associated in approximately 30% of cases [13].

There have been some reports indicating a more serious lower respiratory tract involvement of HCoVs in young children and old people. It is not clear that HCoVs infect the lower respiratory tract but the occurrence of HCoV upper respiratory tract infections coupled with other factors, e.g. in immunocompromised people, may cause more serious disease, including pneumonia [14]. Up to 30% of acute wheezing episodes in asthmatic children may be due to coronavirus infection [15].

A study in a neonatal intensive care unit revealed that all premature infants infected with coronaviruses had symptoms of bradycardia, apnea, hypoxemia, fever or abdominal distention. Chest X-ray revealed diffuse infiltrates in two cases. In a study of nosocomial viral respiratory infections (NVRI) in neonates (up to one month of age) who had been hospitalised, it was concluded that the incidence of NVRI with common respiratory viruses was low, HCoV being the most important pathogen in NVRI in the study [16]. Elderly patients who had been hospitalised because of cardiopulmonary illnesses, and who tested negative for influenza and respiratory syncytial viruses, were examined further. Approximately 8% were identified as having either HCoV 229E or OC43 [17].

Infections with respiratory viruses, of which HCoVs are but one, are commonly associated with asthma exacerbation. Coronavirus was detected in approximately 5% of children [18] and 22% of adults hospitalised because of asthma [19]. Allergic patients with a common cold, associated with a number of viruses, including HCoVs (25%), had prolonged nasal eosinophil influx [20]. Whether that would increase the risk of subsequent allergen-induced hypersensitivity reactions is not known. In this regard it is perhaps worth noting that it has been suggested that the lung pathology observed in human SARS patients might be associated with immunopathology.

Evidence has increased that toroviruses are associated with gastroenteritis in humans. In a case-control study of children, an antigen capture ELISA revealed torovirus in stools from 27% (9/33) of children with acute diarrhoea, 27% (11/41) with persistent diarrhoea and none in controls [21]. Enteraggregative *Escherichia coli* was commonly found in assocation with the torovirus. In another childhood study, electron microscopy revealed a torovirus incidence of 35% (72/206) and 15% in gastroenteritis cases and controls, respectively [22].

What it is to be a coronavirus or torovirus

IBV was the first CoV to be isolated, in 1937, followed about 10 years later by MHV, human coronaviruses being discovered in the mid-1960s. These viruses had a common appearance when visualised with the electron microscope (Fig. 1). This confirmed that they were enveloped viruses, approximately 120 nm in diameter, and showed that they had large (20 nm), club-shaped surface projections (spike protein, S). Toroviruses also have 20 nm spikes. Whilst toroviruses might be seen having a doughnut-shaped internal component (Figs. 1 and 2), this is not always evident, the two types of virus then being easily confused.

When visualised in clinical specimens the quality of image is not always good.

Even with cell culture-grown virus some negatively-stained preparations reveal the spike layer of coronaviruses poorly. Indeed, some virus particles may actually have few spikes. The globular part of the S protein of IBV has a tendency to dissociate from the stalk [23, 24]. Various sedimentation studies have indicated that the mature S protein is a homodimer or homotrimer [25], homodimer [26, 27] or homotrimer [28]. It has two functions; to attach the virus to receptor molecules on host cells, and to activate fusion of the virion membrane with host cell membranes, to release the viral genome into the cell. The structure, variation and functions of the S protein have been reviewed [29–31].

Electron microscopy of BToV revealed few of the 20 nm spikes but rather an intact fringe of smaller spikes, some 7–9 nm in length [32–34]. Toroviruses isolated from human faeces had an intact fringe of 10 nm spikes [33] that resembled those seen on human toroviruses by Beards et al. [35].

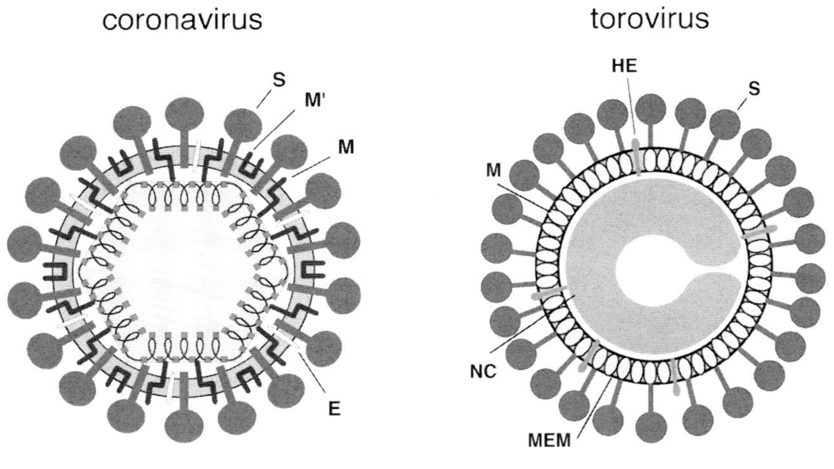

Figure 2. Diagrammatic representation of the virions of a coronavirus and a torovirus. Both types of virus have a lipid membrane (MEM), prominent 20 nm spike proteins (S) and an integral membrane protein (M). Group 2 coronaviruses, and some toroviruses, have an HE protein that forms a layer of 7 nm spikes (not shown). Coronaviruses, but not toroviruses, contain a small number of molecules of an E protein. Cryoelectron microscopy has indicated the presence of a core structure in coronaviruses, comprising a nucleocapsid (NC: N protein plus genomic RNA) and the carboxyterminal endodomain of the M protein (M). In TGEV some of the M molecules (M') have been shown to have both their N- and C-terminal parts on the outer surface of the virion. The nucleocapsid of toroviruses has the appearance of a torus (see Fig. 1). (Reprinted from González et al. 2003 [266] by permission from Springer.)

The latter reported observing the 20 nm spikes only rarely. It is possible that the 10 nm spikes are the haemagglutinin esterase (HE) protein. BToV has a HE protein that forms a fringe of spikes approximately 6 nm in length [32].

Apart from the S protein, all corona- and toroviruses have a smaller membrane glycoprotein (M; reviewed by Rottier [36]) and a protein closely associated with the RNA genome (to form a ribonucleoprotein, RNP), the nucleocapsid protein (N; reviewed by Laude and Masters [37]). The N protein of CoVs is much bigger than that of toroviruses (Tab. 3). Apart from giving some protection to the RNA genome, the N protein may also have roles in RNA replication and transcription, though this awaits demonstration. The N protein of both genera is phosphorylated.

Virions of coronaviruses have low amounts of a very small membrane-associated, non-glycoslyated protein, E (reviewd by Siddell [38]), which is not present in toroviruses (Tab. 3). The E and M proteins are essential for virus particle formation. Non-infectious virus-like particles can be formed in the absence of both the S and N proteins, but not if either E or M is missing [39, 40].

Table 3. Viron-associated proteins of coronaviruses and toroviruses.

Protein		Apparent molecular weight in SDS polyacrylamide gels (kDa)	
		Coronavirus	Torovirus
Spike glycoprotein	S	180–220	200
Integral membrane protein	M	23–35	27
Small envelope protein	E	9–12	Absent
Haemagglutinin-esterase protein	HE	65	65
Nucleocapsid protein	N	50–60	19

Adapted from [264].

It is the N terminus of the M protein, of both coronaviruses and toroviruses, which is exposed at the outer virion surface. Only 20 amino acids or so are exposed, forming the ectodomain, in the case of the coronaviruses. The next 50% or so of the molecule is within the envelope, in the form of three membrane-spanning regions, the remaining, C-terminal, half of the molecule being partly membrane associated and partly within the lumen of the virion i.e. it is amphipathic [36, 41, 42]. Notwithstanding, studies with TGEV have revealed that approximately one-third of the M molecules have both the N- and C-termini exposed at the outer virion surface [43]. The M protein of coronaviruses, but not toroviruses, is glycosylated.

The RNP released from virions had been observed by negative stain electron microscopy as a filamentous helical structure. For many years it was assumed that the RNP was largely independent of the other structural proteins, although probably interacting to some degree with the M protein prior to virus particle formation. Some light on the nature of this interaction has been shed by cryoelectron microscopic studies of TGEV. These have shown that extracellular, infectious coronavirus particles contain a core shell, probably icosahedral [44]. This comprises the RNP intimately associated with the C-terminal half of the M protein [45–47]. This structure can be released intact from virions by appropriate detergents. During this extraction process, the 30% or so of the M molecules that had both their termini at the outer virus surface were released, i.e. were not associated with the core.

M protein molecules interact laterally with each other, through multiple contact sites, particularly in the transmembrane region [48, 49]. The M protein also interacts non-covalently with sequences within the transmembrane region and short, C-terminal, endodomain of the S protein [50, 51]. Mutations to both the transmembrane and amphipathic domains of M interfered with the M-S interaction [52].

The M protein of coronaviruses has one or two glycans, N-linked in the case of groups 1 and 3, O-linked in group 2, on the short externally exposed N-terminal region. Although MHV has four potential glycosylation sites (serine and threonine residues) on the short ectodomain, only one of them is glycoslyated [53]. Glycosylation of M is not actually required for virus particle formation, as shown by the presence of non-glycosylated M within virions, and mutational analysis [48]. The E protein, which is required for the budding process that is part of virus particle formation, is produced in abundance within infected cells, though only a few molecules of E are within virus particles. It has been estimated that the molar ratios of the TGEV E:S:M proteins is 1:20:300 [54]. The E protein is an integral membrane protein, the N-terminal half being buried within the membrane, spanning the membrane once, possibly twice, the C-terminus being within the lumen of virions [55, 56]. Although there is an N-linked glycosylation site near the N-terminus of the IBV E protein, it is not utilised [55]. Toroviruses do not have an E protein.

The group 2 coronaviruses and the toroviruses have an additional structural protein, the HE protein (reviewed by Brian et al. [57]), which forms a layer of short surface projections of approximately 7 nm in length. The HE protein is a neuraminic-O-acetlyesterase. It hydrolyses the 9-*O*-acetylated sialic acid on erythrocytes, thereby reversing haemagglutination induced by HE or S; thus HE is considered to be a receptor-destroying enzyme [31, 58].

Whereas there is virtually no amino acid identity between the S, M and N proteins of the coronaviruses and toroviruses, there is 30% identity between the HE proteins [59]. Moreover, the HE proteins of the *Coronaviridae* have approximately 30% identity with the haemagglutinin esterase fusion (HEF) protein of influenza C virus. This coincidence is believed to have happened as a result of recombination. Whereas the HEF protein is cleaved into two subunits, the HE protein is not cleaved and lacks most of the C-terminal subunit of the HEF protein of influenza C.

Some of these features are summarised within Table 2, together with aspects of the genomes of *Coronaviridae* members that will be discussed later.

Relationships amongst coronaviruses and toroviruses: structural proteins

Coronaviruses have been assigned to three groups (Tab. 1). These were initially devised on the basis of a lack of antigenic relationships between the species of different groups [60]. Sequencing has largely confirmed these groupings, both in terms of amino acid identity and the sequence and location of the accessory non-structural proteins.

Thus within group 2 (MHV, RtCoV, BCoV, HCoV-OC43, for which sufficient sequence data is available) there is at least 61% amino acid identity when comparing the S, E, N and M proteins [61]). In group 3, comparing the E, M and N proteins, IBV and TCoV show identities of ≥ 80%. Fewer genes of PhCoV have been sequenced, but comparison of the accessory proteins encoded by genes 3 and 5 also gave similar percentages.

Group 1 is less homogeneous. The trio of TGEV, CCoV and FCoV have S, E, N and M identities of ≥74%. However, when HCoV 229E and PEDV are included, identities fall to between 23% (E protein) to 42% (S and M proteins). The S2 proteins of PEDV and HCoV 229E have 60% identity [62]. Thus PEDV and HCoV 229E are more related to each other than to the TGEV, CCoV and FCoV subgroup. Indeed, PEDV and HCoV 229E only just "squeeze in" to group 2 on the basis of gene sequences (Fig. 3). Comprehensive antigenic analysis reflects the sequence analysis within group 2 [63–65]. There are many common epitopes in the S, M and N proteins of TGEV, CCoV and FCoV, but no antigenic cross-reaction between these and PEDV/HCoV 229E.

Immune electron microscopy has revealed relationships between the toroviruses of humans, equines and bovines [33, 35]. Much remains to be done to establish the extent of variation among human toroviruses. Viruses similar to EToV would seem to infect a number of ungulate species, as serology has indicated infections with EToV-like viruses in cattle, sheep, goats and pigs [66].

Relationships amongst coronaviruses and toroviruses: non-structural proteins and genome organisation

CoVs and ToVs have the general genome organisation:

5'UTR-polymerase gene – structural protein genes – UTR 3'

where the UTR are untranslated regions (each up to 500 nucleotides in coronaviruses). The structural protein genes of coronaviruses are in the order

(HE)-S-E-M-N

the HE gene only being in group 2 viruses. The corresponding gene order of toroviruses is

S-M-HE-N

where the HE is intact in EToV but a pseudogene in BToV [67].

In addition to sequence differences noted in the preceeding section, the coronaviruses differ with respect to genes that encode proteins that are not structural proteins, i.e. not present in virus particles. The viruses differ with respect to both the number and location of the non-structural protein genes and, in some cases, on the mode of translation of the proteins (Fig. 4; reviewed by Lai and Cavanagh [31]). The toroviruses do not have any non-structural proteins other than those encoded by gene 1.

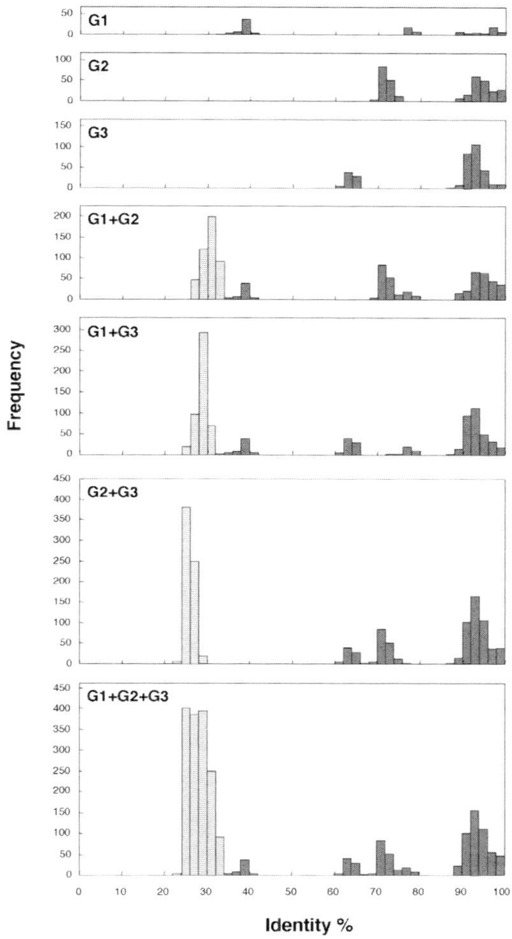

Figure 3. Protein sequence relationships within and between coronavirus groups 1, 2 and 3 (G1, G2 and G3) illustrated by the nucleocapsid protein. The Y-axis shows the frequency distribution of pairwise identity percentages of the N proteins. Histograms of the intra-group scores are in dark grey, those of inter-group scores in light grey. In group 1 the bars with an identity of ~40% correspond to HCoV-229E and PEDV, whereas the other bars in group 1 correspond to TGEV, CECoV and FCoV. In group 3 most of the data is for IBV isolates, the bars with an identity of ~60% corresponding to a group of IBV strains isolated in Australia, significantly different from those isolated on other continents. (Reprinted from González et al. 2003, by permission from Springer.) [266]

Group 2 CoVs are the only ones to have a non-structural protein gene between gene 1 (replicase gene) and the S protein gene. Adjacent to it is the gene encoding the HE structural (though non-essential) protein. In some strains of MHV, which have had multiple passages *in vitro*, the HE gene is

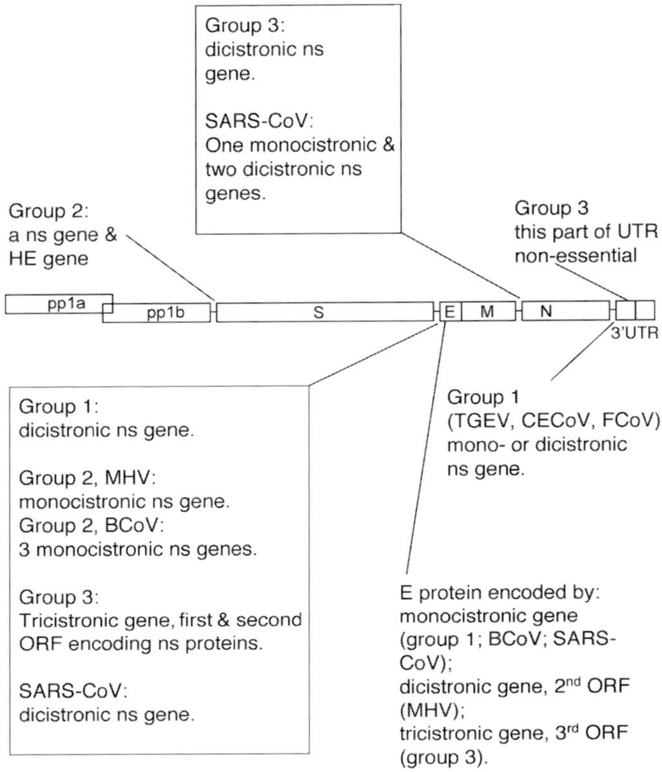

Figure 4. Genome organisation of coronaviruses. The "core" gene complement comprises the genes that encode essential proteins: gene 1, which encodes various proteins derived from polyproteins (pp) 1a and 1b, associated with RNA replication and transcription, and the S, E, M and N proteins, that are found in virus particles. Inserted between these genes, at the points shown, but varying amongst the coronaviruses, are "accessory" genes, which encode proteins that are non-structural (ns) and not essential for replication *per se*, i.e. not required for replication *in vitro*, but which are believed to have roles in host animals i.e. *in vivo*. Gene 1 is not to scale.

incomplete, i.e. it is a pseudogene. Hence such isolates do not have a HE protein in the virions.

All the coronaviruses have open reading frames (ORFs) between the S protein gene and the ORF encoding the E protein. In the case of group 1 and 2 viruses, and SARS-CoV, there is a gene before that encoding the E protein, where a gene means a sequence under the control of a transcription-associated sequence (TAS), which generates a mRNA. This gene may have one, two or three ORFs (Fig. 4). The E protein of group 1 viruses, and SARS-CoV, is encoded by a monocistronic gene, i.e. which encodes a single ORF. In the case of group 2 and 3 viruses, the E protein is encoded by the second and third ORF, of dicistronic and tricistronic genes, respectively.

In all cases (to date) the ORF encoding the E protein is followed by the M protein gene and, for groups 1 and 2, this is followed directly by the N protein gene. In contrast, group 3 viruses and SARS-CoV have one and three genes, respectively, encoding non-structural proteins located between the M and N protein genes (Fig. 4). Finally, TGEV, FCoV and CECoV have a non-structural protein gene (which is mono- or dicistronic) after the N protein gene. Interestingly, the part of the 3' UTR of gene 3 viruses that is adjacent to the N protein gene actually comprises an ORF, though there is no identifiable TAS sequence from which to generate an mRNA [68]. This part of the 3' UTR is not required for viability [69]. It is conceivable that at one time this ORF was part of a gene, encoding a non-structural protein, the TAS sequence having been lost.

Roles of the non-structural proteins

The roles of the non-structural proteins, other than those encoded by gene 1, are not known. Genetically manipulated TGEV [70, 71], MHV [10, 72] and IBV (our unpublished observations) from which the genes encoding these proteins have been deleted or inactivated replicate to more or less normal titres *in vitro*, i.e. in cell culture. Hence they are considered to be non-essential for replication. It is believed that they have roles *in vivo* i.e. within host animals, and have been called "accessory" genes [74]. Deletion of the accessory genes of MHV resulted in attenuation of pathogenicity, to the extent that the mutants were no longer lethal in mice [10]. This is not an inevitable consequence; deletion of the two non-structural protein ORFs of gene 3 of TGEV did not attenuate pathogenicity [75].

There is virtually no amino acid identity between the non-structural proteins of one coronavirus group and another and no identity with any non-coronavirus proteins in public databases. As one might imagine given that these proteins are not required for replication per se, there are variations within some coronavirus species, which tend to be associated with passage of the viruses *in vitro*. For example, some TGEV strains do not have intact ORFs in the gene that precedes the E protein gene. Propagation of SARS-CoV in Vero cells [76] resulted in a 45-nucleotide, in-frame deletion from ORF7b. Most of the SARS-CoV isolates from humans in 2003 had a deletion of 29 nucleotides in gene 8, when compared to the isolates from Himalayan palm civet cats and raccoon dogs, and one of the earliest human isolates [77]. The consequence is that most of the human isolates had two ORFs within gene 8, whereas the animal isolates had a single, longer ORF. Whether this has any functional significance for the pathogenicity of SARS-CoV in humans is not known.

Replication cycle

Coronaviruses and toroviruses have positive-sense genomes; genomic RNA, once released from virions early in infection, acts as an mRNA for translation of gene 1, producing the polymerase. Thereafter this generates mRNAs from the other genes, from which all the other proteins are made. Consequently virions contain only structural proteins, unlike virions of negative-sense RNA viruses that contain proteins involved in RNA replication and transcription. Replication is within the cytoplasm.

Initiation of infection: attachment to receptors

It is the S protein that is responsible for attachment of the virus to host cell receptors, i.e. S is the receptor binding protein. Popova and Zhang [78] have demonstrated that even for group 2 viruses, which have an HE protein, the S protein is sufficient for attachment leading to infection. Earlier Schultze et al. [79] had shown that the S protein of BCoV was more efficient at causing haemagglutination than the HE protein, and had proposed that S was the primary receptor-binding protein. Expression of several coronavirus S proteins from various vectors has shown that it is the S protein that induces membrane fusion, observed as syncytium formation, a prerequisite of which is attachment to a cell (reviewed by Lai and Cavanagh [31]. It is also the major inducer of virus-neutralizing and haemagglutination-inhibiting antibodies (reviewed by Cavanagh [29, 80]).

Cell surface molecules that act as receptors have been identified for MHV, a number of group 2 coronaviruses and, most recently, for SARS-CoV. The part of the S protein that is responsible for attachment to these receptors, the receptor-binding domain, has also been identified for these viruses (Fig. 5). Most studies have been done with *in vitro* material, i.e. cultured cells, as one would expect. In addition there have been some investigations with *ex vivo* material (gut tissue), plus earlier studies with red blood cells. These studies indicate that the attachment process *in vivo* might be more complex than is indicated by *in vitro* studies alone.

The cellular receptor for MHV is CEACAM 1, a member of the carcinoembryonic antigen (CEA) family of glycoproteins in the immunoglobulin superfamily (reviewed by Lai and Cavanagh, [31]). It is a 424-amino acid glycoprotein with four immunoglobulin-like domains (see Lewicki and Gallagher [26]. A soluble form of this protein has been crystallised and an atomic structure deduced [81].

Chen et al. [82] transfected COS-7 cells, which lack a functional receptor for MHV, with genes of human CEACAM and human biliary glycoprotein; the cells were then susceptible to MHV. Experiments with chimaeras of human and murine CEACAM proteins revealed that the immunoglobulin loop of human CEACAM conferred virus-binding specificity. Different

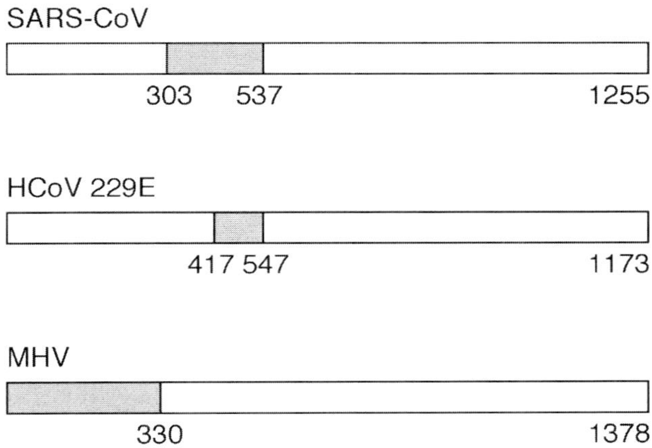

Figure 5. Regions (in grey) of S proteins of three coronaviruses that encompass a receptor-binding domain. The numbers denote amino acid residue positions.

isoforms of murine CEACAMs exist. These have extensive differences in the N-terminal immunoglobulin-like domain to which MHV binds and bind MHV to different extents. Analysis of chimaeras indicated that N-terminal amino acids 38-43 were key elements for binding MHV and activation of its fusion-inducing activity [83], subsequently confirmed [84]. Interestingly, when MHV had established a persistent infection in murine 17 Cl 1 cells, that express very low levels of the CEACAM 1 receptor, there was selection of mutant MHVs that were better able to use other molecules as receptors [85].

The receptor-binding domain of the MHV S protein is formed by sequence within the 330 N-terminal amino acid residues of the S1 protein [86], though the stability of the interaction can be affected by downstream sequence [87] (Fig. 5).

Human aminopeptidase N (APN; also known as CD13) has been identified as a receptor for HCoV-229E [88]. This protein is a metalloprotease located on the surface of epithelial cells, including those of the intestine, lung and kidney. Human cells that were not susceptible to canine coronavirus (CCoV) or FCoV became susceptible when transfected with a human/canine chimaera of APN [89]. The critical, C-terminal domain of the canine APN was formed by amino acids 643 to 841.

The human and porcine APNs do not function as receptors for TGEV and HCoV 229E, respectively. When amino acids 255 to 348 of porcine APN were replaced by amino acids 260 to 353 of human APN, the resulting chimaeric protein was able to function as a receptor for HCoV-229E [90]. Kolb and colleagues [91] went on to show that the human cells became susceptible to FCoV, HCV 229E and TGEV when transfected with a cDNA of the feline APN. Analysis of chimaeric APNs showed that amino acids within the region 132-295 were involved in virus binding. Within this region was a hypervariable stretch of 8 amino acids. When these 8 residues in the porcine APN were replaced with the corresponding amino acids of HCoV 229E, the chimaeric receptor was able to bind HCoV 229E. Human APN with five porcine APN residues from the corresponding region did bind HCV OC43 provided that a glycosylation site with the porcine residues was removed by mutation [92]. The authors concluded that certain differences in glycosylation between coronavirus receptors from different species are critical determinants in the species specificity of infection. Expression of feline APN in rodent cells rendered the cells susceptible not only to FCV but also to HCoV-229E, CCV and TGEV [88]. Various human neuronal and glial cell lines, which were susceptible to HCV 229E, expressed human APN, there being a correlation between the apparent amount of cell surface APN and the level of virus attachment [93].

Not only are there differences amongst APNs with respect to the binding of group 2 coronaviruses, there are also differences with respect to variants within a given coronavirus. Hohdatsu and colleagues [94] have shown that feline APN is a receptor for type II FCoV but not for type I. A monoclonal antibody to feline APN, which blocked infection of primary feline by type II FCoV, CECoV and TGEV did not block infection by type I FCoV. This antibody bound to APN that was recovered from feline intestinal brush-border membrane proteins. Type II FCoVs differ from type I in a number of ways, including that the S protein would appear to have been derived from a FCoV by recombination [95].

Experiments using soluble truncated histidine-tagged S proteins, produced using baculovirus expression vectors, showed that the region of the HCoV-229E S protein from amino acids 417 to 547 was required for binding to its cell receptor [96] (Fig. 5).

The metallopeptidase, angiotensin-converting enzyme 2 (ACE2), on Vero cells has been shown to act as a receptor for SARS CoV [97]. The 293T cell type does not support efficient replication of SARS-CoV but did do so after being transfected with a cDNA expressing ACE2. It was the N-terminal half of the S protein that contained the receptor-binding domain for ACE2. This has been confirmed by Xiao et al. [98], who have shown that the receptor-binding domain of SARS-CoV is formed by residues between positions 303 and 537 (Fig. 5).

The enterotropism of TGEV is associated with the sialic acid-binding activity of the S protein. This virus recognises a mucin-type glycoprotein, in a sialic acid-dependent fashion, extracted from porcine intestinal brush border membranes [99]. The virus was observed to bind to mucin-producing goblet cells in cryosections of the small intestine of suckling piglets. A nonenteropathogenic mutant that did not have a sialic acid-binding activity was unable to bind to the mucin-type glycoprotein or to goblet cells.

Schultze and Herrler [100] had earlier shown that a vital component of the receptor for both the S and HE proteins of BCoV was the glycan component N-acetyl-9-O-acetylneuraminic acid (Neu5,9Ac_2). This residue acted as a receptor not only on erythrocytes but also on susceptible cell cultures. It has also been shown that cell surface sialoglycoproteins act as receptors for TGEV [101, 102]. Sialic acid residues also play a role in the haemagglutination of red blood cells by IBV, the necessary residue being α 2,3-linked N-acetylneuraminic acid [103]. Attachment of coronaviruses might be a two-step (at least) process. Primary attachment might be mediated by a first receptor, e.g. Neu5,9Ac_2 for some coronaviruses, a second receptor e.g. APN or CEACAM proteins, bringing the virus and cell membranes closer together for subsequent membrane fusion. Some receptors might fulfil both functions for some coronaviruses. Although it can mediate binding to erythrocytes, the main function of HE might be to remove neuraminic acid from the virus and cell surface. The esterase activity of the HE, and HEF protein of influenza C, specifically cleaves Neu5,9Ac_2.

Initiation of infection: membrane fusion to release the genome

In order to release the genome into the cytoplasm the coronaviral envelope must fuse with a host cell membrane. This fusion event is brought about by regions in the S2, C-terminal part of the S protein, following attachment mediated by S1. Cleavage of the S polypeptide into S1 and S2 is not a prerequisite for infectivity, and fusion can occur at neutral pH, suggesting that fusion can occur at the cell surface, although some variants require a lower pH, indicating that they would be uncoated in endosomes (reviewed in [29–31]).

That the S protein alone is required for fusion has been demonstrated using viral vectors expressing S protein of FCoV and MHV, at neutral pH [104–106]. Recombination experiments supported the view that S2 is responsible for the promotion of membrane fusion [107, 108]. The S2 polypeptide has a heptad repeat region (HR2) [109], adjacent to the transmembrane region (Fig. 6). There is a second heptad repeat region (HR1), located 170 amino acids upstream in MHV (Fig. 6). The HR2 consists of a leucine zipper motif, highly conserved amongst coronaviruses [110], which is a series of leucine residues repeated every seven amino acids. It is believed that the leucine zipper domain is essential for oligomerization of the S protein, which has a coiled-coil structure in S2 involved in membrane fusion [111, 112] (Fig. 6). Mutations in this region cause defects in oligomerization and reduce fusion capability [113]. The HR1 contains a putative fusion peptide, involved in membrane fusion [114]. Bosch and colleagues

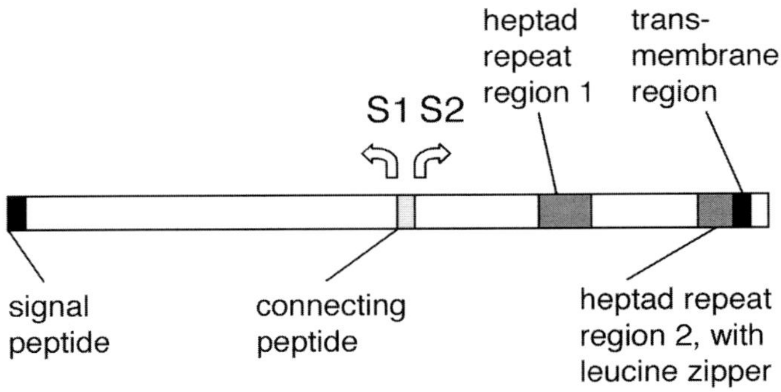

Figure 6. Location of some of the structural features of the S protein of coronaviruses. The S protein of some coronaviruses is not cleaved into S1 and S2 glycopolypeptides; they do not have a basic connecting peptide. Hypervariable region 1 contains the putative fusion peptide responsible for membrane fusion.

[115] made polypeptides corresponding to HR1 (96 amino acids) and HR2 (39 amino acids) which, when mixed, assembled into a stable oligomeric alpha helical complex. The HR1 and HR2 polypeptides associated in an antiparallel fashion, forming 14.5 nm rod-like structures. This would bring the putative fusion peptide in HR1 into close proximity to the transmembrane region.

Components elsewhere in S2, or at least structures formed by other sequences in S2, can affect the fusion process. For example, some monoclonal antibodies that have anti-fusion activity are against epitopes near the N-terminal part of the S2 polypeptide [116, 117]. It has been suggested that binding of these antibodies might destabilise the oligomeric structure of S and thereby interfere with the interaction of the fusogenic region with a cell membrane.

Lysosomotropic agents raise the pH in endosomes. If a virus requires a pH of <7 within endosomes for membrane fusion to occur, these agents prevent or reduce fusion, resulting in fewer cells being successfully infected. Some studies with these reagents led to the conclusion that uncoating of MHV occurs in endosomes (reviewed by [29, 31]). Other studies have shown little effect by these agents, and that the optimum pH for membrane fusion by MHV was 7.4 [118, 119]. The productive infection of cells by the Beaudette strain of IBV was reduced by 90% by ammonium chloride, a lysosomotropic agent, and the optimum pH for cell-cell fusion (syncytium formation) was pH 6.7, indicating that uncoating occurs early after the start of endocytosis [120]. The same authors showed that the ammonium chloride had no effect on another strain of IBV, implying that fusion could occur at the cell surface. The SARS-CoV S protein caused syncytium formation at neutral pH [98].

As few as three amino acid changes in the heptad repeat regions of S2 of MHV resulted in virus that no longer fused optimally at pH 7.0 but required acidic pH (pH 5.5–6.0), and which was adversely affected by lysosomotropic agents [111, 121]. The variants of Gallagher and colleagues [111] had been recovered from a OBL21A neural cell line persistently infected with MHV i.e. the mutants had been selected by replication in this cell type. In conclusion, the weight of evidence is that the S proteins of most coronaviruses can cause membrane fusion a neutral pH, suggesting that fusion of the virus can occur at the cell surface. Notwithstanding, some variants require an acidic pH, indicating that they fuse with an endocytic membrane.

Binding of the S protein to a receptor causes conformational change in the S protein, promoting fusogenic activity [26, 122]. Lewicki and Gallagher [26] produced soluble S1 fragments that were dimers. Binding of these dimers to the CEACAM receptor altered the confirmation of S1, generating alternative disulphide linkages within S1, and inducing separation of S1 and S2. This separation could happen for MHV S protein because, like other group 2 and group 3 coronaviruses, the S protein is cleaved into two subunits, S1 and S2, which are non-covalently associated. Cleavage occurs adjacent to a connecting peptide region that contains one or more pairs of dibasic amino acids, e.g. RRFRR in many isolates of IBV, reviewed in [29, 31]. In some naturally occurring variants of IBV and MHV one of the basic residues has been replaced by histidine, which is weakly basic at neutral pH. Zelus et al. [122] have also shown that the MHV spike protein undergoes conformational changes following binding to soluble receptor at 37 °C. The conformational change occurred not only with MHV S protein that was cleaved into S1 and S2 subunits, but also with a mutant whose S protein was not cleaved.

Initial experiments with MHV indicated that cleavage of S was required for its fusion activity. However, subsequent studies have shown that this is not the case but rather that cleaved S induces fusion more efficiently than uncleaved S [123, 124]. Variant MHVs selected in a persistently infected OBL21A neural cell line required low pH for fusion, in contrast to the wild-type virus. Whereas the latter had the connecting peptide RRAHR, the variants had RRADR, i.e. with an acidic aspartic acid residue in place of the histidine. Revertants, which produced cleaved S and fused cells efficiently at neutral pH, had recovered the connecting peptide RRAHR in most cases, although some revertants had a small, non-charged residue at this position [125].

The coronaviruses of group 1, and SARS-CoV, have an S protein that is not cleaved. Clearly, whatever conformational changes occur following attachment of their S proteins to receptors, the fusion process is not prevented by S being uncleaved.

The S protein of EToV comprises 1,581 amino acids and has a Mr of about 200,000 when glycosylated. It has a highly basic S1-S2 connecting peptide and occurs as two subunits in virions.

Translation of gene 1: transcriptase/replicase proteins

Having a positive-sense RNA genome, a coronavirus has no need of proteins within the virion for the RNA replication and transcription process to start. Rather, the input genomic RNA serves as an mRNA for the transcription of gene 1. This gene accounts for some two-thirds, approximately 20 kb, of the genome. It comprises two very large ORFs, 1a and 1b, the second of which is translated following ribosomal frameshifting. The 1a and 1b polyproteins (pp1a and pp1b) are co-translationally processed by virus-encoded proteases. This topic has been reviewed for toroviruses and arteriviruses in addition to coronaviruses [67].

Gene 1 sequences are available for species within each of the three coronavirus groups plus SARS-CoV. It is within the gene one products that there is the greatest degree of amino acid identity between the coronaviruses, being as high as 70% in parts of pp1b whilst the identity within much, though not all, of pp1a is not more than 30%. It is pp1a that is also the most variable with respect to size; the greater length of the genome of MHV is largely accounted for by a larger pp1a.

A number of functional domains have been identified within pp1a/b. In pp1a of MHV, HCoV 229E and TGEV there are two papain-like proteases (PLP1 and 2), whereas there is only one, equivalent to PLP2, in IBV and SARS-CoV. The PLPs are involved in the processing of the N termini of pp1a. Further downstream is a chymotrypsin/picornavirus 3C-like protease (3CLP). This is responsible for all the other cleavage events necessary to generate the gene one products required for RNA replication and transcription [76, 126, 127]. Within pp1b are an RNA-dependent RNA polymerase, a zinc-finger nucleic acid-binding protein and a nucleoside triphosphate-binding helicase. There are also another ten or so proteolytic cleavage products of pp1a and pp1b.

Translation of pp1b involves ribosomal frameshifting. This mechanism has two essential elements: a slippery site followed by an RNA pseudoknot [128, 129]. At the slippery site (UUUAAAC) the ribosome slips backwards, then proceeds forwards, this time in a –1 frame compared with pp1a.

Transcription

Coronaviruses have several (five for IBV, seven for TGEV and MHV) 3' co-terminal subgenomic mRNAs, the "nested set" (Fig. 7). It is the unique part of each mRNA, i.e. that which is not contained within the next small-

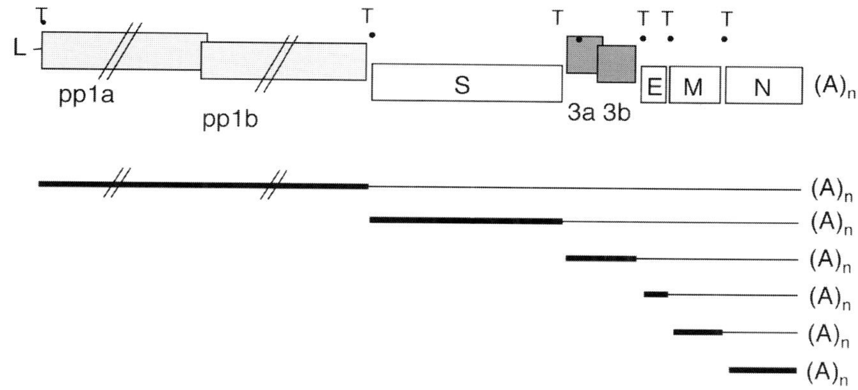

Figure 7. Nested-set arrangement of mRNAs of coronaviruses and toroviruses, illustrated for HCoV-229E. The thick horizontal lines indicate the parts of the mRNAs that are translated. The coronaviruses have a transcription-associated sequence (TAS; T) at the beginning of each gene that is associated with the discontinuous transcription process (see Fig. 8). Toroviruses also have sequences equivalent to the TAS of coronaviruses, though discontinuous transcription is not involved in the production of all the subgenomic RNAs (see legend to Fig. 8; [134]). $(A)_n$, 3' poly(A) tail. L, leader sequence.

est mRNA, that is translated. At the 5' end of each gene is a short sequence common to all the genes, or with only minor variations. These were initially called "consensus sequences" and later "intergenic sequences" because, in MHV, they occur in untranslated regions between genes. However, in IBV most of the genes overlap, such that the consensus sequences are within the ORF of the preceding gene. More appropriate names, therefore, are "transcription-associated sequence" (TAS) or "transcription regulating sequence" (TRS) (Fig. 7). In MHV, IBV and SARS-CoV the core TASs are UCUAAAC, CUUAACAA and ACGAAC, with minor variations. At the 5' end of each mRNA is a sequence (the leader sequence) of 60-90 nucleotides, depending on the species, derived from the 5' end of the genome (Fig. 7). There is a TAS sequence at the 3' end of the leader. The leader and TAS sequences join in the region of the TAS sequences.

A number of mechanisms have been proposed for the production of the subgenomic mRNAs (reviewed in [31]). The TASs play crucial roles in each model [130–132]. Two models involve discontinuous transcription.

In one model (Fig. 8a) each TAS is an attenuator of the polymerisation process during negative-sense RNA synthesis, the leader sequence then being added to the nascent mRNA to produce a negative-sense subgenomic RNA. A positive-sense mRNA is then transcribed from this.

In the other model (Fig. 8b), a TAS is considered to be more like a promoter. In this model the leader sequence is first transcribed from positive-sense genomic RNA, and is then translocated by the polymerase to one or

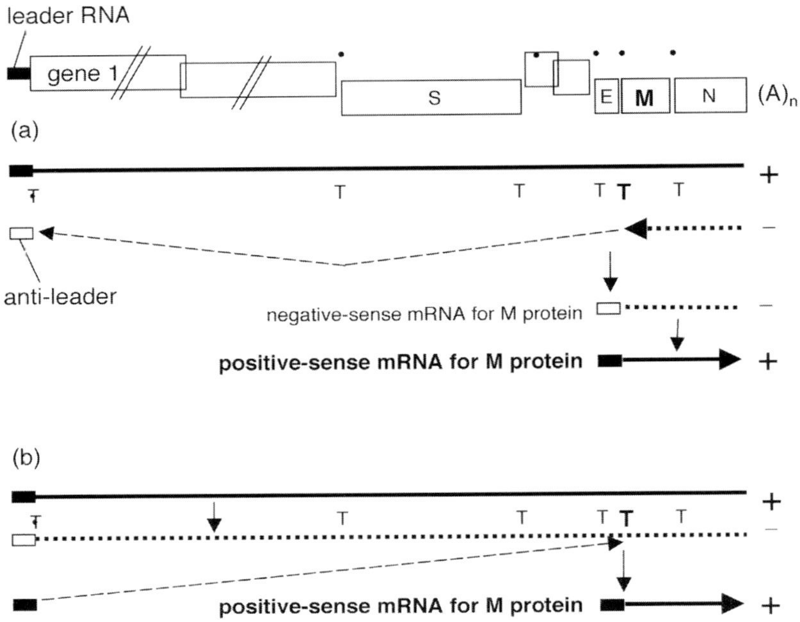

Figure 8. Two models of discontinuous transcription, illustrated for the M gene of HCoV-229E. (a) Discontinuous transcription during negative-strand synthesis, in which the TAS at the beginning of the M gene attenuates progression of the polymerase, which continues transcription at the 5'-terminal TAS at the end of the leader sequence. The resultant negative-sense mRNA is copied into the actual (plus-sense) subgenomic mRNA. (b) Discontinuous transcription during plus-strand synthesis, in which the template for transcription is the full-length, genome negative-sense RNA. In this model the leader sequence is made first, transcription continuing at one or other of the TAS positions, in this case at the M gene TAS, to generate the M gene subgenomic RNA. Transcription of toroviruses has been studied with EToV. Only the S gene mRNA of that virus has a leader sequence derived from the 5' terminus of the genome, from which it has been deduced that production of subgenomic mRNAs of toroviruses is a combination of continuous and discontinuous transcription [134].

other of the TAS, after which transcription continues to produce subgenomic positive-sense mRNAs.

The former model is currently favoured, some evidence for it having been produced by investigation of transcription in arteriviruses which, like coronaviruses, are within the order *Nidovirales*.

The subgenomic mRNAs are not made in equimolar amounts, and the amount of each mRNA does not necessarily decrease in a linear fashion with increasing size of the mRNAs. Sequences adjacent to the TAS sequences affect the efficiency with which a given core TAS operates [133].

Transcription in toroviruses has been best studied with EtoV (Berne virus), as this can be grown in cell culture. Unlike coronaviruses and arteriviruses, both in the order *Nidovirales*, toroviruses were considered not to produce mRNAs by a discontinuous procedure; mRNAs 3, 4 and 5 did not contain a leader sequence. However, mRNA 5 does have a short leader sequence, corresponding to the 5'terminal 18 residues of the genome [134]. Thus EqToV appears to combine discontinuous and non-discontinuous RNA synthesis to produce its subgenomic mRNAs.

Translation of genes downstream from gene 1

The mRNAs for the HE, S and M are translated in a cap-dependent manner from mRNAs that are functionally monocistronic; the 5' region, of their respective mRNA, which is absent from the next smaller mRNA, is that which is translated to produce these proteins. This is mostly the case for the N protein mRNA but in BCoV and MHV there is an internal ORF in addition to that encoding the N protein, i.e. this mRNA is bicistronic. This internal ORF is in a reading frame different from that of the N protein, encodes a non-essential hydrophobic protein and is translated by a leaky ribosomal scanning mechanism [135, 136].

The E protein is translated from a functionally monocistronic mRNA in the case of the group 1 coronaviruses and SARS-CoV but in group 2 and 3 viruses the E proteins is encoded by the second and third ORF, respectively, of bicistronic and tricistronic genes, respectively. Thus the E protein of group 2 and 3 viruses are encoded by ORFs 5b and 3c, respectively. The translation of these ORFs commences after internal initiation of translation by ribsomes, not by read-through by ribosomes that had translated the preceding ORF(s) [137, 138]. This internal initiation is controlled by RNA structures formed by the preceding ORFs which act as internal ribosome entry sites [138, 139].

Synthesis of the structural proteins

The S protein is co-translationally glycosylated with N-linked glycans. Conversion of the high mannose (simple) glycans to complex ones is a slow process, the half-life being one to several hours [27]. The S protein undergoes multiple disulphide linkages to form a more complex structure [140] and oligomerise into a quaternary structure that might be a homodimer or homotrimer [25], homodimer [26, 27] or homotrimer [28]. The S1 and S2 subunits are not held together by disulphide bonds [23]. The S prepropolypeptide is converted to a propolypeptide by removal of the N-terminal signal peptide. Whether the propolypeptide is cleaved to generate S1 and S2 depends on the virus species and strain and, to some extent, on the cell type in which the virus is grown [141]. Essentially the S propolypeptides of the group 2 and 3 CoVs are cleaved at S1-S2 connecting peptides that contain one or more pairs of dibasic residues e.g. RRFRR in many IBV strains [142, 143]. Cleavage of S occurs after conversion of the glycans from simple to complex [144]. The S propolypeptide of group 1 CoVs and SARS-CoV is not cleaved; they do not have dibasic residues in the region corresponding to the location of the connecting peptide of group 2 and 3 viruses. The S2 protein of MHV is acylated, probably involving cysteine residues in the C-terminal hydrophobic tail region of S [145].

Like the S protein, the signal sequence of the HE protein is removed and it has N-linked glycans that are converted to complex ones in the Golgi apparatus. The protein dimerises, the association involving disuphide bonds [146, 147].

There are differences amongst the CoVs regarding post-translational processing of the M proteins. All have one or two glycans at the short N-terminal region exposed on the outer surface of the virion (approximately 20 amino acids). In group 2 viruses the glycans are of the O-linked type whereas in group 1 and 3 CoVs they are N-linked [148, 149]. Unlike the M proteins of groups 2 and 3, which have an internal membrane-insertion sequence, those of the TGEV group have an N-terminal membrane-insertion sequence that is absent from the mature M protein [150], though this signal sequence is not essential [151, 152]. The M protein of TGEV is sulphated [153].

The E protein of MHV has been reported to be acylated [154].

Replication of genomic RNA

RNA sequences involved in the control of genomic RNA replication, and transcription, have been mostly studied using coronaviral defective RNAs, as these were considerably smaller (≤ 9 kb) than genomic RNA [31, 69, 155]. The regulation of coronaviral RNA replication and transcription probably depends on overall RNA confirmation, so the deductions arrived at from experiments with defective RNA must be treated with caution with respect to their applicability to full-size genomic RNA. In the case of MHV, 436 nucleotides at the 3' end of a defective RNA were required for production of positive-strand sequence, whereas only 55 nucleotides were required for negative-strand production. An IBV defective RNA with the 5'-terminal 544 nucleotides, but not as few as 338 nucleotides, and the 3'-terminal 338 nucleotides was replicated [69]. Packaging of the defective IBV RNA into virus particles was poor unless part of gene 1b was present, though no specific part of 1b was required. A packaging signal was present in the 5'-terminal 649 nucleotides of the TGEV genome [155].

The leader sequence of different strains of MHV varies in length, due to different numbers of repeat copies (two to four copies) of the sequence

UCUAA [156]. This sequence is part of the core TAS sequence UCUAAAC that occurs at the 3' end of the leader sequence and at the start of each gene. Interestingly, the copy number of this repeat sequence changes during virus passage [157, 158]. This change in copy number did not occur with BCoV, which only has one UCUAA copy in the leader RNA [159].

Assembly of virus particles

Electron microscope, protein localisation studies and immunofluoresence analysis have revealed that the major location of coronavirus particle formation is the Golgi complex, although early and late in infection budding can also occur in the endoplasmic reticulum-Golgi intermediate compartment (ERGIC) and rough endoplasmic reticulum, respectively (see Fig. 7 in Salanueva et al. [160]). The expression of combinations of coronavirus proteins from cDNAs to produce, or not, virus-like particles (VLPs) has greatly facilitated our understanding of the process by which virions are assembled. The E protein is required for the budding process, i.e. for membranes to curve and ultimately bud off to form vesicles. However, it is the M protein that determines the sites at which virus particle formation occurs; it interacts with the N protein (as part of a ribonucleoprotein complex) and with the S protein (as summarised in the section "What it is to be a coronavirus or torovirus", above). The virus particles are transported through Golgi compartments to secretory vesicles, for subsequent release of virions at the cell surface.

The M protein accumulates in the Golgi complex in homomultimeric complexes [48, 49, 161]. When produced on its own, e.g. by expression from cDNAs or virus vectors, the S protein migrates to the cell surface. Indeed, some does so during infection. However, these molecules are then lost to the process of virus particle formation. Rather, the S molecules that become part of virions are retained in the Golgi complex by interaction with the M protein, *via* C-terminal regions of the S protein [50–52]. Virus-like particles could be formed experimentally when both E and M were expressed together but not if either of them was absent. Neither N nor S proteins were required to form these virus-like particles [39, 40]. When the N protein is present, associated with the genomic RNA to form the RNP, this structure associates with the the C-terminal half of the M protein) to form an icosahedral core structure [47, 162, 163].

Although the M protein is central to the virus assembly process, the E protein, which is also an integral membrane protein, is required to induce membrane curvature that culminates in budding. The effect of the E protein on membranes has been illustrated by Fischer et al. [164] who produced deformed MHV particles when certain parts of the E protein had been mutated. It is the lumenal part of E, i.e. on the inside of the virion, that targets the protein to the Golgi complex [165]. The last six residues, RDKLYS, of the C-terminus of the E protein of IBV were responsible for temporal retention of E in the pre-Golgi compartment [166].

Expression of E and M together resulted in the production of VLPs [39, 40, 167]. However, expression of E protein alone is able to produce, showing that the E protein alone can induce budding [55, 168]. However, the E protein is not absolutely essential for the production of virus particles. Thus mutant MHVs have been made that lack the E protein gene but which still replicate, albeit to a titre of 10^4-fold less than wild type virus [169]. Notwithstanding, it can be said that the E protein greatly enhances virion envelope formation. Kuo and Masters [170] have suggested that E induces membrane curvature whilst M drives the remainder of the virion production process. Lim and Liu [166], using IBV, have expressed various deletions of E and looked for interaction of E and M by immunoprecipitation. The results suggested that the sequence immediately downstream from the putative membrane-spanning region of E interacted with M.

Electron microscope analysis of TGEV-infected cells has revealed two types of virion-related particles [160, 171]. The larger of the two had an electron dense internal periphery and a clear central area. These particles were located at perinuclear regions. Smaller particles were seen to accumulate in secretory vesicles. These smaller particles resembled the virus particles that were released from cells, i.e. they had compact internal cores with polygonal contours. It was concluded that the larger particles were the precursors of the smaller ones, and that the changes occurred during transport through the Golgi complex.

Recombination

Recombination is a feature of coronavirus replication. Chimaeric progeny arise probably by a copy-choice mechanism, i.e. the polymerase periodically falls off the viral RNA template that it is copying and may re-attach on the same or another viral template in the same cell. This probably occurs during replication of a single strain of a coronavirus, which would not usually be apparent. In this circumstance recombination may be a repair mechanism [172]. If a cell is infected by two strains of a given species of coronavirus, then progeny with sequence(s) derived from both parents may result. This phenomenon was discovered with two temperature-sensitive mutants of MHV [173] and has been reviewed [31]. It is sometimes stated that coronavirus recombination occurs at high frequency. This high frequency may only be true of MHV in experimental circumstances [174]. Notwithstanding, recombination is a feature of the evolution of coronaviruses. Recombination between strains of IBV has been demonstrated experimentally [175] whilst sequencing of many field strains has provided convincing evidence that many, possibly all, IBV strains are recombinants between different IBV strains [176–180].

Two forms of FCoV are known, types I and II. FCoV type II is believed to be a recombinant of FCoV type I and CECoV [181], both group 1 CoVs.

In addition to homologous recombination events, i.e. between strains of a given species of coronavirus, or even between different species of coronavirus, non-homologous recombination events have occurred. Thus the HE gene of the group 2 coronaviruses, and the toroviruses, is similar to part of the HEF gene of *influenza C* virus, a negative-strand virus. The HE gene of coronaviruses and toroviruses may have been derived by independent recombination between a coronavirus/torovirus and *influenza C* virus. Comparison between genomic structures of coronavirus and torovirus also suggests that several recombination events may have been involved in rearranging the order of several genes during the evolution of these viruses [182]. For example, the C terminus of pp1a of EToV has 31 to 36% amino acid identity with the N-terminal 190 amino acids of the 30–32 kDa nonstructural 2A protein of coronaviruses.

Evidence for recombination between species of the *Torovirus* genus has been forthcoming from sequence analyses of BToV and *porcine torovirus* (PToV) isolates. For example, all of the newly characterized BToV variants had a 3' end of the HE gene, and the downstream N gene and 3'UTR that more closely resembled those of PToV than older BToVs [66]. Chimaeric HE genes in some PToV and BToVs suggested not only recombination but also the existence of other toroviruses.

There are constraints on the production of viable chimaeric coronaviruses by recombination, especially between different coronavirus species. For example, the structural proteins are not mutually independent of each other. As described above, the M protein interacts with the C-terminal part of S (the transmembrane domain and the cytoplasmic tail), with the N protein and probably with the E protein. Hence viable virus would only ensue from recombination of different coronaviruses within the structural protein gene region if these interactions were not compromised.

Variation in the spike glycoprotein

Within a coronavirus species it is the S protein that generally exhibits the greatest sequence variation. Most differences occur within the amino-terminal part of the molecule, equivalent to the N-terminal S1 glycopolypeptide in the case of those coronaviruses in which the S protein is cleaved into two polypeptides. There appear to be more constraints on the sequence of the S2 polypeptide, this polypeptide being involved in anchoring the protein in the membrane, forming the coiled-coil multimeric mature S protein and activating membrane fusion. By contrast, the function of the S1 subunit would seem to be limited to providing a receptor-binding domain. Provided that is intact, the sequence, and structure, of much of the remainder of S1 would seem not to be as crucial as for S2.

This is most vividly illustrated in the case of IBV, which exists as scores, maybe hundreds, of serotypes. Most IBV serotypes differ from each other by 20 to 25% of S1 amino acids [183, 184], the S2 polypeptides differing by less than half that amount (reviewed in [29]). However, some serotypes differ by 50% of S1 amino acids [185–187]. (Differences between the other IBV proteins are in the range of 10%, rarely exceeding 15% [188, 189]. The differences between the S1 proteins undoubtedly have a selective advantage; generally speaking, the immunity induced by inoculation with one serotype protects poorly against infection with heterologous serotypes (reviewed by Cavanagh [80]). Differences of as few as 2 to 3% of S1 amino acid residues can result in a change in serotype, defined as lack of cross-neutralization using convalescent sera [190-192]. These few differences may contribute to diminished cross-protection in challenge experiments in chickens [193, 228].

Investigation of monoclonal antibody-resistant mutants revealed that many of the amino acids involved in the formation of VN epitopes are located within the first and third quarters of the linear S1 polypeptide [194-196]. Sequence analysis of naturally occurring variants that are genetically very similar (>95% amino acid identity in S1) has shown that most of the differences are within these two regions [185, 190]. Thus these parts of S1 are very tolerant of amino acid changes, changes that probably confer a selective advantage.

Amongst group 2 coronaviruses sequence variation is also greater in S1 than S2, a C-terminal region of S1 being hypervariable (Fig. 9). Indeed, this region is deleted in variants of MHV. Deletions in the N-terminal part of S1 have not been observed with group 2 viruses. This correlates with the finding that the receptor-binding domain of MHV is within the N-terminal 330 residues (Fig. 5; [197]).

In group 1, it is the N-terminal 300 or so residues of S that are most variable. From position 300 to the end of the molecule (at approximately residue number 1450) TGEV, CECoV type II and FCoV type II have ≥94% amino acid identity (80–90% throughout the whole S protein). Within the first 300 residues this falls to ~85% between FCoV type II and CECoV type II, and to ~30% between FCoV type II and TGEV. Moreover, the non-enteropathogenic variant of TGEV, called porcine respiratory coronavirus, has 225 of the first 300 amino acids deleted [198] (for additional references see reviews [29, 199, 200]). This extreme variation at the N-terminal part of S of group 2 viruses correlates with the receptor-binding domain being further down the molecule (Fig. 5; [96]).

The feline and canine coronaviruses of group 1 are not homogeneous. Thus, although the type II FCoVs and type II CECoVs have ~90% identity in the whole S protein, the type I FCoVs and type I CECoVs have only ~45% identity with the type II viruses.

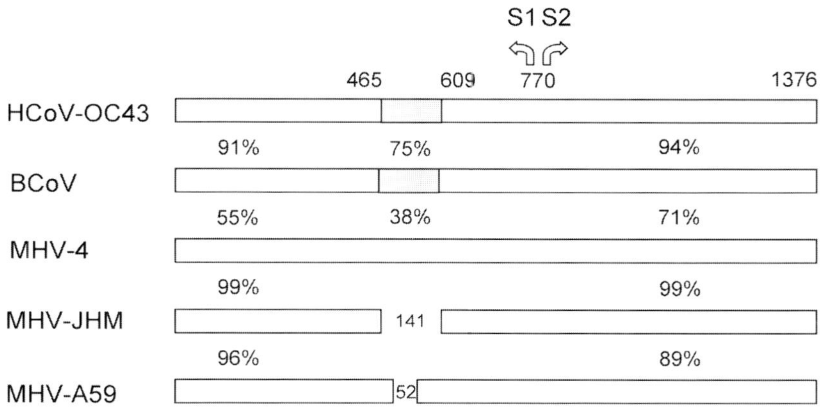

Figure 9. Amino acid identity between three regions of the S proteins of three species of group 2 coronavirus, and between three strains of MHV. Identity between species is greatest in S2. In the C-terminal part of S1 is a hypervariable region (in grey). This is not only the region of least identity between species; it is also a region which has been deleted from some strains of MHV. The amino acid identity between the S protein of BCoV and another isolate of HCoV-OC43 was >98% [202]).

The full-length S proteins of HCoV-229E and PEDV have only ~45% amino acid identity with each other and with the other members of group 1.

Host range of coronaviruses and toroviruses

Although coronaviruses have been described as being fastidious with regard to their hosts, this is true *in vitro* but not *in vivo*. Thus it has been very difficult to obtain cell cultures to grow some coronaviruses. Whereas the HCoV-229E and related strains can be isolated in human embryonic lung fibroblasts, such as W138 and MRC5 cells, HCoV-OC43-related strains usually cannot be grown in cell cultures, at least on initial isolation, and for these strains isolation has been performed in organ cultures of human embryonic tissues (reviewed by Myint, [201]). TCoV can only be grown in embryonated turkey eggs, and to a lesser extent in chicken embros. HToVs have not been grown in culture. However, the host range of coronaviruses, and probably toroviruses [66], is greater *in vivo*.

An HCoV isolate, of the OC43 genotype, had >99% amino acid identity in the S and HE proteins with the corresponding proteins of BCoV [202]. A recently discovered respiratory canine coronavirus is a group 2 coronavirus [203], the S protein of which had 96% and 95% amino acid identity with that of BCoV and HCoV-OC43, respectively. Cross-infection by these viruses has not been studied but a broad host range for them is a possibility. Turkeys are naturally infected with a coronavirus that is genetically very similar to IBV i.e. the same group 3 genome organisation and most proteins with >85% amino acid identity [188]. Notwithstanding, turkeys have been successfully infected with BCoV, a group 2 virus, leading to diarrhoea [204].

Group 1 coronaviruses include TGEV, FCoV and CECoV. CECoV experimentally applied orally to pigs replicated in them, inducing antibodies though not causing disease [205]. When hysterectomy-derived pigs were infected orally by these three viruses, virulent FCoV type I caused villous atrophy in the jejunum and ileum, resulting in clinical signs typical of a virulent TGEV infection, and death of 3/12 pigs. Cell culture-adapted FCoV and virulent CECoV produced less severe lesions and no mortality. Replication of these coronaviruses was confirmed by immunofluorescence.

Given the above, it is not surprising that viruses with >99% nucleotide identity with SARS coronavirus from humans were identified in nearby animals, namely in the Himalayan palm civet cat and racoon dog during the SARS epidemic in China. Experiments have subsequently shown that human isolates of SARS-CoV can replicate, and cause disease, in cynomolgus macaques (*Macaca fascicularis* [206]), in ferrets (*Mustela furo*) and domestic cats (*Felis domesticus* [207]). Several cats and a dog were found to be positive for SARS-CoV in the Amoy Gardens outbreak in Hong Kong.

Most of the known coronaviruses (Tab. 1) are known because they are pathogens of economic importance (e.g. cattle, pigs) or of social importance (cats, dogs, humans), and take their name from their hosts. The SARS epidemic in humans, and the rediscovery of what we already knew about other, long-known coronaviruses (outlined above), tells us that the host range of coronaviruses is much wider than was previously supposed.

Tropisms of coronaviruses

The naming of coronaviruses, like many other viruses, has often been based on the site at which pathology is manifest in a particular host species, e.g. avian infectious bronchitis coronavirus, Murine hepatitis virus. In some cases names have been simplified in recent years, e.g. bovine enteric coronavirus to bovine coronavirus, feline infectious peritonitis virus to feline coronavirus. It has been mooted that murine hepatitis coronavirus should be renamed to simply murine coronavirus. These changes reflect that within a host species a coronavirus replicates in many more tissues than its name would imply. This is well illustrated by IBV, which replicates at a myriad of epithelial surfaces (Fig. 10; reviewed in [80, 208, 209]. TGEV not only replicates at some enteric surfaces, as its name implies, but also in kidneys and lung (reviewed by Garwes [200]). MHV initially replicates in the gut but may then be disseminated to other organs e.g. liver and central nervous system (CNS), where it might cause pathology [210]. FCoV usually causes no more than an enteritis but in some cases, for reasons still not fully under-

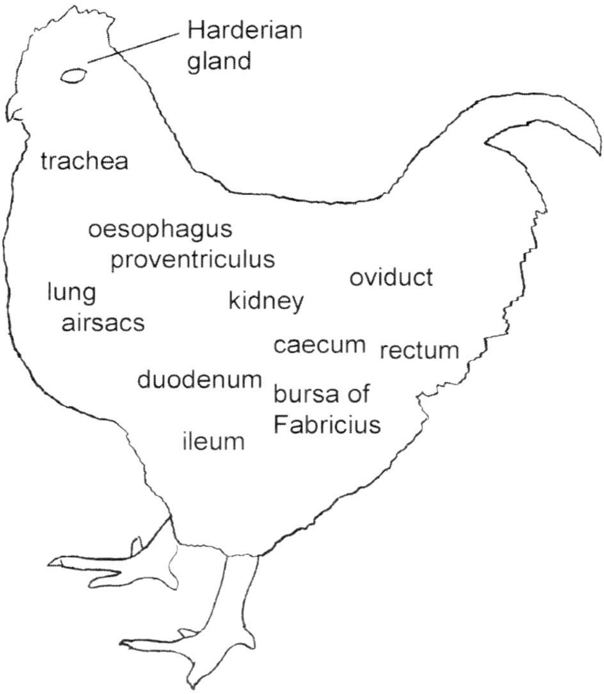

Figure 10. Tissues of the domestic fowl that become productively infected with IBV after inoculation of the nose and by eye-drop. The Harderian gland is a small lymphatic organ behind the eye. The proventriculus is a cranial glandular compartment of the stomach, adjacent to the gizzard, which is the caudal muscular compartment.

stood (but perhaps including the nature of the immune response of the host), it causes infectious peritonitis (actually, a vasculitis; reviewed by de Groot and Horzinek [211], and Addie and colleagues [212, 213]). HEV of pigs initially replicates in the respiratory tract and pharyngeal tonsils, then spreads *via* the peripheral nervous system to the CNS [200].

I have already hinted that strains of a given coronavirus species differ with respect to tropism. Although most strains of IBV replicate in the chicken kidney, only a few are intrinsically nephropathogenic (able to cause kidney-related mortality in experimentally infected chickens), causing up to 44% mortality [214–217]. Recently Yu et al. [218] have studied the pathogenesis of three isolates of IBV that caused proventriculitis, mortality being age-dependent (75–100% in two-week-old birds; 0–25% in 16-week-old chickens).

MHV strains vary with respect to not only whether they cause pathology in the CNS but also in the nature of the pathology e.g. acute or chronic demyelination [210], reviewed by Dales and Anderson [219], Stohlman and Hinton, [220] and Matthews et al. [221]. A number of enveloped and non-enveloped, RNA and DNA viruses have been associated with demyelination in humans and rodents, including coronaviruses [220]. Several studies [222, 223], though not all [224], have resulted in the detection of coronavirus RNA in brain tissue of multiple sclerosis patients. Arbour et al. [222] hypothesized that HCoV RNA might sometimes lead to a low level of viral protein synthesis that could be involved in the stimulation of immune responses within the CNS, exacerbating the effect of coronaviral infection in MS patients. Experiments have shown that both HCoV-OC43 and HCoV-229E can establish acute infections in many human neural cell lines: astrocytoma, neuroblastoma, neuroglioma, oligodendrocyte and microglial cell lines [225]. Persistent infections were established in some of the lines.

Some strains of TGEV do not cause enteritis. Most well known are those that have been called porcine respiratory coronavirus. As would be expected from this name, such variants replicate, as do the classical enteric strains of TGEV, in the respiratory tract, though usually asymptomatically, but replicate to only low levels in the enteric tract (reviewed by Garwes, [200] and Enjuanes and van der Zeijst [199]). The non-enteric strains have a large deletion in the S protein gene, as explained above.

These are just some of the examples of the different tropisms manifest by variants of a given coronavirus species. The pantropism of IBV might be the case for SARS coronavirus, as the latter has not only been associated with pneumonia but also with diarrhoea (though it remains to be demonstrated if the SARS virus is replicating in enteric tissues [227]). A point of difference is that whereas SARS CoV is associated with severe clinical signs in both the respiratory and enteric tracts, IBV is usually limited to disease in the respiratory tract (though the nephropathogenic and proventriculopathogenic strains of IBV are exceptions). Indeed, if it is demonstrated that SARS-CoV was directly responsible for the pathology in both respiratory tract and gut, it will be one of the few cases in which a given strain of a coronavirus has caused serious pathology in both regions.

Before the appearance of SARS there were reports describing coronavirus-like viruses isolated from faecal specimens from humans [33]. Some of these viruses were isolated from infants with necrotizing enterocolitis, patients with non-bacterial gastroenteritis and from homosexual men with diarrhoea who were symptomatic and seropositive for human immunodeficiency virus. Some isolates were shown to be serologically related to HCoV-OC43. The discovery that a protein found in enterocytes functions as a receptor for HCoV-229E strengthens the likelihood that coronaviruses might replicate in the human alimentary tract.

Evidence has increased that toroviruses are associated with gastroenteritis in humans. In a case-control study of children, an antigen capture ELISA revealed torovirus in stools from 27% (9/33) of children with acute diarrhoea, 27% (11/41) with persistent diarrhoea and none in controls [21].

In another childhood study, electron microscopy revealed a torovirus incidence of 35% (72/206) and 15% in gastroenteritis cases and controls, respectively [22].

Determinants of pathogenicity

There are doubtless many positions in the genomes of coronaviruses in which mutations can lead to changes in pathogenicity. For example, when we replaced the S protein gene of an attenuated strain of IBV with that from a pathogenic strain, it remained non-pathogenic [228], although its tropism *in vitro* had been changed [229]. Notwithstanding, the S protein can be a major determinant of pathogenicity. Ballesteros et al. [174] produced recombinants from enteropathogenic and non-enteropathogenic strains of TGEV which had extremely similar genome sequences. Some of the recombinants were non-enteropathogenic, the authors concluding that only one or two amino acid differences in the S protein were associated with the non-enteropathogenic phenotype. The authors produced further support for the role of the S protein in enteropathogenicity by producing recombinant TGEV by targeted recombination [230]. They further suggested that two domains on the S protein might be involved in attachment to enteric cells, one for binding to porcine aminopeptidase N. This receptor is present in lung tissue as well as in enteric tissue; binding to this does not account for the different tropisms. The other domain might be involved in the binding to a coreceptor, not defined, essential for the enteric tropism; differences in this domain affected the tropism of TGEV. The situation might be even more complex, as there is also evidence for the involvement of cell surface sialoglycoproteins as receptors for TGEV [101, 102].

The S protein determines the nature of the neurovirulence of MHV strains. This had been suspected from early sequencing studies (Fig. 10) and has been confirmed by sequencing of mutants arising during replication in persistently infected glial cells [231], and by mutants generated by targeted recombination [232–234]. For example, when the S protein gene of a demyelinating strain of MHV (A59) was replaced with that of a non-demyelinating strain (MHV-2), the resultant recombinant was non-demyelinating [232]. The A59 strain is also hepatotropic, whereas the MHV-4 strain has only minimal effect on the liver. Spike-swapping by targeted recombination showed that the hepatotropism was determined by the S protein [235].

Feline cells *in vitro*, which are normally refractory to infection by MHV, were productively infected by recombinant MHV in which the S protein gene has been replaced by that from FCoV [3]. In other words, MHV was able to replicate well in feline cells provided that it had an S protein capable of initiating infection. Genes other than S affect pathogenicity. The non-structural proteins of coronaviruses, not least SARS-CoV, are attracting attention. Deletion of all the non-structural protein genes of MHV produced virus that replicated in mice but which, unlike the wild-type virus, was non-lethal [10]. Inactivation (whether by deletion or other modification) of individual non-structural protein genes does not necessarily result in reduced pathogenicity. FcoV, unable to make the ORF 7b protein, was still lethal for cats [1]. Removal of gene 3 of TGEV did not diminish its enteropathogenicity [75]. IBV, unable to make non-structural proteins 3a and 3b or 5a and 5b (our unpublished observations), remained lethal for chick embryos.

Persistent infections, asymptomatic shedding

A feature of at least some coronaviruses is that they establish persistent infections not only *in vitro* but also *in vivo*. Chicks that had been experimentally infected with IBV at one day of age re-excreted virus asymptomatically at around 19 weeks of age [236]. It is suspected that the stressor of the start of egg production caused the release of the virus. Similar observations have been made more recently [237]. Approximately 10% of cats that had been naturally infected with FCoV became asymptomatic carriers, excreting virus for over one year [212, 213]. Others excreted virus for periods of several months. Long-term infections of MHV in mice and rats have been known for a long time, associated with neuropathogenesis.

Vaccines

Vaccination against coronavirus infections has been undertaken with respect to IBV, TGEV, CECoV, FCoV and BCoV. Of these, vaccination has been most widely, and arguably most successfully, practised in respect of IBV, for over 50 years [80].

Meat-type chicks (broilers) are usually vaccinated on the day of hatch with live attenuated vaccinal strains applied by spray. Protection of the respiratory tract following a single live attenuated virus vaccination has been found to be short-lived, the number of protected chickens declining after 6 weeks [238, 239]. As explained above, IBV exists as many serotypes, cross-protection between them often being poor. Consequently IBV vaccines have been developed with several serotypes. Vaccination with live attenuated virus is effective not only against respiratory disease but also kidney involement [217].

Inactivated oil-emulsion IBV vaccines were developed during the 1960s and 1970s. The objective was to make a vaccine that would give long-lasting immunity to the hen bird, to protect against drops in egg production. When used without prior priming with live IBV vaccine, killed IBV vaccines produced immunity in too few chickens, even when multiple doses of up to 200 μg of purified, inactivated virus were used [240–242]. The approach commonly used in the poultry industry today is to vaccinate young females two or more times with live vaccine, followed by one dose of inactivated vaccine as the birds come into lay. The live vaccines serve to give protection to the young bird and to prime the immune response to the inactivated vaccine.

Passive administration of convalescent IBV serum to chickens protected against intravenous application of a strain known to produce nephritis [243]. This passive application of immune serum did not protect against respiratory infection, although onset was delayed and was of shorter duration.

The efficacy of vaccination with live vaccine varies amongst inbred lines of chickens i.e. genetic differences between individuals affects the efficacy of the immune response [244–247].

Efforts to make effective vaccines against infectious peritonitis caused by FCoV have been ongoing for many years. A phenomenon that has militated against their widespread application has been that of antibody-dependent enhancement of disease. That is, antibodies induced by a first infection or vaccination may enhance the disease caused by a subsequent infection. Infection of cats by FCoV usually results in an infection confined largely to the digestive tract. In some cases the virus disseminates to other organs, leading to fatal infectious peritonitis. This dissemination is facilitated by macrophages. It is believed that uptake of FCoV by macrophages is enhanced when the virus has immunoglobulins, induced by a prior infection or vaccination, on its surface; the Fc moiety of the immunoglobulin attaches the virus-antibody complex to the surface of the macrophage (reviewd in [211]; see also [212, 213]).

Vaccines have not been developed against human coronaviruses. Immunity following natural infection is short-lived. Re-infection of individuals with the same HCoV serotype often occurs within four months of the first infection, suggesting that homologous HCoV antibodies are protective for about four months [11].

Proteins involved in the induction of protective immunity

There is no doubt that the S protein, when inoculated on its own, can induce protective immunity. The proportion of animals being protected may be dependent on the manner by which the S protein is presented to the host. There is also evidence that the N protein can prime protective immune responses, and a report that the N protein of IBV on its own induced protective immunity.

As would be expected from its global economic importance, there have been several studies on the induction of immunity by IBV (reviewed by Cavanagh, [80]). The S1 subunit induces immunity. S1 produced in a number of ways has been used as an immunogen: by removal from virus by urea (in which event the S1 was no longer multimeric [240]); by removal from virus using non-ionic detergent, followed by affinity chromatography using monoclonal antibodies; by expression in *Spodoptera frugiperda* cells from a recombinant *Autographa californica* baculovirus [242]. Immunisation with these various S1 preparations induced protective immunity against respiratory and kidney disease in a proportion of chickens, up to about 80% after four inoculations of S1. More strikingly, greater protection was achieved following a single oral application of a non-pathogenic fowl adenovirus expressing S1 [248]. Protection, assessed by non-reisolation of challenge virus, was obtained in 90% and 100% of 10 to 13 chickens in two experiments.

Similarly, expression of the MHV S protein from an adenovirus vector protected mice from lethal challenge [249]. Earlier Daniel and Talbot (1990) [267] had shown that immunisation of mice with S recovered from purified virus protected against lethal challenge with MHV.

The first study of the role of the IBV N protein in immunity was by Boots et al. [250]. Although immunisation with N alone did not induce protective immunity, subsequent immunisation with inactivated IBV resulted in greater protection than when the inactivated vaccine alone was administered. The authors concluded that immunisation with the N protein had primed protective immune responses by activation of cytotoxic or helper T cell responses.

More strikingly, two intramuscular immunisations of chickens with a plasmid expressing the N protein, or a fragment of the N protein, induced immune responses that protected the birds from infection by IBV, as evidenced by marked reduction in replication of the challenge virus [251]. A fragment of the N protein comprising the C-terminal 120 amino acid residues contained a major T cell epitope, and was sufficient to induce protection. The immunisation induced cytotoxic T lymphocytes that were deemed to be responsible for the protection. CTL activity was major histocompatibility complex restricted, and lysis was mediated by $CD8^+$ $CD4^-$ cells [252]. Adoptive transfer of IBV infection-induced $\alpha\beta$ T cells bearing CD8 antigen protected chicks from challenge infection [253, 254]. An early and strong T-helper cell response specific for the N protein of MHV has been reported [255]. When mice received N protein-specific $CD4^+$ T cells by adoptive transfer, they were protected against an otherwise lethal challenge with MHV. Further studies have shown the presence of helper and cytotoxic T cell epitopes in the C-terminal part of the MHV N protein [256–259].

Passive administration of monoclonal antibodies against the MHV S and, separately, N, proteins, protected mice against lethal challenge with MHV [260]. Similarly, expression of the MHV S and N proteins, separately, from adenovirus vectors protected mice from lethal challenge [249]. Greater protection was obtained when mice had been immunised simultaneously with both of the adenovirus recombinants.

Final comments

During 2002 PubMed abstracted approximately 130 papers featuring coronaviruses. This rose to approximately 510 in 2003, an increase of almost four-fold. This rise was, of course, a consequence of SARS. The speed with which scientists identified and characterised SARS CoV, and many aspects of its biology, was astounding. The remainder of this book reviews what was revealed in such a short time.

Acknowledgements
The author is supported by the Department for the Environment, Food and Rural Affairs, and the Biotechnology and Biological Sciences Research Council, UK.

References

1 Haijema BJ, Volders H, Rottier PJ (2003) Switching species tropism: an effective way to manipulate the feline coronavirus genome. *J Virol* 77: 4528–4538
2 Koetzner CA, Parker MM, Ricard CS, Sturman LS, Masters PS (1992) Repair and mutagenesis of the genome of a deletion mutant of the coronavirus mouse hepatitis virus by targeted RNA recombination. *J Virol* 66: 1841–1848
3 Kuo L, Godeke GJ, Raamsman MJ, Masters PS, Rottier PJ (2000) Retargeting of coronavirus by substitution of the spike glycoprotein ectodomain: crossing the host cell species barrier. *J Virol* 74: 1393–1406
4 Masters PS (1999) Reverse genetics of the largest RNA viruses. *Adv Virus Res* 53: 245–264
5 Thiel V, Herold J, Schelle B, Siddell SG (2001) Infectious RNA transcribed in vitro from a cDNA copy of the human coronavirus genome cloned in vaccinia virus. *J Gen Virol* 82: 1273–1281
6 Almazán F, González JM, Pénzes Z, Izeta A, Calvo E, Plana-Durán J, Enjuanes L (2000) Engineering the largest RNA virus genome as an infectious bacterial artificial chromosome. *Proc Nat Acad Sci USA* 97: 5516–5521
7 Yount B, Curtis KM, Baric RS (2000) Strategy for systematic assembly of large RNA and DNA genomes: transmissible gastroenteritis virus model. *J Virol* 74: 10600–10611
8 Yount B, Denison MR, Weiss SR, Baric RS (2002) Systematic Assembly of a Full-Length Infectious cDNA of Mouse Hepatitis Virus Strain A59. *J Virol* 76: 11065–11078
9 Yount B, Curtis KM, Fritz EA, Hensley LE, Jahrling PB, Prentice E, Denison MR, Geisbert TW, Baric RS (2003) Reverse genetics with a full-length infectious cDNA of severe acute respiratory syndrome coronavirus. *Proc Natl Acad Sci USA* 100: 12995–13000

10 de Haan CA, Masters PS, Shen X, Weiss S, Rottier PJ (2002) The group-specific murine coronavirus genes are not essential, but their deletion, by reverse genetics, is attenuating in the natural host. *Virology* 296: 177–189
11 Cavanagh D (2004) Coronaviruses and toroviruses. In: AJ Zuckerman JE Banatvala, PD Griffiths, JR Pattison, BD Schoub (eds): *Principles and Practice of Clinical Virology*, 5th ed., John Wiley & Sons Ltd, Chichester, 379–397
12 Makela MJ, Puhakka T, Ruuskanen O, Leinonen M, Saikku P, Kimpimaki M, Blomqvist S, Hyypia T, Arstila P (1998) Viruses and bacteria in the etiology of the common cold. *J Clin Microbiol* 36: 539–542
13 Pitkaranta A, Hayden FG (1998) What's new with common colds? Pathogenesis and diagnosis. *Infections Med* 15: 50–57
14 Pene F, Merlat A, Vabret A, Rozenberg F, Buzyn A, Dreyfus F, Cariou A, Freymuth F, Lebon P (2003) Coronavirus 229E-related pneumonia in immunocompromised patients. *Clin Infect Dis* 37: 929–932
15 McKean MC, Leech M, Lambert PC, Hewitt C, Myint S, Silverman M (2001) A model of viral wheeze in nonasthmatic adults: symptoms and physiology. *Eur Respir J* 18: 23–32
16 Gagneur A, Legrand MC, Picard B, Baron R, Talbot PJ, de Parscau L, Sizun J (2002) Nosocomial infections due to human coronaviruses in the newborn. *Arch Pediatr* 9: 61–69
17 Falsey AR, Walsh EE, Hayden FG (2002) Rhinovirus and coronavirus infection-associated hospitalizations among older adults. *J Infect Dis* 185: 1338–1341
18 Freymuth F, Vabret A, Brouard J, Toutain F, Verdon R, Petitjean J, Gouarin S, Duhamel JF, Guillois B (1999) Detection of viral, *Chlamydia pneumoniae* and *Mycoplasma pneumoniae* infections in exacerbations of asthma in children. *J Clin Virol* 13: 131–139
19 Atmar RL, Guy E, Guntupalli KK, Zimmerman JL, Bandi VD, Baxter BD, Greenberg SB (1998) Respiratory tract viral infections in inner-city asthmatic adults. *Arch Intern Med* 158: 2453–2459
20 van Benten IJ, KleinJan A, Neijens HJ, Osterhaus AD, Fokkens WJ (2001) Prolonged nasal eosinophilia in allergic patients after common cold. *Allergy* 56: 949–956
21 Koopmans MP, Goosen ES, Lima AA, McAuliffe IT, Nataro JP, Barrett LJ, Glass RI, Guerrant RL (1997) Association of torovirus with acute and persistent diarrhea in children. *Pediatr Infect Dis* J 16: 504–507
22 Jamieson FB, Wang EE, Bain C, Good J, Duckmanton L, Petric M (1998) Human torovirus: a new nosocomial gastrointestinal pathogen. *J Infect Dis* 178: 1263–1269
23 Cavanagh D, Davis PJ (1986) Coronavirus IBV: Removal of spike glycopeptide S1 by urea abolishes infectivity and haemagglutination but not attachment to cells. *J Gen Virol* 67: 1443–1448
24 Stern DF, Burgess L, Sefton BM (1982) Structural analysis of virion proteins of the avian coronavirus infectious bronchitis virus. *J Virol* 42: 208–219
25 Cavanagh D (1983) Coronavirus IBV: further evidence that the surface projections are associated with two glycopolypeptides. *J Gen Virol* 64: 1787–1791

26 Lewicki DN, Gallagher TM (2002) Quaternary structure of coronavirus spikes in complex with CEACAM cellular receptors. *J Biol Chem*
27 Vennema H, Heijnens L, Zijderveld A, Horzinek MC, Spaan WJM (1990) Intracellular transport of recombinant coronavirus spike proteins: implications for virus assembly. *J Gen Virol* 64: 339–346
28 Delmas B, Laude H (1990) Assembly of coronavirus spike protein into trimers and its role in epitope expression. *J Virol* 64: 5367–5375
29 Cavanagh D (1995) The coronavirus surface glycoprotein. In: Siddell SG (ed): *The Coronaviridae*. Plenum Press, New York and London, 73–113
30 Gallagher TM, Buchmeier MJ (2001) Coronavirus spike proteins in viral entry and pathogenesis. *Virology* 279: 371–374
31 Lai MMC, Cavanagh D (1997) The molecular biology of coronaviruses. *Adv Virus Res* 48: 1–100
32 Cornelissen LA, Wierda CM, van der Meer FJ, Herrewegh AA, Horzinek MC, Egberink HF, de Groot RJ (1997) Hemagglutinin-esterase, a novel structural protein of torovirus. *J Virol* 71: 5277–5286
33 Duckmanton L, Luan B, Devenish J, Tellier R, Petric M (1997) Characterization of torovirus from human fecal specimens. *Virology* 239: 158– 168
34 Woode GN, Reed DE, Runnels PL, Herrig MA, Hill HT (1982) Studies with an unclassified virus isolated from diarrhoeic calves. *Vet Microbiol* 7: 221–240
35 Beards GM, Hall C, Green J, Flewett TH, Lamouliatte F, Du Pasquier P (1984) An enveloped virus in stools of children and adults with gastroenteritis that resembles the Breda virus of calves. *Lancet* 1: 1050–1052
36 Rottier PJM (1995) The coronavirus membrane glycoprotein. In: Siddell SG (ed): *The Coronaviridae*. Plenum Press, New York and London, 115–139
37 Laude H, Masters PS (1995) The coronavirus nucleocapsid protein. In: Siddell SG (ed): *The Coronaviridae*. Plenum Press, New York and London, 141–163
38 Siddell SG (1995) The small-membrane protein. In: Siddell SG (ed): *The Coronaviridae*. Plenum, Press, New York and London, 181–189
39 Bos EC, Luytjes W, van der Meulen HV, Koerten HK, Spaan WJ (1996) The production of recombinant infectious DI-particles of a murine coronavirus in the absence of helper virus. *Virology* 218: 52–60
40 Vennema H, Godeke GJ, Rossen JWA, Voorhout WF, Horzinek MC, Opstelten DJE, Rottier PJM (1996) Nucleocapsid-independent assembly of coronavirus-like particles by co-expression of viral envelope protein genes. *Embo J* 15: 2020–2028
41 Cavanagh D, Davis PJ, Pappin DJC (1986) Coronavirus IBV glycopolypeptides: locational studies using proteases and saponin, a membrane permeabiliser. *Virus Res* 4: 145–156
42 Rottier P, Armstrong J, Meyer DI (1985) Signal recognition particle-dependent insertion of coronavirus E1, an intracellular membrane glycoprotein. *J Biol Chem* 260: 4648–4652
43 Risco C, Anton IM, Sune C, Pedregosa AM, Martin-Alonso JM, Parra F, Carrascosa JL, Enjuanes L (1995) Membrane protein molecules of transmissible gastroenteritis coronavirus also expose the carboxy-terminal region on the external surface of the virion. *J Virol* 69: 5269–5277

44 Risco C, Anton IM, Enjuanes L, Carrascosa JL (1996) The transmissible gastroenteritis coronavirus contains a spherical core shell consisting of M and N proteins. *J Virol* 70: 4773–4777
45 Escors D, Camafeita E, Ortego J, Laude H, Enjuanes L (2001) Organization of two transmissible gastroenteritis coronavirus membrane protein topologies within the virion and core. *J Virol* 75: 12228–12240
46 Escors D, Ortego J, Laude H, Enjuanes L (2001) The membrane M protein carboxy terminus binds to transmissible gastroenteritis coronavirus core and contributes to core stability. *J Virol* 75: 1312–1324
47 Kuo L, Masters PS (2002) Genetic evidence for a structural interaction between the carboxy termini of the membrane and nucleocapsid proteins of mouse hepatitis virus. *J Virol* 76: 4987–4999
48 de Haan CA, Kuo L, Masters PS, Vennema H, Rottier PJ (1998) Coronavirus particle assembly: primary structure requirements of the membrane protein. *J Virol* 72: 6838–6850
49 de Haan CA, Vennema H, Rottier PJ (2000) Assembly of the coronavirus envelope: homotypic interactions between the M proteins. *J Virol* 74: 4967–4978
50 Godeke GJ, de Haan CA, Rossen JW, Vennema H, Rottier PJ (2000) Assembly of spikes into coronavirus particles is mediated by the carboxy-terminal domain of the spike protein. *J Virol* 74: 1566–1571
51 Opstelten DJ, Raamsman MJ, Wolfs K, Horzinek MC, Rottier PJ (1995) Envelope glycoprotein interactions in coronavirus assembly. *J Cell Biol* 131: 339–349
52 de Haan CA, Smeets M, Vernooij F, Vennema H, Rottier PJ (1999) Mapping of the coronavirus membrane protein domains involved in interaction with the spike protein. *J Virol* 73: 7441–7452
53 de Haan CA, Roestenberg P, de Wit M, de Vries AA, Nilsson T, Vennema H, Rottier PJ (1998) Structural requirements for O-glycosylation of the mouse hepatitis virus membrane protein. *J Biol Chem* 273: 29905–29914
54 Godet M, L'Haridon R, Vautherot J-F, Laude H (1992) TGEV corona virus ORF-4 encodes a membrane protein that is incorporated into virions. *Virology* 188: 666–675
55 Corse E, Machamer CE (2000) Infectious bronchitis virus E protein is targeted to the golgi complex and directs release of virus-like particles. *J Virol* 74: 4319–4326
56 Raamsman MJ, Locker JK, de Hooge A, de Vries AA, Griffiths G, Vennema H, Rottier PJ (2000) Characterization of the coronavirus mouse hepatitis virus strain A59 small membrane protein E. *J Virol* 74: 2333–2342
57 Brian DA, Hogue BG, Kienzle TE (1995) The coronavirus hemagglutinin esterase glycoprotein. In: Siddell SG (ed): *The Coronaviridae*. Plenum Press, New York and London, 165–179
58 Vlasak R, Luytjes W, Spaan W, Palese P (1988) Human and bovine coronaviruses recognise sialic acid-containing receptors similar to those of influenza C viruses. *Proc Natl Acad Sci USA* 85: 4526–4529

59 Snijder EJ, Horzinek MC (1995) The molecular biology of Toroviruses. In: Siddell SG (ed): *The Coronaviridae*. Plenum Press, New York and London, 219–238
60 Pedersen NC, Ward I, Mengeling WL (1978) Antigenic relationships of feline infectious peritonitis virus to coronavirus of other species. *Arch Virol* 58: 45–53
61 Gonzalez JM, Gomez-Puertas P, Cavanagh D, Gorbalenya AE, Enjuanes L (2003) A comparative sequence analysis to revise the current taxonomy of the family Coronaviridae. Arch Virol 148: 2207–2235
62 Duarte M, Tobler K, Bridgen A, Rasschaert D, Ackermann M, Laude H (1994) Sequence analysis of the porcine epidemic diarrhea virus genome between the nucleocapsid and spike protein genes reveals a polymorphic ORF. *Virology* 198: 466–476
63 Correa I, Jimenez G, Sune C, Bullido MJ, Enjuanes L (1988) Antigenic structure of the E2 glycoprotein from transmissible gastroenteritis coronavirus. *Virus Res* 10: 77–93
64 Laude H, Chapsal JM, Gelfi J, Labiau S, Grosclaude J (1986) Antigenic structure of transmissible gastroenteritis virus. I. Properties of monoclonal antibodies directed against virion proteins. *J Gen Virol* 67: 119–130
65 Sanchez CM, Jimenez G, Laviada MD, Correa I, Sune C, Bullido M, Gebauer F, Smerdou C, Callebaut P, Escribano JM et al (1990) Antigenic homology among coronaviruses related to transmissible gastroenteritis virus. *Virology* 174: 410–417
66 Smits SL, Lavazza A, Matiz K, Horzinek MC, Koopmans MP, de Groot RJ (2003) Phylogenetic and evolutionary relationships among torovirus field variants: evidence for multiple intertypic recombination events. *J Virol* 77: 9567–9577
67 de Vries AAF, Horzinek MC, Rottier PJM, de Groot RJ (1997) The genome organisation of the nidovirales: similarities and differences between arteri-, toro- and coronaviruses. *Seminars in Virol* 8: 33–47
68 Sapats SI, Ashton F, Wright PJ, Ignjatovic J (1996) Novel variation in the N protein of avian infectious bronchitis virus. *Virology* 226: 412–417
69 Dalton K, Casais R, Shaw K, Stirrups K, Evans S, Britton P, Brown TD, Cavanagh D (2001) cis-Acting sequences required for coronavirus infectious bronchitis virus defective-RNA replication and packaging. *J Virol* 75: 125–133
70 Ortego J, Sola I, Almazan F, Ceriani JE, Riquelme C, Balasch M, Plana J, Enjuanes L (2003) Transmissible gastroenteritis coronavirus gene 7 is not essential but influences *in vivo* virus replication and virulence. *Virology* 308: 13–22
71 Sola I, Alonso S, Zuniga S, Balasch M, Plana-Duran J, Enjuanes L (2003) Engineering the transmissible gastroenteritis virus genome as an expression vector inducing lactogenic immunity. *J Virol* 77: 4357–4369
72 Ontiveros E, Kuo L, Masters PS, Perlman S (2001) Inactivation of expression of gene 4 of mouse hepatitis virus strain JHM does not affect virulence in the murine CNS. *Virology* 289: 230–238
73 Casais R, Thiel V, Siddell SG, Cavanagh D, Britton P (2001) Reverse genetics

system for the avian coronavirus infectious bronchitis virus. *J Virol* 75: 12359–12369
74 Snijder EJ, Bredenbeek PJ, Dobbe JC, Thiel V, Ziebuhr J, Poon LL, Guan Y, Rozanov M, Spaan WJ, Gorbalenya AE (2003) Unique and conserved features of genome and proteome of SARS-coronavirus, an early split-off from the coronavirus group 2 lineage. *J Mol Biol* 331: 991–1004
75 Sola I, Alonso S, Zuniga S, Balasch M, Plana-Duran J, Enjuanes L (2003) Engineering the transmissible gastroenteritis virus genome as an expression vector inducing lactogenic immunity. *J Virol* 77: 4357–69
76 Thiel V, Ivanov KA, Putics A, Hertzig T, Schelle B, Bayer S, Weissbrich B, Snijder EJ, Rabenau H, Doerr HW, Gorbalenya AE, Ziebuhr J (2003) Mechanisms and enzymes involved in SARS coronavirus genome expression. *J Gen Virol* 84: 2305–15
77 Guan Y, Zheng BJ, He YQ, Liu XL, Zhuang ZX, Cheung CL, Luo SW, Li PH, Zhang LJ, Guan YJ et al (2003) Isolation and characterization of viruses related to the SARS coronavirus from animals in southern China. *Science* 302: 276–278
78 Popova R, Zhang X (2002) The spike but not the hemagglutinin/esterase protein of bovine coronavirus is necessary and sufficient for viral infection. *Virology* 294: 222–236
79 Schultze B, Wahn K, Klenk HD, Herrler G (1991) Isolated HE-protein from hemagglutinating encephalomyelitis virus and bovine coronavirus has receptor-destroying and receptor-binding activity. *Virology* 180: 221–228
80 Cavanagh D (2003) Severe acute respiratory syndrome vaccine development: experiences of vaccination against avian infectious bronchitis coronavirus. *Avian Pathol* 32: 567–582
81 Tan K, Zelus BD, Meijers R, Liu JH, Bergelson JM, Duke N, Zhang R, Joachimiak A, Holmes KV, Wang JH (2002) Crystal structure of murine sCEACAM1a[1,4]: a coronavirus receptor in the CEA family. *Embo J* 21: 2076–2086
82 Chen DS, Asanaka M, Chen FS, Shively JE, Lai MM (1997) Human carcinoembryonic antigen and biliary glycoprotein can serve as mouse hepatitis virus receptors. *J Virol* 71: 1688–1691
83 Rao PV, Kumari S, Gallagher TM (1997) Identification of a contiguous 6-residue determinant in the MHV receptor that controls the level of virion binding to cells. *Virology* 229: 336–348
84 Miura HS, Nakagaki K, Taguchi F (2004) N-terminal domain of the murine coronavirus receptor CEACAM1 is responsible for fusogenic activation and conformational changes of the spike protein. *J Virol* 78: 216–223
85 Schickli JH, Zelus BD, Wentworth DE, Sawicki SG, Holmes KV (1997) The murine coronavirus mouse hepatitis virus strain A59 from persistently infected murine cells exhibits an extended host range. *J Virol* 71: 9499–9507
86 Suzuki H, Taguchi F (1996) Analysis of receptor-binding site of murine coronavirus spike protein. *J Virol* 70: 2632–2636
87 Gallagher TM (1997) A role for naturally occurring variation of the murine

coronavirus spike protein in stabilizing association with the cellular receptor. *J Virol* 71: 3129–3137
88 Tresnan DB, Levis R, Holmes KV (1996) Feline aminopeptidase N serves as a receptor for feline, canine, porcine, and human coronaviruses in serogroup I. *J Virol* 70: 8669–8674
89 Benbacer L, Kut E, Besnardeau L, Laude H, Delmas B (1997) Interspecies aminopeptidase-N chimeras reveal species-specific receptor recognition by canine coronavirus, feline infectious peritonitis virus, and transmissible gastroenteritis virus. *J Virol* 71: 734–737
90 Kolb AF, Maile J, Heister A, Siddell SG (1996) Characterization of functional domains in the human coronavirus HCV 229E receptor. *J Gen Virol* 77: 2515–2521
91 Kolb AF, Hegyi A, Siddell SG (1997) Identification of residues critical for the human coronavirus 229E receptor function of human aminopeptidase N. *J Gen Virol* 78: 2795–2802
92 Wentworth DE, Holmes KV (2001) Molecular determinants of species specificity in the coronavirus receptor aminopeptidase N (cd13): influence of n-linked glycosylation. *J Virol* 75: 9741–9752
93 Lachance C, Arbour N, Cashman NR, Talbot PJ (1998) Involvement of aminopeptidase N (CD13) in infection of human neural cells by human coronavirus 229E. *J Virol* 72: 6511–6519
94 Hohdatsu T, Izumiya Y, Yokoyama Y, Kida K, Koyama H (1998) Differences in virus receptor for type I and type II feline infectious peritonitis virus. *Arch Virol* 143: 839–850
95 Herrewegh AAPM, Smeenk I, Horzinek MC, Rottier PJM, deGroot RJ (1998) Feline coronavirus type II strains 79-1683 and 79-1146 originate from a double recombination between feline coronavirus type I and canine coronavirus. *J Virol* 72: 4508–4514
96 Bonavia A, Zelus BD, Wentworth DE, Talbot PJ, Holmes KV (2003) Identification of a receptor-binding domain of the spike glycoprotein of human coronavirus HCoV-229E. *J Virol* 77: 2530–2538
97 Li W, Moore MJ, Vasilieva N, Sui J, Wong SK, Berne MA, Somasundaran M, Sullivan JL, Luzuriaga K, Greenough TC, Choe H, Farzan M (2003) Angiotensin-converting enzyme 2 is a functional receptor for the SARS coronavirus. *Nature* 426: 450–454
98 Xiao X, Chakrabarti S, Dimitrov AS, Gramatikoff K, Dimitrov DS (2003) The SARS-CoV S glycoprotein: expression and functional characterization. *Biochem Biophys Res Comm* 312: 1159–1164
99 Schwegmann-Wessels C, Zimmer G, Schröder B, Breves G, Herrler G (2003) Binding of transmissible gastroenteritis coronavirus to brush border membrane sialoglycoproteins. *J Virol* 77: 11846–11848
100 Schultze B, Herrler G (1992) Bovine coronavirus uses N-acetyl-9-O-acetylneuraminic acid as a receptor determinant to initiate the infection of cultured cells. *J Gen Virol* 73: 901–906
101 Krempl C, Ballesteros M, Zimmer G, Enjuanes L, Klenk H, Herrler G (2000)

Characterization of the sialic acid binding activity of transmissible gastroenteritis coronavirus by analysis of haemagglutination-deficient mutants. *J Gen Virol* 81: 489–496
102 Schwegmann-Wessels C, Zimmer G, Laude H, Enjuanes L, Herrler G (2002) Binding of transmissible gastroenteritis coronavirus to cell surface sialoglycoproteins. *J Virol* 76: 99
103 Schultze B, Cavanagh D, Herrler G (1992) Neuraminidase treatment of avian infectious bronchitis coronavirus reveals a hemagglutinating activity that is dependent on sialic acid-containing receptors on erythrocytes. *Virology* 189: 792–794
104 De Groot RJ, Van Leen RW, Dalderup MJ, Vennema H, Horzinek MC, Spaan WJ (1989) Stably expressed FIPV peplomer protein induces cell fusion and elicits neutralizing antibodies in mice. *Virology* 171: 493–502
105 Grosse B, Siddell SG (1994) Single amino acid changes in the S2 subunit of the MHV surface glycoprotein confer resistance to neutralization by S1 subunit-specific monoclonal antibody. *Virology* 202: 814–824
106 Pfleiderer M, Routledge E, Siddell SG (1990) Functional analysis of the coronavirus MHV-JHM surface glycoproteins in vaccinia virus recombinants. *Adv Exp Med Biol* 276: 21–31
107 Keck JG, Soe LH, Makino S, Stohlman SA, Lai MMC (1988) RNA recombination of murine coronaviruses: recombination between fusion positive MHV-A59 and fusion negative MHV-2. *J Virol* 62: 1989–1998
108 Yoo D, Parker MD, Song J, Cox GJ, Deregt D, Babiuk LA (1991) Structural analysis of the conformational domains involved in neutralisation of bovine coronavirus using deletion mutants of the spike glycoprotein S1 subunit expressed by recombinant baculoviruses. *Virology* 183: 91–98
109 Luo ZL, Weiss SR (1998) Roles in cell-to-cell fusion of two conserved hydrophobic regions in the murine coronavirus spike protein. *Virology* 244: 483–494
110 Britton P (1991) Coronavirus motif. *Nature* 353: 394
111 Gallagher TM, Escarmis C, Buchmeier MJ (1991) Alteration of the pH dependence of coronavirus induced cell fusion – Effect of mutations in the spike glycoprotein. *J Virol* 65: 1916–1928
112 Routledge E, Stauber R, Pfleiderer M, Siddel SG (1991) Analysis of murine coronavirus surface glycoprotein functions by using monoclonal antibodies. *J Virol* 65: 254–262
113 Luo Z, Matthews AM, Weiss SR (1999) Amino acid substitutions within the leucine zipper domain of the murine coronavirus spike protein cause defects in oligomerization and the ability to induce cell-to-cell fusion. *J Virol* 73: 8152–8159
114 Luo Z, Weiss SR (1998) Roles in cell-to-cell fusion of two conserved hydrophobic regions in the murine coronavirus spike protein. *Virology* 244: 483–494
115 Bosch BJ, van der Zee R, de Haan CAM, Rottier PJM (2003) The coronavirus spike protein is a class I virus fusion protein: structural and functional characterization of the fusion care complex. *J Virol* 77: 8801–8811

116 Luytjes W, Geerts D, Posthumus W, Meloen R, Spaan W (1989) Amino acid sequence of a conserved neutralizing epitope of murine coronaviruses. *J Virol* 63: 1408–1412
117 Routledge E, Stauber R, Pfleiderer M, Siddell SG (1991) Analysis of murine coronavirus surface glycoprotein functions by using monoclonal antibodies. *J Virol* 65: 254–262
118 Kooi C, Cervin M, Anderson R (1991) Differentiation of acid-pH-dependent and acid-pH-nondependent entry pathways for mouse hepatitis virus. *Virology* 180: 108–119
119 Weismiller DG, Sturman LS, Buchmeier MJ, Fleming JO, Holmes KV (1990) Monoclonal-antibodies to the peplomer glycoprotein of coronavirus mouse hepatitis-virus identify 2-subunits and detect a conformational change in the subunit released under mild alkaline conditions. *J Virol* 64: 3051–3055
120 Li D, Cavanagh D (1992) Coronavirus IBV-induced membrane fusion occurs at near-neutral pH. *Arch Virol* 122: 307–316
121 Tsai JC, de Groot L, Pinon JD, Iacono KT, Phillips JJ, Seo SH, Lavi E, Weiss SR (2003) Amino acid substitutions within the heptad repeat domain 1 of murine coronavirus spike protein restrict viral antigen spread in the central nervous system. *Virology* 312: 369–380
122 Zelus BD, Schickli JH, Blau DM, Weiss SR, Holmes KV (2003) Conformational changes in the spike glycoprotein of murine coronavirus are induced at 37 degrees C either by soluble murine CEACAM1 receptors or by pH 8. *J Virol* 77: 830–840
123 Stauber R, Pfleiderer M, Siddell S (1993) Proteolytic cleavage of the murine coronavirus surface glycoprotein is not required for its fusion activity. *Adv Exp Med Biol* 342: 165–170
124 Taguchi F (1993) Fusion formation by the uncleaved spike protein of murine coronavirus JHMV varient cl-2. *J Virol* 67: 1195–1202
125 Gombold JL, Hingley ST, Weiss SR (1993) Fusion-defective mutants of mouse hepatitis virus A59 contain a mutation in the spike protein cleavage signal. *J Virol* 67: 4504–4512
126 Thiel V, Herold J, Schelle B, Siddell SG (2001) Viral replicase gene products suffice for coronavirus discontinuous transcription. *J Virol* 175: 6676–6681
127 Ziebuhr J, Siddell SG (1999) Processing of the human coronavirus 229E replicase polyproteins by the virus-encoded 3C-like proteinase: Identification of proteolytic products and cleavage sites common to pp1a and pp1ab. *J Virol* 73: 177–185
128 Brierley I, Digard P, Inglis SC (1989) Characterization of an efficient coronavirus ribosomal frameshifting signal – requirement for an RNA pseudoknot. *Cell* 57: 537–547
129 Brierley I (1995) Ribosomal frameshifting on viral RNAs. *J Gen Virol* 76: 1885–1892
130 Makino S, Joo M, Makino JK (1991) A system for study of coronavirus mRNA synthesis: a regulated, expressed subgenomic defective interfering RNA results from intergenic site insertion. *J Virol* 65: 6031–6041

131 van der Most RG, de Groot RJ, Spaan WJM (1994) Subgenomic RNA synthesis directed by a synthetic defective interfering RNA of mouse hepatitis virus: a study of coronavirus transcription initiation. *J Virol* 68: 3656–3666
132 van Marle G, Dobbe JC, Gultyaev AP, Luytjes W, Spaan WJ, Snijder EJ (1999) Arterivirus discontinuous mRNA transcription is guided by base pairing between sense and antisense transcription-regulating sequences. *Proc Natl Acad Sci USA* 96: 12056–12061
133 Alonso S, Izeta A, Sola I, Enjuanes L (2002) Transcription regulatory sequences and mRNA expression levels in the coronavirus transmissible gastroenteritis virus. *J Virol* 76: 1293–1308
134 van Vliet AL, Smits SL, Rottier PJ, de Groot RJ (2002) Discontinuous and non-discontinuous subgenomic RNA transcription in a nidovirus. *Embo J* 21: 6571–80
135 Fischer F, Peng D, Hingley ST, Weiss SR, Masters PS (1997) The internal open reading frame within the nucleocapsid gene of mouse hepatitis virus encodes a structural protein that is not essential for viral replication. *J Virol* 71: 996–1003
136 Senanayake SD, Hofmann MA, Maki JL, Brian DA (1992) The nucleocapsid protein gene of bovine coronavirus is bicistronic. *J Virol* 66: 5277–5283
137 Liu DX, Inglis SC (1992) Internal entry of ribosomes on a tricistronic mRNA encoded by infectious bronchitis virus. *J Virol* 66: 6143–6154
138 Thiel V, Siddell SG (1994) Internal ribosome entry in the coding region of murine hepatitis virus mRNA 5. *J Gen Virol* 75: 3041–3046
139 Le SY, Sonenberg N, Maizel JV Jr (1994) Distinct structural elements and internal entry of ribosomes in mRNA3 encoded by infectious bronchitis virus. *Virology* 198: 405–411
140 Opstelten DJ, de-Groote P, Horzinek MC, Vennema H, Rottier PJ (1993) Disulfide bonds in folding and transport of mouse hepatitis coronavirus glycoproteins. *J Virol* 67: 7394–7401
141 Frana MF, Behnke JN, Sturman LS, Holmes KV (1985) Proteolytic cleavage of the E2 glycoprotein of murine coronavirus: host-dependent differences in proteolytic cleavage and cell fusion. *J Virol* 56: 912–920
142 Cavanagh D, Davis PJ, Pappin DJC, Binns MM, Boursnell MEG, Brown TDK (1986) Coronavirus IBV: partial amino terminal sequencing of spike polypeptide S2 identifies the sequence Arg-Arg-Phe-Arg-Arg at the cleavage site of the spike precursor propolypeptide of IBV strains Beaudette and M41. *Virus Res* 4: 133–143
143 Luytjes W, Sturman LS, Bredenbeek PJ, Charite J, Van der Zeijst BA, Horzinek MC, Spaan WJ (1987) Primary structure of the glycoprotein E2 of coronavirus MHV-A59 and identification of the trypsin cleavage site. *Virology* 161: 479–487
144 Vennema H, Heijnen L, Zijderveld A, Horzinek MC, Spaan aWJM (1990) Intracellular transport of recombinant coronavirus spike proteins: Implications for virus assembly. *J Virol* 64: 339–346
145 Schmidt MFG (1982) Acylation of viral spike glycoproteins, a feature of enveloped RNA viruses. *Virology* 116: 327–338
146 King B, Potts BJ, Brian DA (1985) Bovine coronavirus hemaglutinin protein. *Virus Res* 2: 53–59

147 Yoo D, Graham FL, Prevec L, Parker MD, Benko M, Zamb T, Babiuk LA (1992) Synthesis and processing of the haemagglutinin-esterase glycoprotein of bovine coronavirus encoded in the E3 region of adenovirus. *J Gen Virol* 73: 2591–2600
148 Cavanagh D (1983) Coronavirus IBV glycopolypeptides: size of their polypeptide moieties and nature of their oligosaccharides. *J Gen Virol* 64: 1187–1191
149 Stern DF, Sefton BM (1982) Coronavirus proteins: structure and function of the oligosaccharides of the avian infectious bronchitis virus glycoproteins. *J Virol* 44: 804–812
150 Laude H, Rasschaert D, Huet JC (1987) Sequence and N terminal processing of the transmembrane protein E1 of the coronavirus transmissible gastroenteritis virus. *J Gen Virol* 68: 1687–1693
151 Kapke PA, Tung FYT, Hogue BG, Brian DA, Woods RD, Wesley RD (1988) The amino terminal signal peptide on the porcine transmissible gastroenteritis coronavirus matrix protein is not an absolute requirement for membrane translocation and glycosylation. *Virology* 165: 367–376
152 Vennema H, Degroot RJ, Harbour DA, Horzinek MC, Spaan WJM (1991) Primary structure of the membrane and nucleocapsid protein genes of feline infectious peritonitis virus and immunogenicity of recombinant vaccinia viruses in kittens. *Virology* 181: 327–335
153 Garwes DJ, Pocock DH, Pike BV (1976) Isolation of subviral components from transmissible gastroenteritis virus. *J Gen Virol* 32: 283–294
154 Yu X, Bi W, Weiss SR, Leibowitz JL (1994) Mouse hepatitis virus gene 5b protein is a new virion envelope protein. *Virology* 202: 1018–1023
155 Escors D, Izeta A, Capiscol C, Enjuanes L (2003) Transmissible gastroenteritis coronavirus packaging signal is located at the 5' end of the virus genome. *J Virol* 77: 7890–7902
156 Makino S, Soe LH, Shieh C-K, Lai MMC (1988) Discontinuous transcription generates heterogeneity at the leader fusion sites of coronavirus mRNAs. *J Virol* 62: 3870–3873
157 La Monica N, Yokomori K, Lai MMC (1992) Coronavirus mRNA synthesis: Identification of novel transcription initiation signals which are differentially regulated by different leader sequences. *Virology* 188: 402–407
158 Makino S, Lai MMC (1989) Evolution of the 5'-end of genomic RNA of murine coronaviruses during passages *in vitro*. *Virology* 169: 227–232
159 Hofmann MA, Chang R-Y, Ku S, Brian DA (1993) Leader-mRNA junction sequences are unique for each subgenomic mRNA species in the bovine coronavirus and remain so throughout persistent infection. *Virology* 196: 163–171
160 Salanueva IJ, Carrascosa JL, Risco C (1999) Structural maturation of the transmissible gastroenteritis coronavirus. *J Virol* 73: 7952–64
161 Krijnse-Locker J, Ericsson M, Rottier PJ, Griffiths G (1994) Characterization of the budding compartment of mouse hepatitis virus: evidence that transport from the RER to the Golgi complex requires only one vesicular transport step. *J Cell Biol* 124: 55–70
162 Escors D, Camafeita E, Ortego J, Laude H, Enjuanes L (2001) Organization of

two transmissible gastroenteritis coronavirus membrane protein topologies within the virion and core. *J Virol* 75: 12228–12240
163 Escors D, Ortego J, Laude H, Enjuanes L (2001) The membrane M protein carboxy terminus binds to transmissible gastroenteritis coronavirus core and contributes to core stability. *J Virol* 75: 1312–1324
164 Fischer F, Stegen CF, Masters PS, Samsonoff WA (1998) Analysis of constructed E gene mutants of mouse hepatitis virus confirms a pivotal role for E protein in coronavirus assembly. *J Virol* 72: 7885–7894
165 Corse E, Machamer CE (2002) The cytoplasmic tail of infectious bronchitis virus E protein directs Golgi targeting. *J Virol* 76: 1273–1284
166 Lim KP, Liu DX (2001) The missing link in coronavirus assembly. Retention of the avian coronavirus infectious bronchitis virus envelope protein in the pre-Golgi compartments and physical interaction between the envelope and membrane proteins. *J Biol Chem* 276: 17515–17523
167 Baudoux P, Carrat C, Besnardeau L, Charley B, Laude H (1998) Coronavirus pseudoparticles formed with recombinant M and E proteins induce alpha interferon synthesis by leukocytes. *J Virol* 72: 8636–8643
168 Maeda J, Maeda A, Makino S (1999) Release of coronavirus E protein in membrane vesicles from virus- infected cells and E protein-expressing cells. *Virology* 263: 265–272
169 Kuo LL, Masters PS (2003) The small envelope protein E is not essential for murine coronavirus replication. *J Virol* 77: 4597–4608
170 Kuo L, Masters PS (2003) The small envelope protein e is not essential for murine coronavirus replication. *J Virol* 77: 4597–4608
171 Risco C, Muntion M, Enjuanes L, Carrascosa JL (1998) Two types of virus-related particles are found during transmissible gastroenteritis virus morphogenesis. *J Virol* 72: 4022–4031
172 Lai MMC (1992) Genetic recombination in RNA viruses. *Curr Top Microbiol Immunol* 176: 21–32
173 Lai MMC, Baric RS, Makino S, Keck JG, Egbert J, Leibowitz JL, Stohlman SA (1985) Recombination between nonsegmented RNA genomes of murine coronaviruses. *J Virol* 56: 449–456
174 Ballesteros ML, Sanchez CM, Enjuanes L (1997) Two amino acid changes at the N-terminus of transmissible gastroenteritis coronavirus spike protein result in the loss of enteric tropism. *Virology* 227: 378–388
175 Kottier SA, Cavanagh D, Britton P (1995) Experimental evidence of recombination in coronavirus infectious bronchitis virus. *Virology* 213: 569–580
176 Cavanagh D, Davis PJ (1988) Evolution of avian coronavirus IBV: sequence of the matrix glycoprotein gene and intergenic region of several serotypes. *J Gen Virol* 69: 621–629
177 Cavanagh D, Davis PJ, Cook JKA (1992) Infectious-bronchitis virus – evidence for recombination within the massachusetts serotype. *Avian Pathol* 21: 401–408
178 Jia W, Karaca K, Parrish CR, Naqi SA (1995) A novel variant of avian infectious bronchitis virus resulting from recombination among three different strains. *Arch Virol* 140: 259–271

179 Wang L, Junker D, Collisson EW (1993) Evidence of natural recombination within the S1 gene of infectious bronchitis virus. *Virology* 192: 710–716
180 Wang L, Junker D, Hock L, Ebiary E, Collisson EW (1994) Evolutionary implications of genetic variations in the S1 gene of infectious bronchitis virus. *Virus Res* 34: 327–338
181 Herrewegh AA, Smeenk I, Horzinek MC, Rottier PJ, de Groot RJ (1998) Feline coronavirus type II strains 79-1683 and 79-1146 originate from a double recombination between feline coronavirus type I and canine coronavirus. *J Virol* 72: 4508–4514
182 Snijder EJ, Denboon JA, Horzinek MC, Spaan WJM (1991) Comparison of the genome organization of toroviruses and coronaviruses – evidence for two nonhomologous RNA recombination events during berne virus evolution. *Virology* 180: 448–452
183 Adzhar AB, Shaw K, Britton P, Cavanagh D (1995) Avian infectious bronchitis virus: differences between 793/B and other strains. *Vet Rec* 136: 548
184 Kingham BF, Keeler CL Jr, Nix WA, Ladman BS, Gelb J Jr (2000) Identification of avian infectious bronchitis virus by direct automated cycle sequencing of the S-1 gene. *Avian Dis* 44: 325–335
185 Adzhar A, Gough RE, Haydon D, Shaw K, Britton P, Cavanagh D (1997) Molecular analysis of the 793/B serotype of infectious bronchitis virus in Great Britain. *Avian Pathol* 26: 625–640
186 Gelb J, Keeler CL, Nix WA, Rosenberger JK, Cloud SS (1997) Antigenic and S-1 genomic characterization of the Delaware variant serotype of infectious bronchitis virus. *Avian Dis* 41: 661–669
187 Sapats SI, Ashton F, Wright PJ, Ignjatovic J (1996) Sequence analysis of the S1 glycoprotein of infectious bronchitis viruses: Identification of a novel genotypic group in Australia. *J Gen Virol* 77: 413–418
188 Cavanagh D, Mawditt K, Sharma M, Drury SE, Ainsworth HL, Britton P, Gough RE (2001) Detection of a coronavirus from turkey poults in Europe genetically related to infectious bronchitis virus of chickens. *Avian Pathol* 30: 355–368
189 Cavanagh D, Mawditt K, Welchman DdB, Britton P, Gough RE (2002) Coronaviruses from pheasants (Phasianus colchicus) are genetically closely related to coronaviruses of domestic fowl (infectious bronchitis virus) and turkeys. *Avian Pathol* 31: 181–193
190 Cavanagh D, Davis PJ, Cook JKA, Li D, Kant A, Koch G (1992) Location of the amino acid differences in the S1 spike glycoprotein subunit of closely related serotypes of infectious bronchitis virus. *Avian Pathol* 21: 33–43
191 Cook JKA (1984) The classification of new serotypes of infectious bronchitis virus isolated from poultry flocks in Britain between 1981 and 1983. *Avian Pathol* 13: 733–741
192 Cook JKA, Huggins MB (1986) Newly isolated serotypes of infectious bronchitis virus: their role in disease. *Avian Pathol* 15: 129–138
193 Cavanagh D, Ellis MM, Cook JKA (1997) Relationship between sequence variation in the S1 spike protein of infectious bronchitis virus and the extent of cross-protection *in vivo*. *Avian Pathol* 26: 63–74

194 Cavanagh D, Davis PJ, Mockett AP (1988) Amino acids within hypervariable region 1 of avian coronavirus IBV (Massachusetts serotype) spike glycoprotein are associated with neutralization epitopes. *Virus Res* 11: 141–150
195 Kant A, Koch G, van Roozelaar DJ, Kusters JG, Poelwijk FAJ, van der Zeijst BAM (1992) Location of antigenic sites defined by neutralising monoclonal antibodies on the S1 avian infectious bronchitis virus glycopolypeptide. *J Gen Virol* 73: 591–596
196 Koch G, Hartog L, Kant A, van Roozelaar DJ (1990) Antigenic domains of the peplomer protein of avian infectious bronchitis virus: correlation with biological function. *J Gen Virol* 71: 1929–1935
197 Suzuki H, Taguchi F (1996) Analysis of the receptor-binding site of murine coronavirus spike protein. *J Virol* 70: 2632–2636
198 Britton P, Mawditt KL, Page KW (1991) The cloning and sequencing of the virion protein genes from a British isolate of porcine respiratory coronavirus: comparison with transmissible gastroenteritis virus genes. *Virus Res* 21: 181–198
199 Enjuanes L, van der Zeijst BAM (1995) Molecular basis of transmissible gastroenteritis virus epidemiology. In: Siddell SG (ed): *The Coronaviridae*. Plenum Press, New York and London, 337–376
200 Garwes DJ (1995) Pathogenesis of the porcine coronaviruses. In: Siddell SG (ed): *The Coronaviridae*. Plenum Press, New York and London, 377–388
201 Myint SH (1995) Human coronavirus infections. In: Siddell SG (ed): *The Coronaviridae*. Plenum Press, New York, 389–402
202 Zhang XM, Herbst W, Kousoulas KG, Storz J (1994) Biological and genetic characterization of a hemagglutinating coronavirus isolated from a diarrhoeic child. *J Med Virol* 44: 152–161
203 Erles K, Toomey C, Brooks HW, Brownlie J (2003) Detection of a group 2 coronavirus in dogs with canine infectious respiratory disease. *Virology* 310: 216–223
204 Ismail MM, Cho KO, Ward LA, Saif LJ, Saif YM (2001) Experimental bovine coronavirus in turkey poults and young chickens. *Avian Dis* 45: 157–163
205 Woods RD, Wesley RD (1992) Seroconversion of pigs in contact with dogs exposed to canine coronavirus. *Can J Vet Res* 56: 78–80
206 Fouchier RA, Kuiken T, Schutten M, Van Amerongen G, Van Doornum GJ, Van Den Hoogen BG, Peiris M, Lim W, Stohr K, Osterhaus AD (2003) Aetiology: Koch's postulates fulfilled for SARS virus. *Nature* 423: 240
207 Martina BE, Haagmans BL, Kuiken T, Fouchier RA, Rimmelzwaan GF, Van Amerongen G, Peiris JS, Lim W, Osterhaus AD (2003) Virology: SARS virus infection of cats and ferrets. *Nature* 425: 915
208 Cavanagh D, Naqi S (2003) Infectious bronchitis. In: Saif YM, Barnes HJ, Glisson JR, Fadly AM, McDougald LR, Swayne DE (eds): *Diseases of Poultry*. Blackwell, Ames, Iowa, vol 11, 101–119
209 Cook JKA, Mockett APA (1995) Epidemiology of infectious bronchitis virus. In: Siddell SG (ed): *The Coronaviridae*. Plenum Press, New York and London, 317–335

210 Hirano N, Goto N, Ogawa T, Ono K, Murakani T, Fukiwara K (1980) Hydrocephalus in suckling rats infected intracerebrally with mouse hepatitis virus MHV-A59. *Microbiol Immunol* 24: 825

211 de Groot RJ, Horzinek MC (1995) Feline infectious peritonitis. In: Siddell SG (ed): *The Coronaviridae*. Plenum Press, New York and London, 293–315

212 Addie DD, Jarrett O (2001) Use of a reverse-transcriptase polymerase chain reaction for monitoring the shedding of feline coronavirus by healthy cats. Vet Rec 148: 649–53.

213 Addie DD, Schaap IA, Nicolson L, Jarrett O (2003) Persistence and transmission of natural type I feline coronavirus infection. *J Gen Virol* 84: 2735–2744

214 Chen BY, Hosi S, Itakura C (1996) Histopathology and immunohistochemistry of renal lesions due to an infectious bronchitis virus in chicks. *Avian Pathol* 25: 269–283

215 Chen BY, Itakura C (1996) Cytopathology of chick renal epithelia cells experimentally infected with avian infectious bronchitis virus. *Avian Pathol* 25: 675–690

216 Chen BY, Itakura C (1996) Cytopathology of chick renal epithelial cells experimentally infected with avian infectious bronchitis virus. *Avian Pathol* 25: 675–690

217 Pensaert M, Lambrechts C (1994) Vaccination of chickens against a Belgian nephropathogenic strain of infectious bronchitis virus B1648 using attenuated homologous and heterologous strains. *Avian Pathol* 23: 631–641

218 Yu L, Jiang Y, Low S, Wang Z, Nam SJ, Liu W, Kwangac J (2001) Characterization of three infectious bronchitis virus isolates from China associated with proventriculus in vaccinated chickens. *Avian Dis* 45: 416–424

219 Dales S, Anderson R (1995) Pathogenesis and diseases of the central nervous system caused by murine coronaviruses. In: Siddell SG (ed): *The Coronaviridae*. Plenum Press, New York and London, 257–292

220 Stohlman SA, Hinton DR (2001) Viral induced demyelination. *Brain Pathol* 11: 92–106

221 Matthews AE, Weiss SR, Paterson Y (2002) Murine hepatitis virus – a model for virus-induced CNS demyelination. *J Neurovirol* 8: 76–85

222 Arbour N, Day R, Newcombe J, Talbot PJ (2000) Neuroinvasion by human respiratory coronaviruses. *J Virol* 74: 8913–8921

223 Stewart JN, Mounir S, Talbot PJ (1992) Human coronavirus gene expression in the brains of multiple sclerosis patients. *Virology* 191: 502–505

224 Dessau RB, Lisby G, Frederiksen JL (2001) Coronaviruses in brain tissue from patients with multiple sclerosis. *Acta Neuropathol (Berl)* 101: 601–604

225 Arbour N, Cote G, Lachance C, Tardieu M, Cashman NR, Talbot PJ (1999) Acute and persistent infection of human neural cell lines by human coronavirus OC43. *J Virol* 73: 3338–3350

226 Enjuanes L, Smerdou C, Sanchez CM, Sune C, Kelly S, Curtiss R 3rd, Torres JM (1995) Induction of transmissible gastroenteritis coronavirus specific immune responses using vectors with enteric tropism. *Adv Exp Med Biol* 1535–1541

227 Peiris J, Lai S, Poon L, Guan Y, Yam L, Lim W, Nicholls J, Yee W, Yan W, Cheung M et al (2003) Coronavirus as a possible cause of severe acute respiratory syndrome. *Lancet* 361: 1319–1325
228 Hodgson T, Casais R, Dove B, Britton P, Cavanagh D (2004) Recombinant infectious bronchitis coronavirus Beaudette with the spike protein gene of the pathogenic M41 strain remains attenuated but induces protective immunity. *J Virol* 78: 13804–13811
229 Casais R, Dove B, Cavanagh D, Britton P (2003) Recombinant avian infectious bronchitis virus expressing a heterologous spike gene demonstrates that the spike protein is a determinant of cell tropism. *J Virol* 77: 9084–9089
230 Sanchez CM, Izeta A, Sanchez-Morgado JM, Alonso S, Sola I, Balasch M, Plana-Duran J, Enjuanes L (1999) Targeted recombination demonstrates that the spike gene of transmissible gastroenteritis coronavirus is a determinant of its enteric tropism and virulence. *J Virol* 73: 7607–7618
231 Leparc-Goffart I, Hingley ST, Chua MM, Jiang X, Lavi E, Weiss SR (1997) Altered pathogenesis of a mutant of the murine coronavirus MHV-A59 is associated with a Q159L amino acid substitution in the spike protein. *Virology* 239: 1–10
232 Das Sarma J, Fu L, Tsai JC, Weiss SR, Lavi E (2000) Demyelination determinants map to the spike glycoprotein gene of coronavirus mouse hepatitis virus. *J Virol* 74: 9206–9213
233 Phillips JJ, Chua MM, Lavi E, Weiss SR (1999) Pathogenesis of chimeric MHV4/MHV-A59 recombinant viruses: the murine coronavirus spike protein is a major determinant of neurovirulence. *J Virol* 73: 7752–7760
234 Phillips JJ, Chua M, Seo SH, Weiss SR (2001) Multiple regions of the murine coronavirus spike glycoprotein influence neurovirulence. *J Neurovirol* 7: 421–431
235 Navas S, Seo SH, Chua MM, Sarma JD, Lavi E, Hingley ST, Weiss SR (2001) Murine coronavirus spike protein determines the ability of the virus to replicate in the liver and cause hepatitis. *J Virol* 75: 2452–2457
236 Jones RC, Ambali AG (1987) Re-excretion of an enterotropic infectious bronchitis virus by hens at point of lay after experimental infection at day old. *Vet Rec* 120: 617–618
237 Naqi S, Gay K, Patalla P, Mondal S, Liu R (2003) Establishment of persistent avian infectious bronchitis virus infection in antibody-free and antibody-positive chickens. *Avian Dis* 47: 594–601
238 Darbyshire JH, Peters RW (1984) Sequential development of humoral immunity and assessment of protection in chickens following vaccination and challenge with avian infectious bronchitis virus. *Res Vet Sci* 37: 77–86
239 Gough RE, Alexander D (1979) Comparison of duration of immunity in chickens infected with a live infectious bronchitis vaccine by three different routes. *Res Vet Sci* 26: 329–332
240 Cavanagh D, Davis PJ, Darbyshire JH, Peters RW (1986) Coronavirus IBV: virus retaining spike glycopolypeptide S2 but not S1 is unable to induce virus-neutralizing or haemagglutination-inhibiting antibody, or induce chicken tracheal protection. *J Gen Virol* 67: 1435–1442

241 Ignjatovic J, Galli L (1994) The S1 glycoprotein but not the N or M proteins of avian infectious bronchitis virus induces protection in vaccinated chickens. *Arch Virol* 138: 117–134
242 Song CS, Lee YJ, Lee CW, Sung HW, Kim JH, Mo IP, Izumiya Y, Jang HK, Mikami T (1998) Induction of protective immunity in chickens vaccinated with infectious bronchitis virus S1 glycoprotein expressed by a recombinant baculovirus. *J Gen Virol* 79: 719–723
243 Macdonald JW, Randall CJ, McMartin DA, Dagless MD, Gazdzinski P (1981) Active and passive immunisation against nephritis induced by an avian infectious bronchitis virus. *Avian Pathol* 10: 121–129
244 Bumstead N, Huggins MB, Cook JKA (1989) Genetic differences in susceptibility to a mixture of avian infectious bronchitis virus and *Escherichia coli*. *Brit Poultry Sci* 30: 39–48
245 Cook JKA, Smith HW, Huggins MB (1986) Infectious bronchitis immunity: its study in chickens experimentally infected with mixtures of infectious bronchitis virus and Escherichia coli. *J Gen Virol* 67: 1427–1434
246 Otsuki K, Huggins MB, Cook JKA (1990) Comparison of the susceptibility to avian infectious bronchitis virus infection of two inbred lines of White Leghorn chickens. *Avian Pathol* 19: 467–475
247 Smith HW, Cook JKA, Parsell ZE (1985) The experimental infection of chickens with mixtures of infectious bronchitis virus and Escherichia coli. *J Gen Virol* 66: 777–786
248 Johnson MA, Pooley C, Ignjatovic J, Tyack SG (2003) A recombinant fowl adenovirus expressing the S1 gene of infectious bronchitis virus protects against challenge with infectious bronchitis virus. *Vaccine* 21: 2730–2736
249 Wesseling JG, Godeke G-J, Schijns VECJ, Prevec L, Graham FL, Horzinek MC, Rottier PJM (1993) Mouse hepatitis virus spike and nucleocapsid proteins expressed by adenovirus vectors protect mice against a lethal infection. *J Gen Virol* 74: 2061–2069
250 Boots AMH, Benaissatrouw BJ, Hesselink W, Rijke E, Schrier C, Hensen EJ (1992) Induction of antiviral immune-responses by immunization with recombinant-DNA encoded avian coronavirus nucleocapsid protein. *Vaccine* 10: 119–124
251 Seo SH, Wang L, Smith R, Collisson EW (1997) The carboxyl-terminal 120-residue polypeptide of infectious bronchitis virus nucleocapsid induces cytotoxic T lymphocytes and protects chickens from acute infection. *J Virol* 71: 7889–7894
252 Pei J, Briles WE, Collisson EW (2003) Memory T cells protect chicks from acute infectious bronchitis virus infection. *Virology* 306: 376–384
253 Collisson EW, Pei J, Dzielawa J, Seo SH (2000) Cytotoxic T lymphocytes are critical in the control of infectious bronchitis virus in poultry. *Dev Comp Immunol* 24: 187–200
254 Seo SH, Pei J, Briles WE, Dzielawa J, Collisson EW (2000) Adoptive transfer of infectious bronchitis virus primed alphabeta T cells bearing CD8 antigen protects chicks from acute infection. *Virology* 269: 183–189
255 Korner H, Schliephake A, Winter J, Zimprich F, Lassmann H, Sedgwick J,

Siddell S, Wege H (1991) Nucleocapsid or spike protein-specific cd4+ lymphocytes-t protect against coronavirus-induced encephalomyelitis in the absence of cd8+ cells-t. *J Immunol* 147: 2317–2323
256 Bergmann C, McMillan M, Stohlman S (1993) Characterization of the Ld-restricted cytotoxic T-lymphocyte epitope in the mouse hepatitis virus nucleocapsid protein. *J Virol* 67: 7041–7049
257 Stohlman SA, Kyuwa S, Cohen M, Bergmann C, Polo JM, Yeh J, Anthony R, Keck JG (1992) Mouse hepatitis-virus nucleocapsid protein-specific cytotoxic lymphocytes-t are L(d) restricted and specific for the carboxy terminus. *Virology* 189: 217–224
258 Stohlman SA, Kyuwa S, Polo JM, Brady D, Lai MMC, Bergmann C (1993) Characterization of mouse hepatitis virus specific cytotoxic T cells derived from the central nervous system of mice infected with the JHM strain. *J Virol* 67: 7050–7059
259 Wege H, Schliephake A, Korner H, Flory E, Wege H (1993) An immunodominant $CD4^+$ T-cell site on the nucleocapsid protein of murine coronavirus contributes to protection against encephalomyelitis. *J Gen Virol* 74: 1287–1294
260 Nakanaga K, Yamanouchi K, Fuziwara K (1986) Protective effect of monoclonal antibodies on lethal mouse hepatitis virus infection in mice. *J Virol* 59: 168–171
261 Evermann JF, Heeney JL, McKeirnan AJ, Obrien SJ (1989) Comparative features of a coronavirus isolated from a cheetah with feline infectious peritonitis. *Virus Res* 13: 15–28
262 Heeney JL, Evermann JF, McKeirnan AJ, Marker-Kraus L, Roelke ME, Bush M, Wildt DE, Meltzer DG, Colly L, Lukas J et al (1990) Prevalence and implications of feline coronavirus infections of captive and free-ranging cheetahs (Acinonyx jubatus). *J Virol* 64: 1964–1972
263 Cavanagh D, Brian DA, Brinton M, Enjuanes L, Holmes KV, Horzinek MC, Lai MMC, Laude H, Plagemann PGW, Siddell S et al (1994) Revision of the taxonomy of the coronavirus, torovirus and arterivirus genera. *Arch Virol* 135: 227–237
264 Enjuanes L, Brian D, Cavanagh D, Holmes K, Lai MMC, Laude H, Masters P, Rottier P, Siddell SG, Spaan WJM et al (2000) Coronaviridae. In: van Regenmortel MHV, Fauquet CM, Bishop DHL, Carstens EB, Estes MK, Lemon S, Maniloff J, Mayo M, McGeoch DJ, Pringle CR, Wickner RB (eds): *Virus Taxonomy. Classification and Nomenclature of Viruses*. Academic Press, San Diego, 835–849
265 Duckmanton L, Luan B, Devenish J, Tellier R, Petric M (1997) Characterization of torovirus from human faecal specimens. *Virology* 239: 158–168
266 González JM, Gomez-Puertas P, Cavanagh D, Gorbalenya AE, Enjuanes L (2003) Taxonomical relations within the family *Coronaviridae* based on sequence identity analysis. *Arch Virol* 148: 2207–2235
267 Daniel C, Talbot PJ (1990) Protection from lethal coronavirus infection by affinity-purified spike glycoprotein of murine hepatitis virus, strain-A59. *Virology* 174: 87–94

Coronaviruses with Special Emphasis on First Insights Concerning SARS
ed. by A. Schmidt, M.H. Wolff and O. Weber

Coronavirus infections in veterinary medicine

Olaf Weber[1] and Axel Schmidt[2]

[1] *Institute of Molecular Medicine and Experimental Immunology, Rheinische Friedrich-Wilhelms-University Bonn, Sigmund-Freud-Str. 25, 53105 Bonn, Germany*
[2] *Institute of Microbiology and Virology, University Witten/Herdecke, Stockumer Str. 10, 58448 Witten, Germany*

Introduction

The evidence that the "SARS-virus" could be an animal coronavirus and/or could originate from an animal coronavirus has increased the level of interest for coronavirus infections in animals. It was reported during the outbreak of SARS that researchers from HongKong University examined 25 animals representing eight species in a live animal market in southern China and found the virus in six palm civets. The same investigators also found the "SARS-virus" in a badger and a raccoon dog (Yahoo on Friday, May 23rd; The Wall Street Journal, May 27th). It is noteworthy that food handlers represented more than 30% of the early SARS cases. It is still not clear yet whether the virus was transmitted from animals to humans or *vice versa*.

Coronavirus infections have been recognized as causative agents for deadly diseases or important economic factors for a long time (see Tab. 1).

Coronaviruses are distributed worldwide. Many coronaviruses are propagated in the respiratory or the intestinal tract and are accordingly transmitted by the aerogenic or by fecal-oral route. Most coronaviruses cause clinical signs in the infected animals.

A natural or artificial transmission into other species than the natural host has been described for many coronaviruses although the virus preferably spreads within one host species.

Coronaviruses and the toroviruses represent separate genera within the *Coronaviridae* family (see the chapter by Cavanagh in this book; [1–3]). The *Coronaviridae* are named after their relatively unique virion morphology. In addition, coronaviruses have unique genome features and a replication strategy that distinguishes them from other RNA viruses.

Together with the *Arteriviridae*, *Coronaviridae* belong to the order of *Nidovirales*. These viruses have plus-strand RNA genomes that are transcribed to yield a nested set of overlapping sub-genomic mRNAs with a common 3'end. One of the most intriguing aspects of coronavirus replica-

Table 1. Overview of coronaviruses most relevant in veterinary medicine: their natural hosts and associated diseases and clinical manifestations.

Virus	Host	Disease
Feline infectious peritonitis virus (FIPV, FCoV)	Cat	Peritonitis
Transmissible gastroenteritis virus of swine (TGEV)	Swine	Gastroenteritis
Avian infectious bronchitis virus (IBV)	Chicken	Bronchitis
Mouse hepatitis virus (MHV)	Mouse	Hepatitis
Canine enteric coronavirus (CECoV)	Dog	Gastroenteritis
Turkey bluecomb coronavirus (TCoV)	Turkey	"Bluecomb disease"
Bovine coronavirus (BCoV)	Cattle	Gastroenteritis Respiratory symptoms
Rat coronavirus	Rat	Respiratory symptoms
Sialodacryadenitis virus (SDAV)	Rat	Sialodacryadenitis
Porcine epizootic diarrhea virus (PEDV)	Swine	Gastroenteritis
Porcine haemagglutinating encephalomyelitis virus (HEV)	Swine	Encephalomyelitis
Porcine respiratory coronavirus (PRCoV)	Swine	Respiratory symptoms
Feline enteritic coronavirus (FCoV)	Cat	Gastroenteritis

tion is high frequency RNA recombination [4]. This strategy might be important for the crossing of species barriers for many important animal coronaviruses as well as the "SARS-CoV". The members of the *Nidovirales* order, however, especially differ with respect to their envelopes and nucleocapsids [5].

The biology of coronaviruses has been described in detail in other chapters. Therefore, this chapter focuses on clinical and economical aspects of coronavirus infections in companion (pets), live-stock (farm) and laboratory animals.

Based on phylogenetic analysis and antigenic cross reactivity, three groups can be distinguished in the *Coronaviridae* family. Some important viruses that are discussed below belong to group I and include the canine enteric coronavirus (CECoV), the transmissible gastroenteritis virus (TGEV) of swine, the porcine epidemic diarrhoea virus (PEDV), the porcine respiratory coronavirus (PRCoV) and the feline coronaviruses (FCoVs).

Most coronaviruses are enzootic and/or endemic in the respective host species. The vast majority of infections occur with inapparent clinical signs. The virus usually infects and replicates in epithelia and outbreaks of gastrointestinal and/or respiratory diseases are often seasonal. Clinical signs are in general more severe in younger animals. Immunocompromised animals and infected adults also serve as a major virus reservoir.

Genomic recombination appears to be a very common event *in vitro* and *in vivo* [6] in coronaviruses also relevant in animal health. Therefore, interactions of different coronaviruses can lead to new types and novel clinical entities [7, 8].

Specific infections

Coronavirus infections in swine

Porcine coronaviruses include i) TGEV; ii) PRCoV which is a mutant of TGEV; iii) PEDV I and II; and iv) haemagglutinating encephalomyelitis virus (HEV). The latter belongs to the coronavirus group II.

TGEV and PEDV are highly infectious and highly contagious enteric viruses of swine. PEDV and TGEV infections are considered difficult to distinguish clinically and also histopathologically [9–11] but can be distinguished by using modern, up-to-date techniques such as PCR and/or specific sequencing [12]. TGE is an economically important disease that might result in high mortality and was first described in the 1940s. While older animals generally recover by time, piglets under the age of three weeks usually die from the infection. The TGEV genome consists of a single-stranded, positive-sense 28.5-kb RNA. The viral membrane contains three transmembrane proteins: the S protein (220 kDa), M protein (29 to 36 kDa), and minor E protein (10-kDa). The S surface protein initiates the infection by binding to the cell surface. It also mediates the subsequent fusion between the viral and cellular membranes. The S protein binds to aminopeptidase N and to sialic acid. Aminopeptidase N binding is required for TGEV to initiate the infection of cells [13]. Recognition of sialic acids appears to be important for both, the haemagglutinating activity and the enteropathogenicity of TGEV [14].

The enteric tropism of TGEV presumably also requires the binding to a co-receptor that maps around amino acid 219 of the S protein as well as other additional co-factors [15, 16]. The importance of sialic acid binding for entropathogenicity is supported by the fact that the non-enteropathogenic PRCoV lacks sialic acid binding activity. This can be explained by a large deletion in the S gene that results in a truncated spike protein [17, 18]. PRCoV causes a mostly mild and moderate epizootic respiratory disease and might have worked like a vaccine against TGE in a number of swine populations.

TGEV is transmitted either directly or indirectly through contact with feces of infected pigs or *via* vector animals such as dogs and cats. Like other coronaviruses, TGEV is fragile and highly sensitive to disinfectants as further detailed in the chapter by Wolff et al. Epidemic peaks mostly occur during the cold season. After an incubation period of one to three days, symptoms of TGEV-associated disease emerge that include watery diarrhea, typical foul smelling yellowish-green feces that often contains flecks of undigested milk, vomiting, and loss of appetite. While the mortality rate is high in suckling piglets – up to 100% in piglets under two weeks of age – clinical symptoms in older piglets and adults are often mild and these animals will survive if especially their hydration status is adequate and ensured. The mortality rate is generally lower in these animals and will largely depend on additional factors such as secondary bacterial infections, cardiovascular decompensation, chilling and dampness. Outbreaks usually only last a couple of weeks with occurrence of specific neutralizing antibodies in mucosa, blood and milk. Further, lactating sows are highly susceptible. Clinical signs may include vomiting, severe diarrhea, malnutrition, and cease of lactation. In large herds the disease can persist for some time, often contributing to post-weaning diarrhea. The clinical symptoms of endemic/enzootic TGE are usually less severe in the older pigs, making a clinical differentiation between TGE and other infectious enteric diseases, like that caused by rotaviruses and/or clostridia, impossible. Upon histopathological examination, villous atrophy is frequently found in both rotaviral and enzootic TGE infections. Mixed infections are possible and underscore the importance of a strict disease management and/or prevention regimen. TGE represents a reportable disease also in EU member states. There is no specific treatment available yet, however, electrolytes, nursing and enhanced management of the piglets may reduce mortality and lethality. In smaller herds cross-suckling of affected piglets onto recovered sows would offer a biological treatment. It is critical to almost impossible to assess general hygiene measures in prevalently infected herds. Modified live vaccines are available and immunization of pregnant swine is a common vaccination strategy.

Coronavirus infections in dogs

CECoV is associated with moderate to severe enteritis in young puppies. The genome contains the open reading frames (ORFs) 1a and 1b, encoding polyproteins leading to the viral replicase formation. Downstream of ORF 1b are ORFs encoding the coronavirus structural proteins S (ORF 2), E (ORF 4), M (ORF 5) and the nucleocapsid (N) protein [19]. The E protein has a function for virus assembly [20], the M protein is a type III glycoprotein [21]. ORF 2 encodes the spike (S) protein, a glycoprotein ranging from 1,160 to 1,452 amino acids (aa) in length [19]. This large protein has three structural domains. The large external domain at the N-terminus is furthermore organized into two sub-domains S1 and S2 with the S1 sub-domain including the N-terminal half of the molecule and forming the globular portion of the spikes. S1 contains sequences responsible for binding specific cellular receptors. S1 sequences are extremely variable, and mutations in the S1 region have been associated with problems of altered antigenicity and pathogenicity/virulence. In contrast, S2 sequences are genetically much more conserved and contain two heptad repeat motifs that suggest a coiled-coil structure [22].

Sequence analyses of CECoV detected in fecal samples that were collected from dogs with diarrhea showed mutations accumulating over the M gene [23]. A genetic drift to FCoV type II was also observed in the sequence of CECoV detected in the faeces of puppies infected naturally during the late stages of long-term viral shedding. Infection by mixed populations of genetically different CECoV and recombination *in vivo* might, therefore, be common events [24].

The clinical signs of these coronavirus infections vary. They commonly include vomiting, diarrhea and "unspecific" symptoms such as depression, anorexia, and fever. Puppies most obviously die from severe dehydration. The majority of dogs that are not severely affected recover without any treatment. Animals with severe symptoms of dehydration need supportive care stabilizing the hydration status. Antibiotic/antibacterial treatment may be indicated in order to prevent exacerbations of bacterial superinfections. Although vaccination may be indicated in kennels, sanitation is also the economically most effective way to control these coronavirus infections and, therefore, should be maintained by keeping the kennels free of feces and cleaning the environment by an appropriate desinfection regimen.

Feline coronavirus infection

FCoV is commonly associated with mild enteric infections but is also associated with feline infectious peritonitis (FIP). FIP is a routinely fatal disease in both wild and domestic *Felidae*. FCoV can be distinguished into two serotypes: I and II, on the basis of a virus neutralization assay *in vitro* using both type-specific feline sera and monoclonal antibodies directed against the S protein [25–27]. The prevalence of these two serotypes is uncertain; type II FCoVs may account for up to thirty percent of the FIP cases in cats in Japan [26]. The S protein of the type II FCoV shares immunodominant neutralization epitopes with the S protein of canine coronavirus [25]. The S proteins of type II FCoV strains show great amino acid sequence identity to those of CECoV (approximately 91%) and TGEV (approximately 81%) but not to several type I strains (approximately 45%) [28, 29].

In the first phase of the infection the symptoms are extremely unspecific. A mild upper respiratory disease, as evidenced by watery eyes and sneezing, might be diagnosed. A high percentage of primarily infected cats clear the virus; some of them, however, become long-term virus carriers. Only a small percentage of exposed cats – higher, up to twenty percent in kennels – develop FIP, months or years after primary infection. It is still unclear whether an endogenous reactivation could also be responsible for this pathomechanism. The clinical signs of FIP usually gradually increase in severity over a period of several months, starting with rather unspecific signs such as inappetence, depression, rough fur, weight loss and fever. The forms of the lethal FIP may be effusive (wet) and/or non-effusive (dry and/or proliferative). Combinations of both clinical manifestations are rather common. The most characteristic clinical sign of wet FIP is ascites. Other symptoms may be rather unspecific like swollen lymph nodes, ocular symptoms with conjunctivitis and/or corneal ulcers. As the name suggests, fluid accumulation is minimal in the dry form of FIP. Instead, other, rather unspecific symptoms dominate. The dry form progresses slowly, often making clinical diagnosis difficult. Weight loss, depression, anemia, and fever, are frequently observed symptoms. Signs of severe kidney and/or liver failure, pancreatic, neurological or ocular disorders are observed in various combinations. A characteristic granulomatous inflammation is mostly observed by biopsy or in pathological examinations if performed. A cure does not exist yet. The therapy should provide supportive care and to alleviate the self-destroying inflammatory response of the disease. Short-term remissions in a small percentage of patients have been described. A combination of corticosteroids, cytostatic drugs and antibiotics may be helpful in some cases despite the often fatal overall prognosis pro vitam.

Virulence of FCoV strains appears to correlate to their ability to infect macrophages [30]. The clinical symptoms are induced by immune complex reactions. Antibodies are not only not protective, they might even accelerate the onset and the course of the disease in form of an antibody-enhanced infection (AEI) such as observed in Dengue fever in humans [31]. The pathogenesis of the lesions, however, is not yet fully understood in its complexity. On the one hand there is evidence that immune complexes and subsequent activation of complement factors play an important role in the pathogenesis of FIP [32]. On the other hand, abnormal cytokine or chemokine secretion patterns – i.e. in infected immunocompetent cells – could also play a pathogenic role in the development of typical FIP lesions like in granulomas [5].

Bovine coronavirus infections and the possibility of transmission to humans

Bovine coronavirus (BCoV) is an important cause of neonatal calf diarrhea [33] but may also infect the respiratory tract and has been recognized as the causing agent especially for winter dysentery in adult cattle. Enteric and respiratory virus strains are antigenically related [34] but differ genetically [35]. Amino acid alterations in the S1 subunit of the S protein (e.g. residues 113, 115, 118, 146, 148, 501, 510 and 531) of respiratory isolates conferred significant changes to the structure of the protein compared with the BCoV strains that cause winter dysentery and calf diarrhea.

BCoV was first reported in 1972 [35–37]. The zoonotic potential of BCoV remains to be determined although a case of transmission to humans has been reported [38]. BCoV possesses a single-stranded, enveloped, nonsegmented RNA genome of positive polarity [39]. The mature virion contains five major structural proteins – the nucleocapsid (N) protein, the transmembrane (M) protein, the haemagglutinin/esterase (HE) glycoprotein, the spike (S) protein, and a small membrane (E) protein [40, 41]. HE fulfills receptor binding and detachment functions. The S glycoprotein also recognizes the 9-O-acetylated sialic acid, apparently with a higher affinity than HE [42, 43]. The S protein is proposed to be responsible for the primary attachment of BCoV to other cell surface receptors [42]. Variations in the S glycoprotein are most likely responsible for host specificity and tissue tropism [44].

BCoV is distributed worldwide and antibodies can be detected in the vast majority of cattle [45, 46]. BCoV infects calves/cattle by both the oral and/or respiratory route. Although the virus can be detected in healthy animals, the most common source of enteric infection is diarrhoeic faeces from other infected animals. The virus infection of the enteritic tract starts in the small intestine and spreads after an initial replication throughout the gastrointestinal (GI) tract. Since the virus replicates in the surface distal villi of the epithelial cells of the GI tract, these cells will eventually be destroyed, leading to fusions of adjacent villi in the small intestine and to atrophy of the colonic ridges [33]. The severity of clinical signs varies with the age and especially the immunological status. Usually, a yellowish diarrhea is observed that lasts for about three to seven days. It is difficult to distinguish between rota- and coronavirus-associated infection based on clinical signs solely. If diarrhea is severe, calves become pyrexic and dehydrated.

Infections with respiratory BCoV often appear after stress such as shipment and/or environmental disturbances. Infected animals will develop clinical signs of respiratory distress including wheezing and nasal discharge three to four days after infection. Bacterial superinfections often complicate the clinical status. Respiratory disease was induced experimentally after oral inoculation in colostrum-deprived calves [47]. As for other coronaviruses, seasonal changes in temperature, environmental factors but also the immune status play an important role in the transmission of the virus and the clinical outcome of the infection. Different virus isolates have been reported to have differences in tissue tropism [48]. These authors report that about 50% of the infections in calves involve the respiratory tract in parallel and the enteric tract, whereas each 25% only involve either the respiratory or the GI tract.

As for other coronaviruses, diagnosis/diagnostics requires detection of specific nucleic acids. Virus isolation may be difficult and mostly not practicable in all day diagnostics. Alternatively, nasal swabs might be used for detection of BCoV antigen by immunofluorescence tests or other appropriate immunological methods.

Interestingly, a fragment amplified from "SARS-CoV" (BNI109 fragment) showed 75% homology with BCoV and mouse hepatitis virus (MHV) at the amino acid level [49].

Avian infectious bronchitis

Infectious bronchitis virus (IBV) is a major cause of disease in domestic fowl and causes an acute, highly contagious disease of the respiration and sometimes also urogenital tract [50]. The IBV genome consists of approximately 27 kb [51] and codes for the spike (S) glycoprotein, the membrane (M) glycoprotein, and the nucleocapsid (N) phosphoprotein [52]. IBV is distributed worldwide, and different variants have been isolated [53–58]. IBV strains within a geographic region might be unique and distinct, examples are Europe, the USA, and Australia, i.e. for avian IBV [59]. The different antigenic types make the use and possible efficacy of a single vaccine extremely questionable.

The natural hosts for IBV are chicken and pheasants. IBV infections represent an important economic threat for the poultry industry. Infected animals of all ages show signs of an acute, highly contagious respiratory disease. It is characterized by coughing, sneezing, and a nasal discharge. The major production loss results from the reduction in egg production and inferior egg quality. In younger birds there may be a high death rate, weight losses, or problems in weight development. Some virus strains may also induce primary infectious kidney lesions. The lethality in these animals may be up to 25%. As for other coronavirus infections, only a virological examination, mainly based on serological techniques, can lead to the appropriate diagnosis. Other important respiratory diseases include Newcastle disease (ND) and infectious laryngotracheitis (ILT). According to regulations of many EU member states, ND is a disease that requires immediate reporting and action by veterinary authorities. ILT is also a reportable animal disease. There is no specific treatment for infectious bronchitis. Antibiotic treatment might help to prevent or reduce secondary, i.e. bacterial superinfections. Strict hygienic management and/or isolation of the flock may help to interrupt the disease cycle. Different live virus vaccines have been developed and are currently in use; however, the use of live vaccines complicates especially serological diagnostics. Sequencing of the S1 glycoprotein gene is the method recommended by the OIE (Office International des Epizooties) to discriminate between different IBV strains.

Coronavirus infections in turkeys – "bluecomb disease"

Turkey coronavirus (TCoV) causes acute and highly contagious enteritis of significant economical importance in turkeys [60]. The clinical signs usually appear at seven to 30 days of age in turkeys under six weeks of age and consist of diarrhea, litter eating, decreased feed efficiency and decreased weight development. Morbidity is high, although mortality might be low. TCoV is difficult to eradicate. TCoV-induced enteritis has been described to be Minnesota's most costly turkey disease from 1951 to 1971 [61]. TCoV treatments of the disease are often unsuccessful and there are currently no effective vaccines and/or other medications to prevent this disease. The local immune system of the mucosa of the gastrointestinal tract plays a major role in the protection against an infection and modulates clinical signs as well. Recent studies indicate that neutralizing, intestinal secretory mucosal IgA antibodies to TCoV are elicited in turkeys following infection with TCoV and that local mucosal antibodies may provide protective immunity for infected turkeys to recover from TCoV infection [62].

As for other coronaviruses, mechanical vectors play an important role in the transmission of the virus: it was demonstrated recently that house flies can transmit TCoV [63].

TCoV from intestinal contents of diarrheal poults could be propagated in a human adenocarcinoma line and one-day-old turkey poults inoculated orally with tissue culture-adapted TCoV isolates developed mild to severe diarrhea [64]. However, the passaging of TCoV could not be reproduced by other investigators so far [65, 66]. This viral enteritis is different from haemorrhagic enteritis (HE), another economically important disease of turkeys that is caused by a type II adenovirus (reviewed by Sharma 1991 [67]). In contrast to bluecomb disease, turkeys younger than four weeks of age are clinically "resistant" to HE. In addition to the enteritis, a pathological frequent finding is hepatosplenomegalia. Bursectomy and/or splenectomy abrogate clinical HE [68].

Coronavirus infections in mice – "mouse hepatitis"

MHV belongs to the *Coronaviridae* family and represents one of the most important pathogens of the laboratory mouse. MHV is serologically related to other coronaviruses of rats, pigs, cattle, and also humans. It is a very well-studied virus, because of its adverse influence on several research approaches and consecutively also results. About 25 different MHV strains have been reported so far. Some strains are polytropic; they infect a variety of tissues and cause symptoms in various organs. Other strains are more specifically organotropic, e.g. enterotropic, and cause villus attenuation, syncytia formation and mucosal necrosis of the terminal small intestine and the colon.

MHV is very contagious; transmission occurs by aerosol, faeces and many other contacts/transmission routes. There are usually no clinical symptoms in infected adult mice. Clinical signs such as weakness, diarrhea, wasting and weight loss are observed in young mice. The mortality rate varies but might be high. Since laboratory animals almost always come from controlled breeding providers/animal environment (e.g. SPF = specifically pathogen free), serology is a highly reliable method to detect the target infection.

Considering the costs of modern biomedical research, infection with MHV is an economically important disease in small laboratory animals. The effects of the MHV infection on immunocompromised mice include enhanced phagocytic activities of macrophages, rejection of xenograft tumors [69], abnormal tumor growth patterns [70], altered response to chemical carcinogens [71], and impaired liver regeneration. Pharmcokinetics of test compounds might also be altered due to a change of enzyme activities. In immunocompetent mice, effects observed include immunoestimulation and, later on, immunodepression [72, 73]. Macrophage function is altered in infected mice [74], and effects on other immune competent cells are frequently found in infected mice as well. Often the best solution for infected facilities is to eliminate the entire affected stock with a consecutive appropriate desinfection regimen.

Host range mutants of MHV strains were isolated from mixed cultures containing progressively increasing concentrations of non-permissive Syrian baby hamster kidney (BHK) cells. The mutant virus was polytrophic, replicating efficiently in normally non-permissive BHK cells, Syrian and Chinese hamster (DDT-1 and CHO) cells, human adenocarcinoma (HRT), primate kidney (VERO) and in murine 17Cl-1 cell lines [75].

References

1 Cavanagh D, Brian DA, Brinton MA, Enjuanes L, Holmes KV, Horzinek MC, Lai MM, Laude H, Plagemann PG, Siddell SG (1993) The *Coronaviridae* now comprises two genera, coronavirus and torovirus: Report of the *Coronaviridae* Study Group. *Adv Exp Med Biol* 342: 255–257

2 Cavanagh D (1997) *Nidovirales*: A new order comprising *Coronaviridae* and *Arteriviridae*. *Arch Virol* 142: 629–633

3 González JM, Gomez-Puertas P, Cavanagh D, Gorbalenya AE, Enjuanes L (2003) A comparative sequence analysis to revise the current taxonomy of the family *Coronaviridae*. *Arch Virol* 148: 2207–2235

4 Makino S, Keck JG, Stohlman SA, Lai MMC (1986) High-frequency RNA recombination of murine coronaviruses. *J Virol* 57: 729–739

5 Horzinek MC (1999) Molecular evolution of corona- and toroviruses. *Adv Exp Med Biol* 473: 61–72

6 Brian DA, Spaan WJM (1998) Recombination and coronavirus defective interfering RNAs. *Semin Virol* 8: 101–107

7 Blau DM, Holmes KV (1999) Human coronavirus 229E enters susceptible cells *via* the endocytic pathway. *Mol Biol Cell* 10: 220

8 McIntosh K (1996) Coronaviruses. In: Fields BN, Knipe DM, Howley PM, Griffin DE, Lamb RA, Martin MA, Roizman B, Strais SE (eds): *Fields Virology*. Lippincott-Raven, Philadelphia, 1192–1204

9 Phillip SF, Cartwright SF, Scott AC (1971) The size and morphology of trans-

missible gastroenteritis and vomiting and wasting disease viruses of pigs. *Vet Res* 88: 311–312
10 Pensaert MB, Debouck P (1978) A new coronavirus-like particle associated with diarrhea in swine. *Arch Virol* 58: 243–247
11 Debouck P, Pensaert M (1980) Experimental infection of pigs with a new porcine enteric coronavirus, CV777. *Am J Vet Res* 41: 219–223
12 Jung K, Kim J, Kim O, Kim B, Chae C (2003) Differentiation between porcine epidemic diarrhea virus and transmissible gastroenteritis virus in formalin-fixed paraffin-embedded tissues by multiplex RT-nested PCR and comparison with *in situ* hybridization. *J Virol Method* 108: 41–47
13 Delmas B, Gelfi J, L'Haridon R, Vogel LK, Sjostrom H, Noren O, Laude H (1992) Aminopeptidase N is a major receptor for the entero-pathogenic coronavirus TGEV. *Nature* 357: 417–420
14 Krempl C, Schultze B, Laude H, Herrler G (1997) Point mutations in the S protein connect the sialic acid binding activity with the enteropathogenicity of transmissible gastroenteritis coronavirus. *J Virol* 71: 3285–3287
15 Sánchez CM, Izeta A, Sánchez-Morgado JM, Alonso S, Sola I, Balasch M, Plana-Durán J, Enjuanes L (1999) Targeted recombination demonstrates that the spike gene of transmissible gastroenteritis coronavirus is a determinant of its enteric tropism and virulence. *J Virol* 73: 7607–7618
16 Ballesteros ML, Sánchez CM, Enjuanes L (1997) Two amino acid changes at the N-terminus of transmissible gastroenteritis coronavirus spike protein result in the loss of enteric tropism. *Virology* 227: 378–388
17 Rasschaert D, Duarte M, Laude H (1990) Porcine respiratory coronavirus differs from transmissible gastroenteritis virus by a few genomic deletions. *J Gen Virol* 71: 2599–2607
18 Saif LJ (1993) Coronavirus immunogens. *Vet Microbiol* 37: 285–297
19 Enjuanes L, Bria D, Cavanagh D, Holmes K, Lai MMC, Laude H, Masters P, Rottier P, Siddell S, Spaan WJM (2000) *Coronaviridae*. In: Van Regenmortel MHV, Fauquet CM, Bishop DHL, Carstens EB, Estes MK, Lemon SM, Maniloff J, Mayo MA, McGeoch DJ, Pringle CR (eds): *Virus Taxonomy, Classification and Nomenclature of Viruses*. Academic Press, New York, 835–849
20 Raamsman MJB, Locker JK, de Hooge A, de Vries AAF, Griffiths G, Vennema H, Rottier PJM (2000) Characterization of the coronavirus mouse hepatitis virus strain A59 small membrane protein. *Eur J Virol* 74: 2333–2342
21 Rottier PJM (1995) The coronavirus membrane protein. In: Siddell SG (ed): *The Coronaviridae*. Plenum Press, New York, 115–139
22 Lai MMC, Holmes KV (2001) *Coronaviridae*: The viruses and their replication. In: Knipe DM, Howley PM, Griffin DE, Lamb RA, Martin MA, Roizman B, Strais SE (eds): *Fields Virology*. Lippincott – Williams & Wilkins, Philadelphia, 1163–1185
23 Pratelli A, Martella V, Elia G, Decaro N, Aliberti A, Buonavoglia D, Tempesta M, Buonavoglia C (2001) Variation of the sequence in the gene encoding for

transmembrane protein M of canine coronavirus (CCV). *Mol Cell Probes* 15: 229–233
24 Pratelli A, Elia G, Martella V, Tinelli A, Decaro N, Marsilio F, Buonavoglia D, Tempesta M, Buonavoglia C (2002) M gene evolution of canine coronavirus in naturally infected dogs. *Vet Res* 151: 758–761
25 Herrewegh AAPM, Smeenk I, Horzinek MC, Rottier PJM, De Groot RJ (1998) Feline coronavirus type II strains 79-1683 and 79-1146 originate from a double recombination between feline coronavirus type I and canine coronavirus. *J Virol* 72: 4508–4514
26 Hohdatsu T, Okada S, Koyama H (1991) Characterization of monoclonal antibodies against feline infectious peritonitis virus type II and antigenic relationship between feline, porcine, and canine coronaviruses. *Arch Virol* 117: 85–95
27 Hohdatsu T, Okada S, Ishizuka Y, Yamada H, Koyama H (1992) The prevalence of types I and II feline coronavirus infections in cats. *J Vet Med Sci* 54: 557–562
28 Motokawa K, Hohdatsu T, Aizawa C, Koyama H, Hashimoto H (1995) Molecular cloning and sequence determination of the peplomer protein gene of feline infectious peritonitis virus type I. *Arch Virol* 140: 469–480
29 Wesseling JG, Vennema H, Godeke G, Horzinek MC, Rottier PJM (1994) Nucleotide sequence and expression of the spike (S) gene of canine coronavirus and comparison with the S proteins of feline and porcine coronaviruses. *J Gen Virol* 75: 1789–1794
30 Stoddard CA, Scott FW (1989) Intrinsic resistance of feline macrophages to coronavirus infection correlates with *in vivo* virulence. *J Virol* 63: 436–440
31 Pedersen NC (1987) Virologic and immunologic aspects of feline infectious peritonitis virus infection. *Adv Exp Med Biol* 218: 529–550
32 Jacobse-Geels HE, Daha MR, Horzinek MC (1982) Antibody, immune complexes, and complement activity fluctuations in kittens with experimentally induced feline infectious peritonitis. *Am J Vet Res* 43: 666–670
33 Clark MA (1993) Bovine coronavirus. *Br Vet J* 149: 51–70
34 Zhang X, Herbst W, Kousoulas KG, Storz J (1994) Comparison of the S genes and the biological properties of respiratory and enteropathogenic bovine coronavirus. *Arch Virol* 134: 421–426
35 Hasoksuz M, Sreevatsan S, Cho KO, Hoet AE, Saif LJ (2002) Molecular analysis of the S1 subunit of the spike glycoprotein of respiratory and enteric bovine coronavirus isolates. *Virus Res* 84: 101–109
36 Mebus CA, White RG, Stair EL, Rhodes MB, Twiehaus MJ (1972) Neonatal calf diarrhea: Results of a field trial using a reo-like virus vaccine. *Vet Med / Small Anim Clin* 67: 173–178
37 Mebus CA, Stair FL, Rhodes MB, Twiehaus MJ (1973) Neonatal calf diarrhea: Propagation, attenuation and characteristics of a coronavirus-like agent. *Am J Vet Res* 34: 145–150
38 Storz J, Rott R (1981) Reactivity of antibodies in human serum with antigens of an enteropathogenic bovine coronavirus. *Med Microbiol Immunol* 169: 169–178
39 De Vries AAF, Horzinek MC, Rottier PJM, De Groot RJ (1997) The genome

organization of the *Nidovirales*: Similarities and differences between arteri-, toro-, and coronaviruses. *Semin Virol* 8: 33–47
40 Chouljenko VN, Kousoulas KG, Lin X, Storz J (1998) Nucleotide and predicted amino acid sequences of all genes encoded by the 3' genomic portion (9.5 kb) of respiratory bovine coronaviruses and comparisons among respiratory and enteric coronaviruses. *Virus Genes* 17: 33–42
41 Lai MMC, Cavanagh D (1997) The molecular biology of coronaviruses. *Adv Virus Res* 48: 1–100
42 Schultze B, Gross HJ, Brossmer R, Herrler G (1991) The S protein of bovine coronavirus is a haemagglutinin recognizing 9-O-acetylated sialic acid as a receptor determinant. *J Virol* 65: 6232–6237
43 Schultze B, Herrler G (1994) Recognition of N-acetly-9-O-acetylneuraminic acid by bovine coronavirus and haemagglutinating encephalomyelitis virus. In: Laude H, Vautherot JF (eds): *Coronaviruses*. Plenum Press, New York, 299–304
44 Gallagher TM, Buchmeier MJ (2001) Coronavirus spike proteins in viral entry and pathogenesis. *Virology* 279: 371–374
45 Hajer I, Storz J (1978) Antigens of bovine coronavirus strain LY and their diagnostic properties. *Am J Vet Res* 39: 441–444
46 Rodak I, Babiuk LA, Acres SD (1982) Detection by radioimmunoassay and enzyme-linked immunosorbent assay of coronavirus antibodies in bovine serum and lacteal secretions. *J Clin Microbiol* 16: 34–40
47 Kapil S, Pomeroy KA, Goyal SM, Trent AM (1991) Experimental infection with a virulent pneumoenteric isolate of bovine coronavirus. *J Vet Diagn Invest* 3: 88–89
48 Kapil S, Basaraba RJ (1997) Infectious bovine rhinotracheitis, parainfluenza-3 and respiratory coronavirus. *Vet Clin North Am Food Anim Pract* 13: 455–469
49 Yang J, Wang ZH, Chen JJ, Hou JL (2003) Clinical detection of polymerase gene of SARS-associated coronavirus. *Di Yi Jun Yi Da Xue Xue Bao* 23: 424–427
50 King DJ, Cavanagh D (1991) Infectious bronchitis. In: Calnek BW, Barnes HJ, Beard CW, Reid WM, Yoder HWJr (eds): *Disease of Poultry*. Iowa State University Press, Ames, IA, 471–484
51 Boursnell ME, Brown TD, Foulds IJ, Green PF, Tomley FM, Binns MM (1987l) Completion of the sequence of the genome of the coronavirus avian infectious bronchitis virus. *J Gen Virol* 68: 57–77
52 Siddle S, Wege H, ter Meulen V (1982) The structure and replication of coronaviruses. *Curr Top Microbiol Immunol* 99: 131–163
53 Cook JKA (1984) The classification of new serotypes of infectious bronchitis virus isolated from poultry flocks in Britain 1981 and 1983. *Avian Pathol* 13: 733–741
54 Davelaar FG, Kouwenhoven B, Burger AG (1984) Occurrence and significance of infectious bronchitis virus variant strains in egg and broiler protection in The Netherlands. *Vet Q* 6: 114–120
55 King DJ (1988) Identification of recent infectious bronchitis virus isolated that are serologically different from current vaccine strains. *Avian Dis* 32: 362–364

56 Wang CH, Hsieh MC, Chang PC (1996) Isolation, pathogenicity, and H120 protection efficacy of infectious bronchitis viruses isolated in Taiwan. *Avian Dis* 40: 620–625
57 Wang CH, Tsai CT (1996) Genetic grouping for the isolates of avian infectious bronchitis viruses in Taiwan. *Arch Virol* 141, 1677–1688
58 Wang HN, Wu QZ, Huang Y, Liu P (1997) Isolation and identification of infectious bronchitis virus from chickens in Sichuan, China. *Avian Dis* 41: 279–282
59 Ignjatovi J, Sapats S (2000) Avian infectious bronchitis virus. *Rev Sci Tech Off Int Epiz* 19: 493–508
60 Nagaraja KV, Pomeroy BS (1997) Coronaviral enteritis of turkeys (bluecomb disease). In: Calnek BW, Barnes HJ, Beard CW, McDougald LR, Saif YM (eds): *Diseases of Poultry*. Iowa State University Press, Ames, IA, 686–692
61 Pomeroy BS, Nagaraja KV (1991) Coronaviral enteritis pf turkeys (bluecomb disease). In: Calnek BW, Barnes J, Beard CW, Reid WM, Yoder HW Jr (eds): *Diseases of Poultry*. Iowa State Univ. Press, Ames, IA, 239–246
62 Loa CC, Lin TL, Wu CC, Bryan T, Hooper T, Schrader D (2002) Specific mucosal IgA immunity in turkey poults infected with turkey coronavirus. *Vet Immunol Immunopathol* 88: 57–64
63 Calibeo-Hayes D, Denning SS, Stringham SM, Guy JS, Smith LG, Watson DW (2003) Mechanical transmission of turkey coronavirus by domestic houseflies (Musca domestica LINNAEAUS). *Avian Dis* 47: 149–153
64 Dea S, Garzon S, Tijssen P (1989) Isolation and trypsin-enhanced propagation of turkey enteric (bluecomb) coronaviruses in a continuous human rectal adenocarcinoma cell line. *Am J Vet Res* 50: 1310–1318
65 Guy JS, Barnes HJ, Smith LG, Breslin J (1997) Antigenic characterization of a turkey coronavirus identified in poultry enteritis- and mortality syndrome-affected turkeys. *Avian Dis* 41: 583–590
66 Ali A, Reynolds DL (1998) The *in vitro* propagation of stunting syndrome agent. *Avian Dis* 42: 657–666
67 Sharma JM (1991) Haemorrhagic enteritis of turkeys. *Vet Immunol Immunopathol* 30: 67–71
68 Ossa JE, Alexander J, Schurig GG (1983) Role of splenectomy in prevention of haemorrhagic enteritis and death from hemorrhagic enteritis virus in turkeys. *Avian Dis* 27: 1106–1111
69 Kyriazis AP, Di Persio L, Michael JG, Pesce AJ (1979) Influence of the mouse hepatitis virus (MHV) infection on the growth of human tumors in the athymic mouse. *Intl J Cancer* 23: 402–409
70 Akimaru K, Stuhlmiller GM, Seigler HF (1981) Influence of mouse hepatitis virus on the growth of human melanoma in the peritoneal cavity of the athymic mouse. *J Surg Oncol* 17: 327–339
71 Barthold SW (1986) Research complications and state of knowledge of rodent coronaviruses. In: Hamm TF (ed): *Complications of Viral and Mycoplasmal Infections in Rodents to Toxicology Research Testing*. Hemisphere, Washington DC, 53–89
72 Virelizier JL, Virelizier AM, Allison AC (1976) The role of circulating interfer-

on in the modifications of the immune responsiveness to mouse hepatitis virus (MHV-3). *J Immunol* 117: 748–753
73 Baker DG (1998) Natural patogens of laboratory mice, rats and rabbits and their effects on research. *Clin Microb Rev* 11: 231–266
74 Boorman GA, Luster MI, Dean JH, Cambell ML, Lauer LA, Talley FA, Wilson RE, Collins MJ (1982) Peritoneal and macrophage alterations caused by naturally occurring mouse hepatitis virus. *Am J Pathol* 106: 110–117
75 Hensley LE, Holmes KV, Beauchemin N, Baric RS (1998) Virus-receptor interactions and interspecies transfer of a mouse hepatitis virus. *Adv Exp Med Biol* 440: 33–41

ed. by A. Schmidt, M.H. Wolff and O. Weber

Severe acute respiratory syndrome: clinical features

Princess Margaret Hospital SARS Study Group: Po Oi Lee, Ping Tim Tsui, Tak Yin Tsang, Tai Nin Chau, Chi Pong Kwan, Wai Cho Yu, Sik To Lai

Department of Medicine & Geriatrics, 2–10 Princess Margaret Hospital Road, Hong Kong Special Administrative Region, China

Introduction

The incubation period of severe acute respiratory syndrome (SARS) ranges from 2 to 10 days. The clinical features and key laboratory parameters on presentation are summarised in Tables 1 and 2. The majority of patients with SARS present with abrupt onset of high fever of more than 38 °C with or without chills. Flu-like symptoms of malaise, myalgia, headache and dizziness are rather common. While the respiratory system is predominantly affected, other organs are also involved.

Respiratory tract

Many SARS patients do not have upper respiratory tract symptoms of sore throat or running nose. Cough may not be present even in patients with radiological evidence of pneumonitis and is usually not associated with sputum production. Some of them may already have shortness of breath and tachypnoea on presentation. Chest sign is usually minimal. Inspiratory crackles may be heard at lung bases. Chest radiography is the primary imaging tool for diagnosis and follow up assessment of treatment response. High resolution computer tomography (HRCT) of the thorax is performed when initial chest radiograph is negative despite high clinical suspicion. It is also helpful in detecting complication and in defining nature and extent of lung damage.

Chest radiography

Chest radiography can serve as a screening tool in the correct clinical setting. In a prospective study conducted in a SARS screening clinic for hospital staff, patients and their relatives, chest radiological changes were found to have the highest odds ratio of all the predictors [7]. The authors concluded that chest radiography should be mandatory for all patients screened for the disease. At the peak of the epidemic, patients with flu-like symptoms attending outpatient clinic were asked to take a chest radiograph before being interviewed for history-taking and physical examination [8].

Most patients have abnormal chest radiographs on presentation. Lee et al. noted that 78% of SARS patients had abnormal chest radiographs at the onset of fever, all showing air-space consolidation [4]. In a cluster of 10 epidemiologically linked patients, all except one showed abnormal initial chest radiographs [9]. In another retrospective study of 51 patients with probable SARS, abnormal findings were noted in 80% of initial chest films [10].

The initial changes are indistinguishable from those with other causes of atypical or viral pneumonia. All patients with abnormal initial chest radiograph present with air-space opacification [4, 9, 10]. This can be focal, unilateral or bilateral multifocal involvement (Fig. 1). The lower zones and peripheral lung fields are commonly affected [4,11]. Grinblat et al. reported similar findings of predominant peripheral consolidation in middle and lower zones in a review of 40 patients in Toronto [12]. Relevant negative findings are lack of cavitation, calcification, reticular or nodular pattern of opacification and pleural effusion.

For those with normal initial chest radiographs, follow-up films were found to become abnormal after an average of 3 days [7]. It can however remain falsely negative until late in the course of the disease [13].

Serial radiographs showed one of the four patterns in the review by Antonio et al. [7]:

1. Appearance deteriorates for a week followed by improvement in 70.3%.
2. Appearance fluctuates with at least one intervening period of significant improvement followed by deterioration and later recovery in 17.4%.
3. Relatively static for 10 days followed by improvement in 7.2%.
4. Progressive deterioration leading to death in 5.1%.

Radiographic deterioration takes on the form of multifocal unilateral or bilateral opacification in most patients. Resolution of lung opacities can be demonstrated with successful treatment response. Confluent consolidation compatible with adult respiratory distress syndrome (ARDS) is associated with a grave prognosis.

HRCT

Both conventional CT and HRCT have been performed on patients with suspected SARS early in the outbreak. Only HRCT is now required with increasing knowledge on the radiographic and CT features of the disease. It can reveal parenchymal disease in patients whose radiographs are nor-

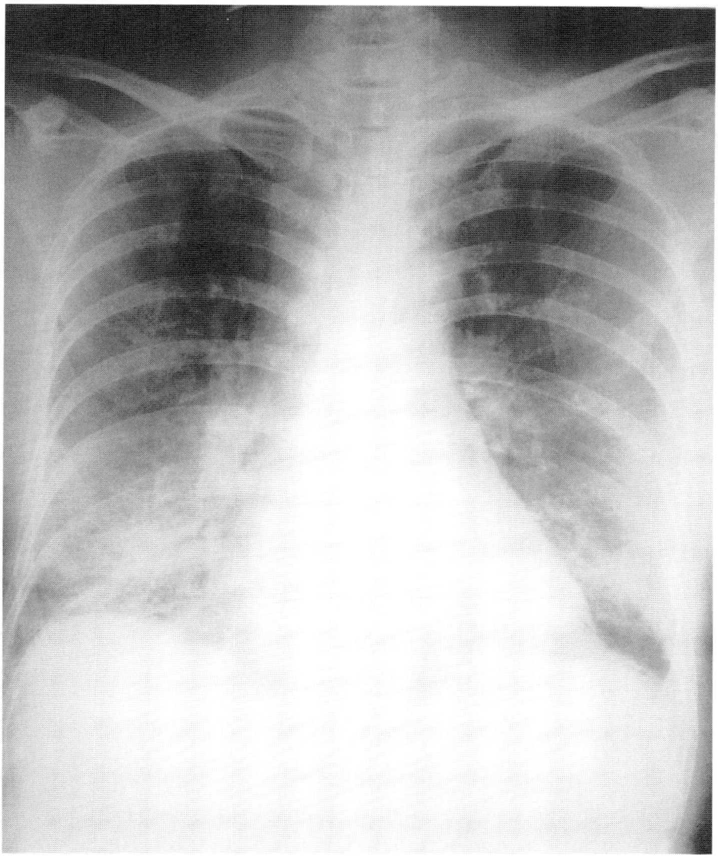

Figure 1. Frontal chest radiograph showing bilateral multifocal consolidation in lower zones

mal [13,14]. The abnormality can either be very small, or in the paraspinal region hidden by the heart or mediastinal structures, or in the posterior costophrenic angles [7].

Lee et al. reviewed the CT findings in 25 patients [4]. The typical finding was ill defined ground glass opacification in the periphery usually in a subpleural location, an appearance similar to that seen in bronchiolitis obliterans organizing pneumonia (BOOP). No bronchial dilatation was noted. Wong et al. reviewed the CT findings in 73 patients exposed to or with the disease [15]. Common findings included ground glass opacification, sometimes with consolidation, interlobular septal and intralobular interstitial thickening (Fig. 2). Lower lobe and peripheral distribution were again noted. Cavitation, calcification, reticular or nodular pattern of opacification, lymphadenopathy, or pleural effusion are not features of this disease [7].

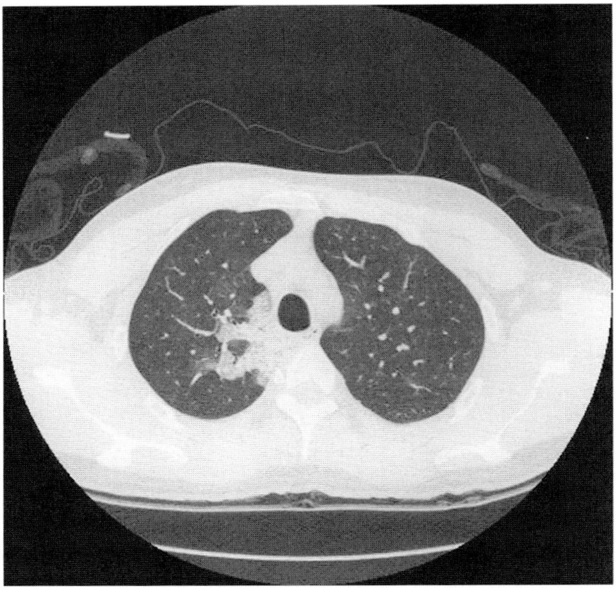

Figure 2. High resolution computed tomography of thorax showing consolidation in right upper lobe

Chan et al. reviewed the HRCT findings in 27 patients [16]. Ground glass density and crazy paving pattern were found to be the key features in the first week of the disease. The ground glass opacity could be as small as 5 mm, and in a perihilar, central or peripheral location. Crazy paving pattern which consisted of thin reticular shadow superimposed on ground glass opacity, again showed no specific pattern of distribution. Other findings included a sharp line of demarcation between normal and abnormal lungs, and subpleural sparing. Small localized pleural effusion was noted in 7 out of 27 patients (25.9%), usually with extensive disease.

Serial HRCT show a shifting pattern of air-space opacification, with resolution of the original lesion and appearance of a new lesion in the adjacent lung [17]. Progressive decrease in the extent of ground glass opacity and consolidation occurs with resolution of symptoms. Spontaneous pneumomediastinum is found in a substantial proportion of patients, usually during or just after completion of drug treatment [16–18]. This is unrelated to the use of positive end-expiratory pressure ventilation. Possible causes like peribronchiolar abscess formation leading to interstitial pulmonary emphysema, and the presence of subpleural blebs have been proposed. Subcutaneous emphysema and pneumothorax may develop as a result of pneumo-mediastinum.

Findings consistent with fibrosis have been described in a small percentage of patients [17, 18]. Muller et al. reviewed the HRCT findings in 29 patients [18]. Reticulation with associated architectural distortion and traction bronchiectasis was present in eight patients. The longest follow up HRCT was 27 days after hospital admission. Further follow up is required to determine whether these changes are reversible.

The role of imaging is to provide radiological evidence for diagnosis and to monitor disease progress and treatment response. The radiographic and CT appearances are not specific and clinical information is vital in establishing the diagnosis. HRCT should be limited to patients with high clinical suspicion and normal chest radiographs, and for detecting complications. While radiography is routinely performed using a portable machine at the bedside, CT scanners are often located in the main radiology department. Strict infection control is necessary to minimize cross infection. Mobile CT may be an alternative for seriously ill patients requiring strict isolation during an outbreak [19].

Gastrointestinal tract

Gastrointestinal symptoms of nausea, vomiting and diarrhea may be prominent presenting features of SARS (Tab. 1). Diarrhea is common (38-73%) during the whole course of illness [3, 5, 20]. It is more frequently observed during the first week of illness and usually self limiting [20]. Some patients may have protracted diarrhea leading to dehydration. Cheng et al. found that higher viral load in nasopharyngeal specimens was significantly associated with diarrhea and death [21].

There are other possible explanations of the high incidence of diarrhea reported in SARS. Most SARS patients in Hong Kong received a course of amoxicillin/clavulanic acid, clarithromycin and ribavirin, which had been reported to cause diarrhea. In studies using a combination of amoxicillin and clarithromycin for one week to eradicate *Helicobacter pylori*, diarrhea was reported in 3–34% of cases [22–24]. *Clostridium difficile* toxin could not be detected in stool of SARS patients treated with broad spectrum antibiotics [20].

Coronaviruses are a diverse group of enveloped RNA viruses that are known to cause a wide spectrum of diseases including respiratory and gastrointestinal systems in animals. Enteric coronavirus has been described to cause diarrhea in children and subjects with acquired immunodeficiency syndrome [25]. Recently, Leung et al. reported histological features of five post-mortem examinations of bowel and one colonic biopsy in SARS patients [20]. Light microscopic results were unremarkable with little inflammatory changes. Electron microscopy showed presence of virus particles in dilated endoplasmic reticulum and on the luminal surface of microvilli. This suggests viral shedding into the lumen of the gastrointestinal tract. SARS-associated coronavirus (SARS-CoV) could also be isolated from intestinal tissue by cell culture. Nonetheless, in view of the limited

Table 1. Clinical features of SARS on presentation

	Donnelly et al. [1]	Booth et al. [2]
Number of patients	1425	144
Fever (%)	94	99
Chills (%)	65	28
Malaise (%)	64	NR
Myalgia (%)	51	49
Headache (%)	50	35
Dizziness (%)	31	NR
Sore throat (%)	23	13
Running nose (%)	25	2
Cough (%)	50	69
Sputum production (%)	28	5
Shortness of breath (%)	31	NR
Nausea (%)	22	NR
Vomiting (%)	14	NR
Diarrhea (%)	27	24

NR, not reported

architectural disturbance, there is still no solid evidence that the SARS-CoV is the cause of diarrhea. Protein or toxins released from SARS-CoV was postulated to cause diarrhea but this theory remains speculative [20]. The gastrointestinal tract is the only organ other than the lungs where SARS-CoV could be isolated by cell culture.

Diarrhea poses a significant infection control problem because SARS-CoV RNA can be identified in stool of a majority of cases [5]. Although stool culture for SARS-CoV has not been successful, fecal-oral transmission of SARS-CoV remains a distinct possibility. The outbreak of SARS in a densely populated private housing complex of Hong Kong was traced to a 33 year-old SARS patient with watery diarrhea. It was postulated that the virus-laden aerosols were spread via a faulty sewage system [26].

Liver

Twenty-three to 35% of patients had an elevated alanine transaminase on presentation (Tab. 2). Wong et al. reported a drop of albumin level and an elevation of globulin and serum bilirubin levels on serial measurements [27]. Seventy-six percent of patients developed liver dysfunction during the course of illness. They also found that the time to peak of alanine transaminase or bilirubin level correlated with the time to worst chest radiographic scores. These findings were not shared by the control group of age- and sex-matched patients with community-acquired pneumonia. Tsang et al. reported that higher alanine transaminase levels were found among patients with positive reverse transcriptase-polymerase chain reaction (RT-PCR) for SARS-CoV in nasopharyngeal aspirate [28]. This suggests a rela-

Table 2. Key laboratory findings of SARS at presentation

	Choi et al. [3]	Booth et al. [2]	Lee et al. [4]	Peiris et al. [5]	Vu et al. [6]
Number of patients	267	144	138	75	62
Leucopenia (%)	27	NR	34	7	19
Lymphopenia (%)	73	85	70	75	79
Thrombocytopenia (%)	50	NR	45	37	40
Hyponatraemia (%)	NR	NR	20	NR	30
Elevated ALT (%)	31	NR	23	29	35
Elevated CK (%)	19	39	32	36	NR
Elevated LDH (%)	47	87	71	NR	NR

ALT, alanine transaminase; CK, creatine kinase; LDH, Lactate dehydrogenase; NR, not reported

tionship between hepatic dysfunction and viral load. SARS-CoV is a novel virus of which hepatotropism is unknown. Mouse hepatitis virus, a group 2 coronavirus, can cause liver damage ranging from minimal change to fulminant hepatitis. Liver histology provides important clues as to the cause of liver dysfunction. Autopsy findings of SARS patients showed features of fibrinoid necrosis, and infiltration of monocytes and lymphocytes into the vessel, suggestive of systemic vasculitis while others showed apoptosis and fatty degeneration in liver. However, most of these findings belonged to patients with respiratory failure and multi-organ failure, hence the changes in the liver might not be solely due to SARS-CoV. Chau et al. reported liver biopsy results of three patients with marked hepatic dysfunction [29]. Prominent mitotic figures of hepatocytes were noted in two and apoptosis in all three patients. Conspicuous mitosis may be related to cell cycle arrest as a result of SARS-CoV infection. Furthermore, RT-PCR also showed evidence of SARS-CoV in liver tissues, though electron microscopy could not identify viral particles.

Hematology system

The majority of patients presented with lymphopenia with normal or low total white cell count (Tab. 2). Wong et al. found that both CD4 and CD8 lymphocytes were depleted on presentation while their ratio remained normal [30]. The B lymphocytes counts were normal. The lymphocyte counts might further fall or remain low as the disease progressed and 153 out of 157 (98%) patients had lymphopenia during the whole course of illness. On the other hand, thrombocytopenia is also a common presenting feature (Tab. 2). Reactive thrombocytosis may occur in some patients. Lee et al. reported that prolonged activated partial-thromboplastin time and elevated D-dimer levels were found in 43% and 45% of patients on presentation, respectively [4]. The prothrombin time remained normal. Both thrombocytopenia and deranged clotting profile did not cause clinically significant bleeding. Neutrophilia may develop and can be partly attributed to the use of steroids and secondary nosocomial infection. Hemoglobin may drop secondary to hemolysis in patients receiving ribavirin.

Other systems

Both creatine kinase and lactate dehydrogenase may be elevated on presentation and they continue to rise as the disease progresses (Tab. 2). The lactate dehydrogenase level reflects tissue destruction or hemolysis secondary to ribavirin treatment. Wang et al. reported three cases of rhabdomyolysis associated with probable SARS [31]. The patients had very high peak creatine kinase levels and developed myoglobinuria leading to acute renal failure; two of them died. Muscle biopsies showed degenerative changes and necrosis of muscle fibers in the most severe cases. Cardiac-specific troponin levels are usually normal. Sub-clinical diastolic dysfunction without systolic impairment in heart had been reported in SARS and was reversible as the patients recovered [32]. Post-mortem examination did not reveal direct invasion of myocardium by the virus. Lau et al. reported a pregnant woman with SARS who developed generalized convulsion without an obvious explanatory cause [33]. She was found RT-PCR positive for SARS-CoV in cerebrospinal fluid. This raises the possibility of central nervous system invasion by the SARS-CoV. Recent experimental evidence showed neurotropism and neuroinvasion of human coronavirus and its link with multiple sclerosis [34]. Electrolyte disturbances including hypokalemia may develop during the course of illness secondary to diarrhea, use of ribavirin and steroids.

Atypical presentation

Subclinical infection by SARS-CoV is rare. Lee et al. performed serological screening of asymptomatic healthcare workers who had taken care of SARS patients [35]. Only one out of 101 subjects was tested positive for SARS-CoV. Chow et al. found that none of the 84 exposed healthcare workers in whom SARS did not develop had seroconversion [36]. Mild infection by SARS-CoV without florid pulmonary involvement has been described. Lin et al. reported a 28-year-old physician who had close contact with SARS patients and presented with fever, malaise and myalgia without apparent pneumonitis by chest radiography [37]. His serum was later found to be positive for immunoglobulin G against SARS-CoV. These findings raise a possibility of genetic predisposition or susceptibility to SARS-CoV infection. Preliminary research by Li et al. found that the human leukocyte antigen system might be linked to the severity of SARS-CoV infection [38].

SARS runs a milder and shorter course in children under the age of 12 [39]. Hon et al. reported that four out of five teenagers but none of the younger children required supplemental oxygen therapy [40]. Two teenagers required assisted ventilation.

Atypical presentation of SARS in geriatric patients is a diagnostic challenge. The clinical picture is often confounded by multiple co-existing diseases that apparently could explain the illnesses [41]. Epidemiological history of contact may not be obvious. Fever may be low grade, self limiting or even absent in elderly patients infected with SARS-CoV. Clinicians may have mistaken spontaneous resolution of fever as response to antibiotics and misdiagnosed SARS as bacterial pneumonia. Cough may be absent because of suppressed cough reflex in elderly.

Clinical course and prognosis

The clinical outcome and prognostic factors are summarized in Table 3. Peiris et al. found that the viral load peaked at around day 10 after onset of symptoms [5]. The majority of patients had a fall in temperature after ribavirin and steroids combination therapy. However, 85% of patients developed recurrence of fever and progression of pneumonitis despite fall in viral load; 20% developed ARDS. Immunological damage secondary to cytokine deregulation was postulated to be the underlying pathogenetic mechanism. Twenty to 34% of patients were in intensive care while 13–26% required assisted ventilation (Tab. 3). Non-invasive positive pressure ventilation has been tried successfully in SARS patients, alleviating the need of intubation and mechanical ventilation. Nosocomial chest infection is an important problem in patients who depend on ventilator support and receive steroid therapy. Superinfection with *Aspergillus fumigatus* was reported in patients receiving high dose steroids with broad-spectrum antibiotics [44]. Acute renal or mutli-organ failure may further complicate the clinical course and compromise the chance of survival in critically ill SARS patients.

The case fatality rate varied widely among different affected regions. According to the World Health Organization (WHO), the overall worldwide case fatality rate was 9.6% and ranged from 7 to 17% in individual countries with major outbreak [45]. The rates stated in major published data ranged from 3.6 to 12%. The figures should be interpreted with care. The study populations might not be comparable. Studies with longer follow-up time have higher case fatality rate. The case definition of SARS in many studies was based only on clinical parameters instead of serological criteria. The sensitivity and specificity of the WHO criteria for the diagnosis of SARS-CoV infection was only 26% and 96%, respectively [46]. The pre-morbid risk profile of SARS patients may also affect the case fatality rate. SARS-CoV could be the principal cause of death or one of the contributing factors in patients with multiple underlying diseases.

Table 3. Clinical outcome and prognostic factors in SARS

Study	Number of patients	Median or mean (SD) age	Case fatality rate (%)	ICU care (%)	Assisted ventilation (%)	Adverse outcomes	Clinical correlates of adverse outcomes	Odds ratio or relative risk (95% CI)
Tsui et al. [42]	323	41 (14)	NR	21	13	Death or ICU care	Age (per 10-year increase) Admission neutrophil count (per 1×10^9/L increase) Initial LDH level (per 100 IU/L increase)	1.57 (1.26–1.95) 1.28 (1.13–1.46) 1.35 (1.11–1.64)
Choi et al. [3]	267	39	12 (3 months)	26	21	Death	Age > 60 LDH > 3.8 μkat/L at presentation	5.1 (2.3–11.31) 2.2 (1.03–4.71)
Booth et al. [2]	144	45	6.5 (21 days)	20	13.9	Death, ICU care or assisted ventilation	Diabetes mellitus Other comorbid conditions	3.1 (1.4–7.2) 2.5 (1.1–5.8)
Lee et al. [4]	138	39 (16.8)	3.6 (21 days)	23.2	13.8	Death or ICU care	Advanced age (per 10-year increase) High absolute neutrophil count on presentation High peak LDH level	1.8 (1.16–2.81) 1.6 (1.03–2.5) 2.09 (1.28–3.42)
Chan et al. [43]	115	41 (14.8)	10 (21 days)	34	26	Death	Age >60 Diabetes mellitus or heart disease Another coexisting condition	3.5 (1.2–10.2) 9.1 (2.8–29.1) 5.2 (1.4–19.7)
Peiris et al. [5]	75	40 (12.2)	7 (25 days)	NR	NR	Development of ARDS	Age of 61–80 Positive test for hepatitis B surface antigen	28.0 (3.1–253.3) 18.0 (3.2–101.3)

NR, not reported; ICU, intensive care unit; ARDS, adult respiratory distress syndrome; LDH, Lactate dehydrogenase; CI, confidence interval

Prognostic factors

Identification of prognostic factors is key to risk stratification and planning of management in SARS patients, although no treatment has yet been proven in randomized trial to be efficacious in the combat of SARS. Prognostic factors varied among different research centers depending on the variables included under study and case-mix. Advanced age [4, 42], especially those over the age of 60 [3, 5, 43], concurrent medical illnesses [2, 43], particularly diabetes mellitus [2, 43] are consistently established as independent clinical prognostic indicators for adverse clinical outcomes comprising death, intensive care admission or assisted ventilation (Tab. 3). High neutrophil counts [4, 42] and lactate dehydrogenase level [30, 42] on presentation, low CD4 and CD8 lymphocyte counts [30], hypoxemia and thrombocytopenia [47] are also associated with poor outcomes.

High viral load [21] or positivity of RT-PCR for SARS-CoV in nasopharyngeal aspirate [28] is also a prognostic factor. The development of quantitative, real-time, nested RT-PCR assay for SARS-CoV in upper respiratory tract or serum offers hope for early detection of SARS and monitoring of viral load [48, 49]. Higher serum SARS-CoV concentration predicts intensive care unit admission [48].

Chest radiography also carries prognostic information. Paul et al. [10] reviewed the chest radiographs of 51 patients. Four radiographic patterns were seen: normal (group 1) in 19.6% (10/51), focal opacity (group 2) in 39.2% (20/51), multifocal opacities (group 3) in 27.5% (14/51), and diffuse air-space opacification (group 4) in 13.7% (7/51). Radiographic progression occurred in 38.8% of the patients in group 1–4. There was no death in group 1 and 2. Mortality was 7.7% in group 3 and 71.4% in group 4. Diffuse air-space opacification was noted on the last radiographs for all patients who died. The authors concluded that patients presenting with normal findings or focal air-space opacity on chest radiograph had a good clinical outcome. Patients with multifocal opacities that progressed to diffuse opacification and patients presenting with diffuse air-space opacification had a high fatality rate. Chau et al. found that initial chest radiographic score was an independent prognostic factor among the clinical, laboratory and chest radiography variables studied [50].

References

1 Donnelly CA, Ghani AC, Leung GM, Hedley AJ, Fraser C, Riley S, Abu-Raddad LJ, Ho L, Thach T, Chau P et al (2003) Epidemiological determinants of spread of causal agent of severe acute respiratory syndrome in Hong Kong. *Lancet* 361: 1761–1766

2 Booth CM, Matukas LM, Tomlinson GA, Rachlis AR, Rose DB, Dwosh HA, Walmsley SL, Mazzulli T, Avendano M, Derkach P et al (2003) Clinical features

and short-term outcomes of 144 patients with SARS in the greater Toronto area. *JAMA* 289: 2801–2809

3 Choi KW, Chau TN, Tsang O, Tso E, Chiu MC, Tong WL, Lee PO, Ng TK, Ng WF, Lee KC et al (2003) Outcomes and prognostic factors in 267 patients with severe acute respiratory syndrome in Hong Kong. *Ann Intern Med* 139: 715–723

4 Lee N, Hui D, Wu A, Chan P, Cameron P, Joynt GM, Ahuja A, Yung MY, Leung CB, To KF et al (2003) A major outbreak of severe acute respiratory syndrome in Hong Kong. *N Engl J Med* 348: 1986–1994

5 Peiris JS, Chu CM, Cheng VC, Chan KS, Hung IF, Poon LL, Law KI, Tang BS, Hon TY, Chan CS et al (2003) Clinical progression and viral load of coronavirus pneumonia in a community outbreak: a prospective study. *Lancet* 361: 1767–1772

6 Vu HT, Leitmeyer KC, Le DH, Miller MJ, Nguyen QH, Uyeki TM, Reynolds MG, Aagesen J, Nicholson KG, Vu QH et al (2004) Clinical description of a completed outbreak of SARS in Vietnam, February–May 2003. *Emerg Infect Dis* 10: 334–338

7 Antonio GE, Wong KT, Chu WC, Hui DS, Cheng FW, Yuen EH, Chung SS, Fok TF, Sung JJ, Ahuja AT (2003) Imaging of severe acute respiratory syndrome in Hong Kong. *AJR* 81: 11–17.

8 Young DYN, Lau BWK (2003) An outcome analysis of chest x-ray examination for detecting severe acute respiratory syndrome in general practice. *HK Pract* 25: 357–362

9 Tsang KW, Ho PL, Ooi GC Yee WK, Wang T, Chan-Yeung M, Lam WK, Seto WH, Yam LY, Cheng TM et al (2003) A cluster of cases of severe acute respiratory syndrome in Hong Kong. *N Engl J Med* 348: 1977–1985.

10 Paul NS, Chung T, Konen E, Roberts HC, Rao TN, Gold WL, Mehta S, Tomlinson GA, Boylan CE, Grossman H et al (2004) Prognostic significance of the radiographic pattern of disease in patients with severe acute respiratory syndrome. *AJR* 182: 493–498

11 Wong KT, Antonio GE, Hui DS, Lee N, Yuen EH, Wu A, Leung CB, Rainer TH, Cameron P, Chung SS et al (2003) Severe acute respiratory syndrome: radiographic appearances and pattern of progression in 138 patients. *Radiology* 228: 401–406

12 Grinblat L, Shulman H, Glickman A, Matukas L, Paul N (2003) Severe acute respiratory syndrome: radiographic review of 40 probable cases in Toronto, Canada. *Radiology* 228: 802–809

13 Rao TNA, Paul N, Chung TB, Mazzulli T, Walmsley S, Boylan CE, Provost Y, Herman SJ, Weisbrod GL, Roberts HC et al (2003) Value of CT in assessing probable severe acute respiratory syndrome. *AJR* 181: 317–319

14 Muller NL, Ooi GC, Khong PL, Nicolaou S (2003) Severe acute respiratory syndrome: radiographic and CT findings. *AJR* 181: 3–8

15 Wong KT, Antonio GE, Hui DS, Lee N, Yuen EH, Wu A, Leung CB, Rainer TH, Cameron P, Chung SS (2003) Thin-section CT of severe acute respiratory

syndrome: evaluation of 73 patients exposed to or with the disease. *Radiology* 228: 395–400
16 Chan MS, Chan IY, Fung KH, Poon E, Yam LY, Lau KY et al (2004) High-resolution CT findings in patients with severe acute respiratory syndrome: a pattern-based approach. *AJR* 182: 49–56
17 Hui JY, Cho DH, Yang MK, Wang K, Lo KK, Fan WC, Chan CC, Chu CM, Loke TK, Chan JC et al (2003) Severe acute respiratory syndrome: spectrum of high-resolution CT findings and temporal progression of the disease. *AJR* 181: 1525–1538
18 Muller NL, Ooi GC, Khong PL, Zhou LJ, Tsang KW, Nicolaou S (2004) High-resolution CT findings of severe acute respiratory syndrome on presentation and after admission. *AJR* 182: 39–44
19 Parmar HA, Lim TC, Goh JS, Tan JT, Sitoh YY, Hui F (2004) Providing optimal radiology service in the severe acute respiratory syndrome outbreak: use of mobile CT. *AJR* 182: 57–60
20 Leung WK, To KF, Chan PK, Chan HL, Wu AK, Lee N, Yuen KY, Sung JJ (2003) Enteric involvement of severe acute respiratory syndrome-associated coronavirus infection. *Gastroenterology* 125(4): 1011–1017
21 Cheng VC, Hung IF, Tang BS, Chu CM, Wong MM, Chan KH, Wu AK, Tse DM, Chan KS, Zheng BJ et al (2004) Viral replication in the nasopharynx is associated with diarrhea in patients with severe acute respiratory syndrome. *Clin Infect Dis* 38: 467–475
22 Sung JJ, Chan FK, Wu JC, Leung WK, Suen R, Ling TK, Lee YT, Cheng AF, Chung SC (1999) One-week ranitidine bismuth citrate in combinations with metronidazole, amoxycillin and clarithromycin in the treatment of *Helicobacter pylori* infection: the RBC-MACH study. *Aliment Pharmacol Ther* 13(8): 1079–1084
23 Sung JJ, Leung WK, Ling TK, Yung MY, Chan FK, Lee YT, Cheng AF, Chung SC (1998) One-week use of ranitidine bismuth citrate, amoxicillin and clarithromycin for the treatment of *Helicobacter pylori*-related duodenal ulcer. *Aliment Pharmacol Ther* 12(8): 725–730
24 Veldhuyzen Van Zanten SJO, Bradette M, Farley A, Leddin D, Lind T, Unge P, Bayerdorffer E, Spiller RC, O'morain C, Sipponen P et al (1999) The DU-MACH study: eradication of *Helicobacter pylori* and ulcer healing in patients with acute duodenal ulcer using omeprazole based triple therapy. *Aliment Pharmacol Ther* 13(3): 289–295
25 Schmidt W, Schneider T, Heise W, Weinke T, Epple HJ, Stoffler-Meilicke M, Liesenfeld O, Ignatius R, Zeitz M, Riecken EO et al (1996) Stool viruses, coinfections, and diarrhea in HIV-infected patients. Berlin Diarrhoea/Wasting Syndrome Study Group. *J Acquir Immune Defic Syndr Hum Retrovirol* 13: 33–38
26 Department of Health, HKSAR (2003) Outbreak of severe acute respiratory syndrome (SARS) at Amoy Gardens, Kowloon Bay, Hong Kong. Available from: http://www.info.gov.hk/info/ap/pdf/amoy_e.pdf (accessed June 2 2003)
27 Wong WM, Ho JC, Hung IF, Ng W, Lam YM, Tam WO, Wong BC, Wong PC,

Lai CL, Lam WK et al (2003) Temporal patterns of hepatic dysfunction and disease severity in patients with SARS. *JAMA* 290: 2663–2665
28 Tsang OT, Chau TN, Choi KW, Tso YK, Lim W, Chiu MC, Tong WL, Lee PO, Lam BH, Ng TK et al (2003) Coronavirus-positive nasopharyngeal aspirate as predictor for severe acute respiratory syndrome mortality. *Emerg Infect Dis* 9: 1381–1387.
29 Chau TN, Lee KC, Yao H, Tsang TY, Chow TC, Yeung YC, Choi KW, Tso YK, Lau T, Lai ST et al (2004) SARS-associated viral hepatitis caused by a novel coronavirus: report of three cases. *Hepatology* 39(2): 302–310
30 Wong RS, Wu A, To KF, Lee N, Lam CW, Wong CK, Chan PK, Ng MH, Yu LM, Hui DS et al (2003) Haematological manifestations in patients with severe acute respiratory syndrome: retrospective analysis. *BMJ* 326: 1358–1362
31 Wang JL, Wang JT, Yu CJ, Chen YC, Hsueh PR, Hsiao CH, Kao CL, Chang SC, Yang PC (2003) Rhabdomyolysis associated with probable SARS. *Am J Med* 115: 421–422
32 Li SS, Cheng CW, Fu CL, Chan YH, Lee MP, Chan JW, Yiu SF (2003) Left ventricular performance in patients with Severe Acute Respiratory syndrome-a 30-day echocardiographic follow-up study. *Circulation* 108: 1798–1803
33 Lau KK, Yu WC, Chu CM, Lau ST, Sheng B, Yuen KY (2004) Possible central nervous system infection by SARS coronavirus. *Emerg Infect Dis* 10: 342–344
34 Arbour N, Talbot PJ (1998) Persistent infection of neural cell lines by human coronaviruses. *Adv Exp Med Biol* 440: 575–581
35 Lee HK, Tso EY, Chau TN, Tsang OT, Choi KW, Lai TS (2003) Asymptomatic severe acute respiratory syndrome-associated coronavirus infection. *Emerg Infect Dis* 9: 1491–1492
36 Chow PK, Ooi EE, Tan HK , Ong KW, Sil BK, Teo M, Ng T, Soo KC (2004) Healthcare worker seroconversion in SARS outbreak. *Emerg Infect Dis* 10: 249–250
37 Li G, Zhao Z, Chen L, Zhou Y (2003) Mild severe acute respiratory syndrome. *Emerg Infect Dis* 9: 1182–1183
38 Lin M, Tseng HK, Trejaut JA, Lee HL, Loo JH, Chu CC, Chen PJ, Su YW, Lim KH, Tsai ZU et al (2003) Association of HLA class 1 with severe acute respiratory syndrome coronavirus infection. Available from: http://www.biomedcentral.com/1471–2350/4/9 (Accessed Dec 6, 2003)
39 Chiu WK, Cheung PC, Ng KL, Ip PL, Sugunan VK, Luk DC, Ma LC, Chan BH, Lo KL, Lai WM (2003) Severe acute respiratory syndrome in children: experience in a regional hospital in Hong Kong. *Pediatr Crit Care Med* 4: 279–283
40 Hon KL, Leung CW, Cheng WT Chan PK, Chu WC, Kwan YW, Li AM, Fong NC, Ng PC, Chiu MC et al (2003) Clinical presentations and outcome of severe acute respiratory syndrome in children. *Lancet* 361: 1701–1703
41 Tee AK, Oh HML, Hui KP, Lien CT, Narendran K, Heng BH, Ling AE (2004) Atypical SARS in geriatric patient. *Emerg Infect Dis* 10:261–264
42 Tsui PT, Kwok ML, Yuen H, Lai ST (2003) Severe acute respiratory syndrome: clinical outcome and prognostic correlates. *Emerg Infect Dis* 9:1064–1069
43 Chan JW, Ng CK, Chan YH, Mok TY, Lee WH, Lee S, Chu SY, Law WL, Lee

MP, Li PCl (2003) Short term outcome and risk factors for adverse clinical outcomes in adults with severe acute respiratory syndrome (SARS). *Thorax* 58: 686–689
44 Wang H, Ding Y, Li X, Yang L, Zhang W, Kang W (2003) Fatal aspergillosis in a patient with SARS who was treated with corticosteroids. *N Engl J Med* 349: 507–508
45 World Health Organization (2003) Summary of probable SARS cases with onset of illness from 1 Nov 2002 to 31 July 2003. Available from: http://www.who.int/csr/sars/country/table2004_04_21/en/ (Accessed Dec 6, 2003)
46 Rainer TH, Cameron PA, Smit D, Ong KL, Ng AW, Chan DP, Ahuja AT, Chan LY, Sung YY et al (2003) Evaluation of WHO criteria for identifying patients with severe acute respiratory syndrome out of hospital: prospective observational study. BMJ 326: 1354–1358
47 Zou Z, Yang Y, Chen J, Xin S, Zhang W, Zhou X, Mao Y, Hu L, Liu D, Chang B et al (2004) Prognostic factors for severe acute respiratory syndrome: a clinical analysis of 165 cases. *Clin Infect Dis* 38: 483–489
48 Ng EK, Hui DS, Chan KC, Hung EC, Chiu RW, Lee N, Wu A, Chim SS, Tong YK, Sung JJ et al (2003) Quantitative analysis and prognostic implication of SARS coronavirus RNA in the plasma and serum of patients with severe acute respiratory syndrome. *Clin Chem* 49: 1976–1980
49 Grant PR, Garson JA, Tedder RS, Chan PK, Tam JS, Sung JJ (2003) Detection of SARS Coronavirus in Plasma by Real-Time RT-PCR. *N Engl J Med*. 349: 2468–2469
50 Chau TN, Lee PO, Choi KW, Lee CM, Ma KF, Tsang TY, Tso YK, Chiu MC, Tong WL, Yu WC et al (2004) Value of initial chest radiographs for predicting clinical outcomes in patients with severe acute respiratory syndrome. *Am J Med* 117(4): 249–254

SARS coronavirus infection: pathology and pathogenesis of an emerging virus disease

Sherif R. Zaki and Cynthia S. Goldsmith

Infectious Disease Pathology Activity, Division of Viral and Rickettsial Diseases, National Center for Infectious Diseases, Centers for Disease Control and Prevention (CDC), Atlanta, GA 30333, USA

Introduction

Severe acute respiratory syndrome (SARS) was first recognized during a global outbreak of severe pneumonia that first occurred in late 2002 in Guangdong Province, China, and then erupted in February 2003 with cases in more than two dozen countries in Asia, Europe, North America, and South America. The disease causes an influenza-like illness with fever, cough, dyspnea, and headache, and in severe cases, it can cause human death. Person-to-person transmission, combined with international travel of infected persons, accelerated the worldwide spread of the illness, and by the time the outbreak was contained, 8,098 probable cases resulting in 774 deaths were reported [1–4]. During the outbreak, a global network of 11 laboratories was established by the World Health Organization (WHO) to identify the causal agent. Early in the investigation, the clinical, pathologic, and laboratory studies focused on previously known agents of respiratory illness. Subsequently, however, a previously unknown virus was isolated from the oropharynx of a SARS patient and identified by ultrastructural characteristics as belonging to the family *Coronaviridae* [5–7]. These findings shifted the focus of the investigation toward verification of the role played by this newly recognized coronavirus. A vast array of laboratory approaches was utilized in this investigation, including pathologic, serologic, and molecular assays [6–10]. Within weeks, infection of non-human primates was achieved, thus establishing an animal model for SARS coronavirus (SARS-CoV) [11].

This chapter presents the morphologic characteristics of SARS-CoV grown in tissue culture and the histopathologic changes, electron microscopic findings, and cellular localization of the virus in tissues from human patients and experimentally infected animals. In addition, the pathophysiology of this newly emergent virus will be discussed.

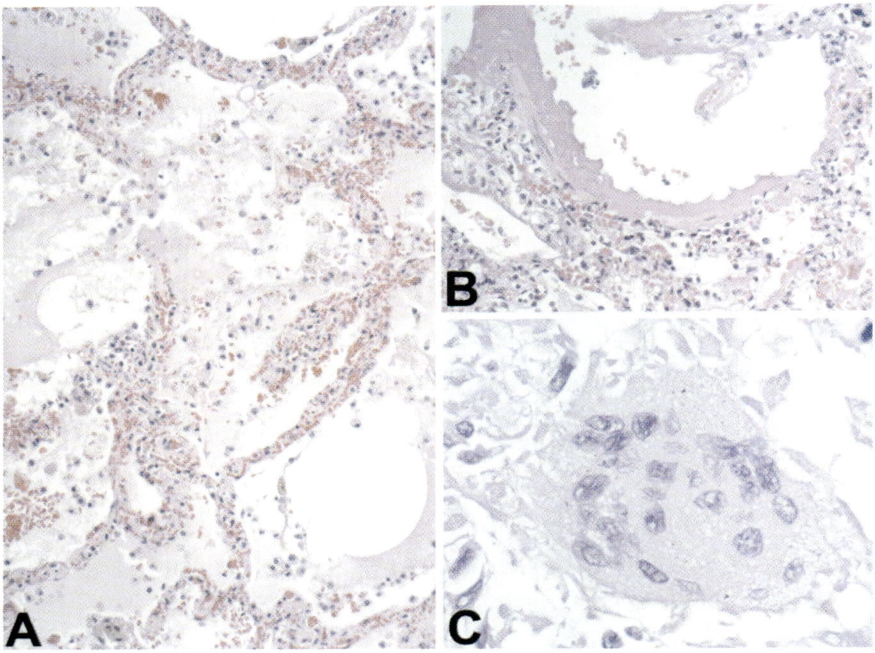

Figure 1. Histopathology of SARS in fatal human cases. (A) Low-power photomicrograph of lung showing interstitial pneumonia and intra-alveolar edema. (B) Higher power photomicrograph showing diffuse alveolar damage with prominent hyaline membranes. (C) Multinucleated syncytial giant cells are seen in some cases of fatal SARS. Note absence of discernable viral inclusions. Original magnifications, A, 20×; B, 40×; C, 100×.

Histopathology

Several reports have described diffuse alveolar damage with various levels of progression and severity as the main histopathologic findings in SARS patients [6, 12–17]. Lungs typically show changes in the proliferative phase of diffuse alveolar damage, with hyaline-membrane formation, desquamation of epithelial cells, fibrin deposit in the alveolar space, and hyperplasia of type 2 pneumocytes (Fig. 1A, B). Increased mononuclear infiltrate in the interstitium can be seen in some cases. Other findings identified in some patients included focal intra-alveolar hemorrhage, necrotic inflammatory debris in small airways, and organizing pneumonia. In addition, multinucleated syncytial cells were seen in the intra-alveolar spaces of some patients who died 14 days or more after onset of illness (Fig. 1C). These cells contained abundant vacuolated cytoplasm with cleaved and convoluted nuclei. No obvious intranuclear or intracytoplasmic viral inclusions were identified.

Virus isolation and morphogenesis

Ultrastructural characteristics of SARS-CoV have been described in recent reports [18, 19]. Maturation is similar to features previously described for other coronaviruses [20–22]. Virions form by alignment of the helical nucleocapsids along the membranes of the endoplasmic reticulum or Golgi complex and by budding into the lumina of the cisternae (Fig. 2A). These vesicles become filled with virions and progress to the cell surface for release of the virus particles; large numbers of particles remain adherent to the plasma membrane at the cell surface (Fig. 2B). Other cytoplasmic structures associated with infection include double-membrane vesicles, which are the proposed replication complex for the virus [23, 24], and nucleocapsid inclusions (Fig. 2C). Immunogold electron microscopy, using a hyperimmune mouse ascitic fluid, was used to confirm the viral nature of the particles and inclusions (Fig. 2D). Infection of Vero E6 cells with SARS-CoV produces characteristic syncytial cells similar to those sometimes observed in lungs of patients who died. By light microscopy, abundant viral antigens can be detected in the cytoplasm of these cells grown in tissue culture (Fig. 2E).

Tissue distribution and cellular targets

In situ hybridization (ISH) and immunohistochemical (IHC) studies of tissues from SARS patients demonstrated coronavirus infection of upper airway bronchiolar epithelium [12, 25–27]. Infected ciliated columnar epithelial cells can be seen focally in lining epithelium of trachea and larger bronchi (Fig. 3A). Many of these infected cells slough off the epithelium and can be observed by using ISH within the bronchial lumen (Fig. 3B). Similarly, ultrastructural examination of bronchiolar lavage from a SARS patient showed numerous coronavirus-infected cells (Fig. 3C).

Abundant viral antigens can also be found distributed focally in parenchyma of lungs of some patients and are seen predominantly in cytoplasm of pneumocytes (Fig. 4A), in occasional macrophages (Fig. 4B) and in association with intra-alveolar necrotic debris and fibrin (Fig. 4C). Double-stain studies revealed that most SARS-CoV-infected cells are type 2 pneumocytes (co-labeled with surfactant), with occasional macrophages (co-labeled with CD68). Double-stain studies also detected viral nucleic acids with a distribution similar to that seen in IHC studies, mainly in pneumocytes and some macrophages [26]. Electron microscopic examination of lung tissues selected from areas with abundant IHC staining showed numerous coronavirus particles and nucleocapsid inclusions (Fig. 4D–F). Virions were seen in cytoplasmic vesicles and along the cell membranes of pneumocytes, in phagosomes of macrophages, and associated with fibrin in alveolar spaces. Because coronavirus particles may be confused morpho-

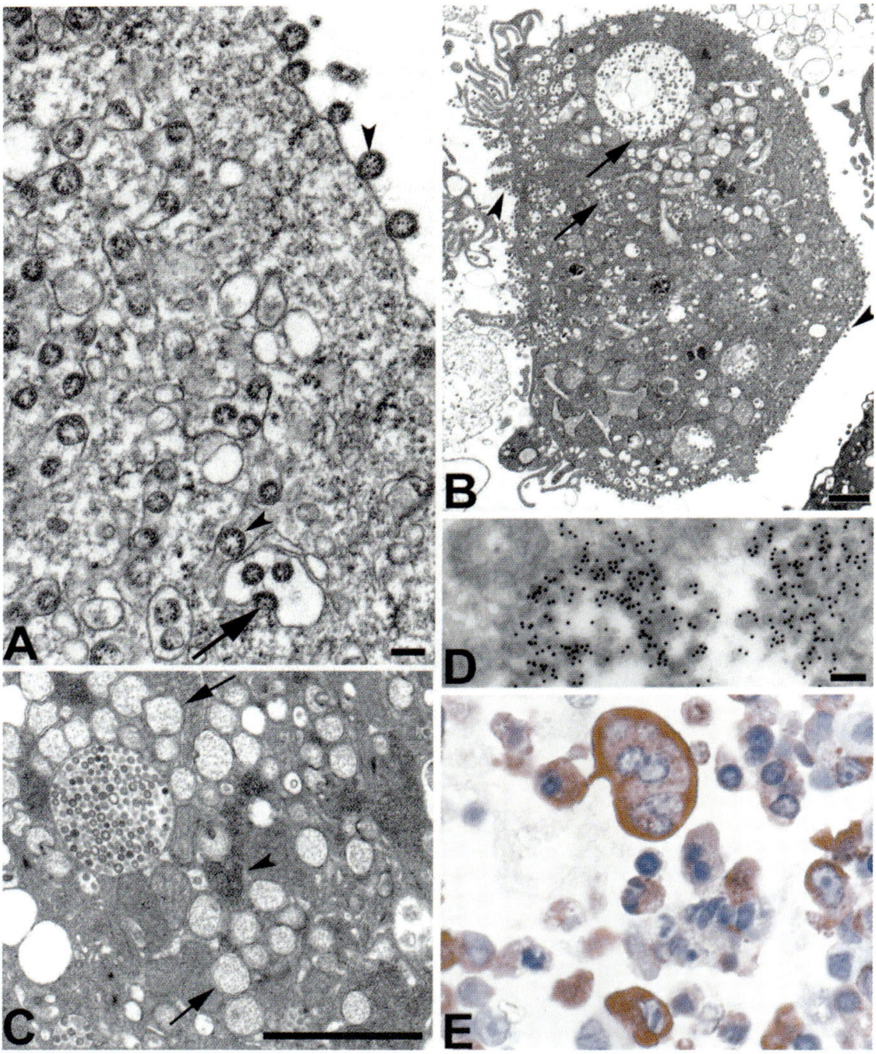

Figure 2. SARS-CoV-infected Vero E6 cells. (A) Virus particles form upon cytoplasmic membranes (arrow) and accumulate in vesicles as they progress to the cell surface. Cross-sections of the viral nucleocapsids (arrowheads) are evident in the virions. More virus particles are seen attached at the plasma membrane. (B) Low-magnification electron micrograph shows virus particles adherent to the plasma membrane (arrowheads) and within small and large vesicles (arrows) in the cytoplasm. (C) Cytoplasm of infected cell containing double-membrane vesicles (arrows), nucleocapsid inclusions (arrowhead), and virus particles within membrane-bound vesicles. (D) Immunogold labeling of intracellular virions. (Mouse hyperimmune ascitic fluid; goat anti-mouse conjugated to 12 nm gold.) (E) Immunohistochemical detection of SARS-CoV antigens in infected Vero E6 cells, using mouse anti-coronavirus. (Immunoalkaline phosphatase with napthol fast red substrate and hematoxylin counterstain.) Bars, A, B, C, 1 μm; D, 100 nm. Original magnification, E, 100×.

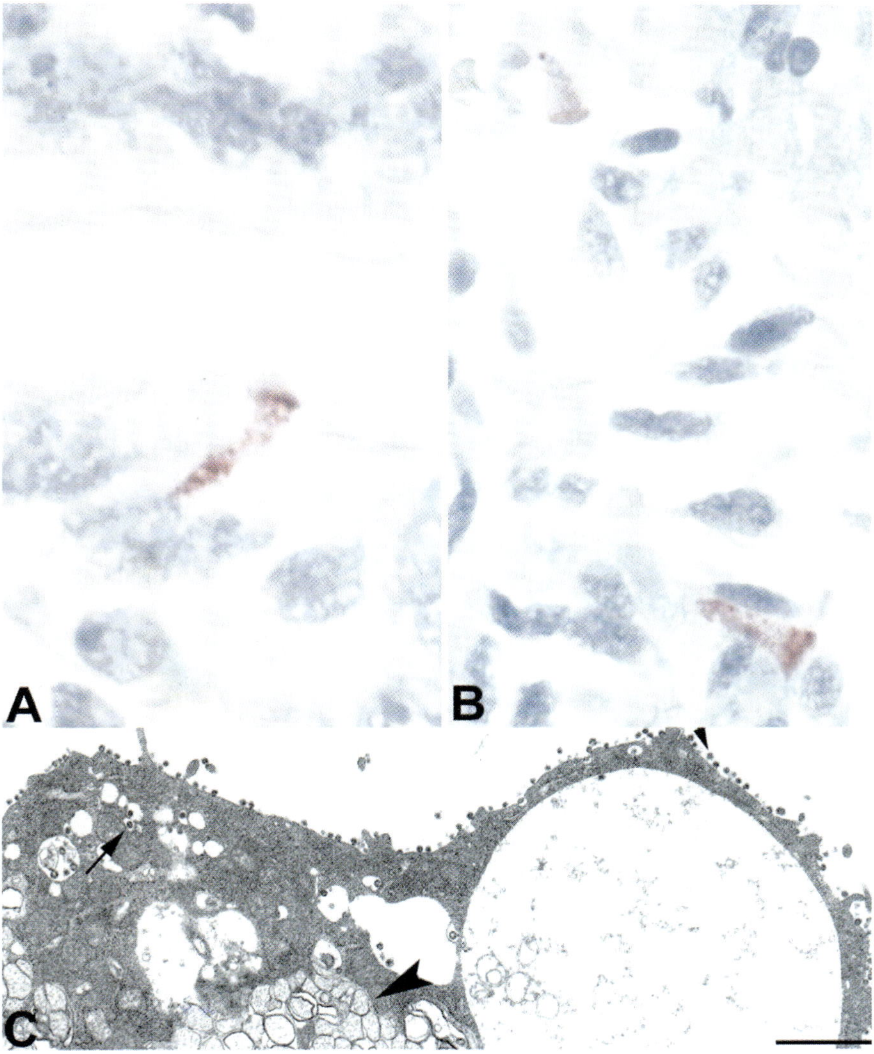

Figure 3. Cellular targets of infection in upper airways. (A) ISH of surface epithelium from a fatal human case. (B) ISH of infected cells that sloughed off into the lumen of a large bronchus. (C) Infected cells, presumed to be sloughed-off pneumocytes, are seen in a bronchial alveolar lavage obtained early in infection. Virus particles (arrows) are found along the cell surface and within cytoplasmic vesicles. Double-membrane vesicles (arrowhead) are also present. Original magnifications, A, B, 100×. Bar, C, 1 μm.

logically with other non-viral cellular components, definitive ultrastructural identification can be achieved by using immunogold labeling electron microscopy (IEM) (Fig. 4G).

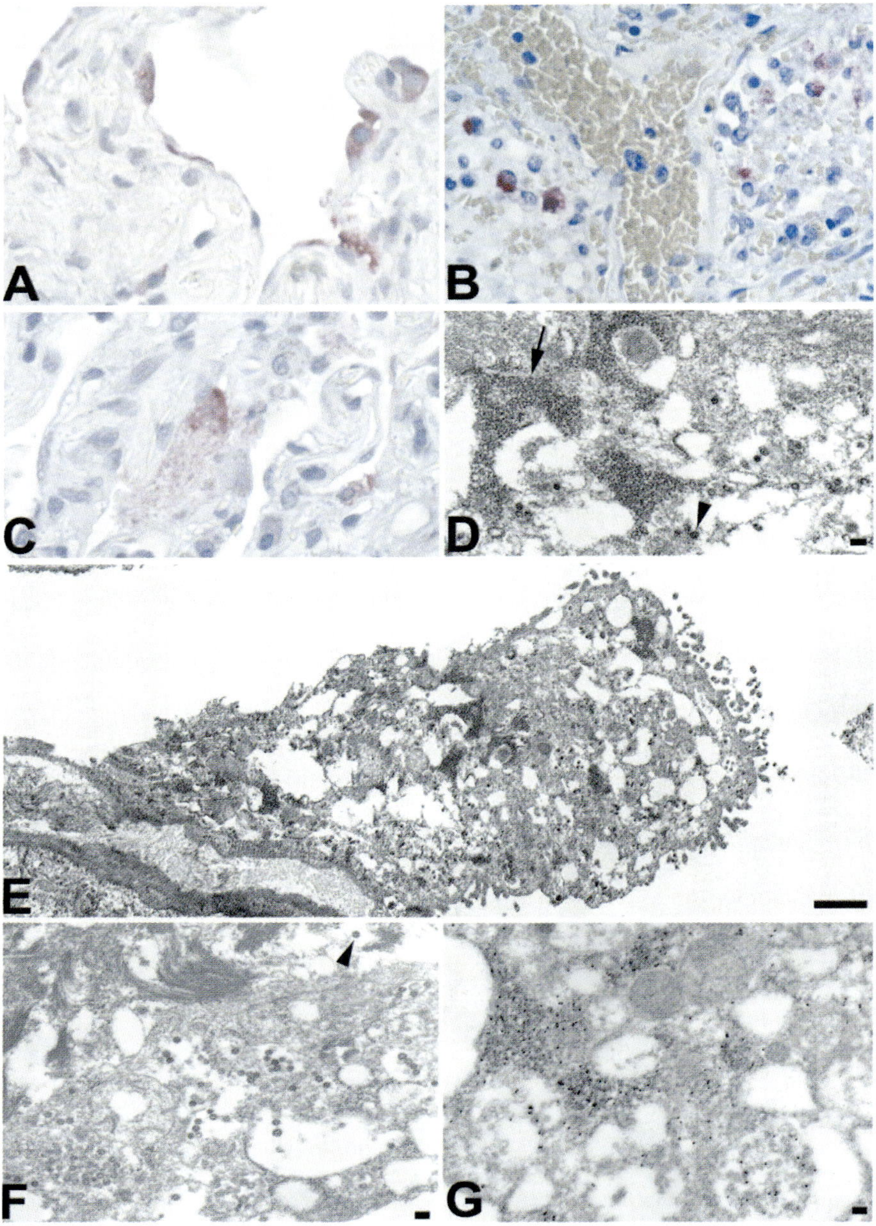

Figure 4. Cellular targets of infection in lower airways. (A) Type 2 pneumocytes containing viral antigens by IHC. (B) Intra-alveolar macrophages containing viral antigens as seen by IHC. (C) Antigen associated with intra-alveolar fibrin as seen by IHC. (D) High magnification of cell in figure (E), showing nucleocapsid inclusions (arrows) and virus particles (arrowhead). (E) Infected pneumocyte, attached at one edge to the basement membrane. (F) Virus particles

Pathogenesis and animal models

The primary histopathologic lesions seen in the lungs of patients who died from SARS are somewhat nonspecific and can also be seen in acute lung injury cases that can be caused by infectious agents, trauma, drugs, or toxic chemicals [28]. Multinucleated syncytial cells similar to those seen in some SARS patients can also be found in a number of virus infections, including measles, parainfluenzaviruses, respiratory syncytial virus, and Nipah virus infections [28–30]. In an early study of four human SARS patients [6], we were not able to demonstrate viral antigens in the lung by IHC. The most likely explanation is that all tissue samples in the study were from patients with a clinical course averaging more than 2 weeks. For many virus infections, viral antigens and nucleic acids are cleared within 2 weeks of disease onset by the host immune response. It is also possible that the pulmonary damage associated with SARS is not caused directly by the virus but represents a secondary effect of cytokines or other factors induced by the virus infection. In influenza virus infections, viral antigens are seen predominantly in respiratory epithelial cells of large airways and are only rarely identified in pulmonary parenchyma despite concomitant and occasionally severe interstitial pneumonitis [31]. In recent reports by Shieh et al. [32] and Chong et al. [12], the temporal relationship between the duration of illness and clearance of SARS-CoV in human lung tissue was examined. Viral antigens and nucleic acids were detected only in pulmonary tissues of patients who died early in the disease. The development of specific IHC, ISH, and IEM assays to identify SARS-CoV in formalin-fixed, paraffin-embedded samples also allowed for the assessment of the cellular tropism of SARS-CoV infection in human lung tissues. Localization of SARS-CoV in the lung occurs mainly in the cytoplasm of pneumocytes, primarily type 2, and occasionally in alveolar macrophages. Type 2 pneumocytes are known to secrete pulmonary surfactant, resulting in reduced surface tension and preservation of the integrity of the alveolar space. These cells also play an important role in tissue restitution following lung damage. Moreover, there is mounting evidence to support their contribution to the development of acute inflammatory lung injury following exposure to biological or chemical agents. Additional studies are needed to further define the role of type 2 pneumocytes and alveolar macrophages in SARS-CoV infection.

The severe morbidity and mortality associated with SARS make it imperative that effective means to prevent and treat the disease be devel-

---

(arrowhead) among fibrin fibers adjacent to an infected pneumocyte. (G) Immunogold labeling confirms the viral nature of the nucleocapsid inclusions and the particles in membrane-bound vesicles. Original magnifications, A, B, C, 63×; Bars, D, F, G, 100 nm; E, 1 μm. (A, B, and C: immunoalkaline phosphatase with napthol fast red substrate and hematoxylin counterstain; G: mouse hyperimmune ascitic fluid and goat anti-mouse conjugated to 12 nm gold.)

oped and evaluated, especially since it is not known whether the virus will reappear and exhibit a seasonal pattern of circulation like other respiratory virus pathogens or whether it will be independently reintroduced into the human population. Cynomolgus macaques have been reported to develop pathologic findings of pneumonia and have been proposed as an animal model for SARS [11]. Haagmans et al. [33] showed extensive SARS-CoV antigen expression in experimentally infected cynomolgus macaques 4 days after infection. The antigens were mainly in alveolar lining epithelial cells with morphologic characteristics of type 1 pneumocytes, indicating type 1 pneumocytes are the primary target for SARS-CoV infection early in the disease. Type 1 pneumocytes normally represent 90% of the alveolar epithelial cell volume and are easily damaged during pulmonary infections or other types of injury. In a recent study on non-human primates [34], evidence was found of infection of mainly type 1 pneumocytes in addition to some type 2 pneumocytes and macrophages.

Small animal models, such as rodents, would be very useful for evaluating vaccines, immunotherapies, and antiviral drugs, and recently the mouse has been identified as an animal model for this purpose [35]. In those studies, microscopic examination of trachea, bronchus, lung, thymus, and heart on day 2 after infection revealed mild and focal peribronchiolar mononuclear inflammatory infiltrates (Fig. 5A) with no significant histopathologic change in other organs. Viral antigens and nucleic acids were focally distributed in bronchiolar epithelial cells (Fig. 5B), and virions were found in these same areas by ultrastructural analysis (Fig. 5C, D). Data indicate that SARS-CoV replicates to high enough titer in mice that we will be able to evaluate vaccines and antivirals in this model. The mouse and other small animal models [36] might also be used to test the ability of the virus to replicate and cause disease and, thus, facilitate identification of host-immune mechanisms that contribute to the resolution of SARS-CoV infection.

Conclusions

The emergence of SARS-CoV has posed a major threat to global health. A specific etiologic diagnosis is particularly important during such outbreaks because of the impact on hospital infection control and other public health measures. The discovery of this new virus occurred through a broad-based and multidisciplinary effort by clinical, epidemiologic, and laboratory investigators and speaks to the power of a global collaborative effort to address the ever-present threat of emerging infectious diseases. The identification of this novel coronavirus relied on classic tissue-culture isolation to amplify the pathogen, on electron-microscopic studies to identify the type of virus, and on molecular studies to confirm the identity of the virus, characterize its unique nature, and help link it to the disease. The discovery of this previously unknown virus, a member of the family

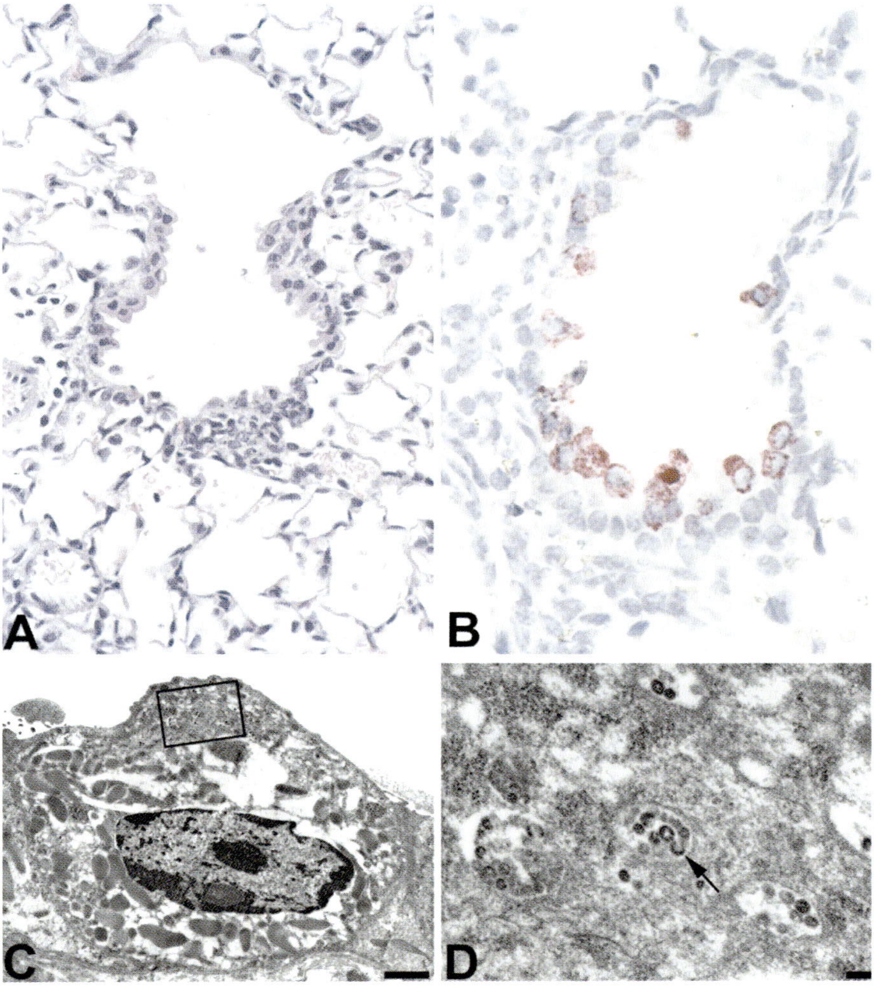

Figure 5. Mouse animal model of SARS. (A) Hematoxylin and eosin-stained tissue showing mild inflammation in peribronchiolar areas. (B) Viral antigens in bronchial epithelial cells as seen by using IHC. (Immunoalkaline phosphatase with napthol fast red substrate and hematoxylin counterstain.) (C) Virus as seen in bronchial epithelial cells by electron microscopy. (D) Higher magnification of boxed area in C, showing numerous spherical particles (arrow) in cytoplasmic vesicles. Original magnifications, A, 20×; B, 63×. Bars, C, 1 μm; D, 100 nm.

Coronaviridae, underscores the importance of versatile laboratory techniques, such as virus isolation and electron microscopy, in identifying etiologic pathogens. As with previous outbreak investigations, electron microscopy proved to be a rapid technique that did not require specific reagents nor prior knowledge of a particular agent but that could nevertheless categorize a pathogen on the basis of its appearance and morphogenesis. This technique was combined with other traditional methods, including virus isolation in suckling mice and cell culture, histopathologic examination, and serologic analysis. Molecular techniques of polymerase chain reaction (PCR), reverse-transcription PCR, and real-time PCR were also used and were invaluable for the characterization and discovery of this novel virus.

In summary, since the clinical features of SARS-CoV infection can be similar to those of many other respiratory infections, a definitive diagnosis can only be made by laboratory confirmation. Traditional pathologic methods in association with more contemporary molecular pathologic methods should help enhance the pathologic diagnosis and further our understanding of the pathogenesis of SARS-CoV infection.

Acknowledgements

The authors thank Wun-Ju Shieh, Chris Paddock, and Jeannette Guarner for pathologic evaluation; Kathleen Tatti for *in situ* hybridization studies; Tom Ksiazek for virus isolates; Pierre Rollin for antibodies; Kanta Subbarao for animal model collaborations; and Claudia Chesley for editorial assistance.

References

1 Anonymous (2003) Acute respiratory syndrome. China, Hong Kong Special Administrative Region of China, and Viet Nam. *Wkly Epidemiol Rec* 78: 73–74

2 Anonymous (2003) WHO issues consensus document on the epidemiology of SARS. *Wkly Epidemiol Rec* 78: 373–375

3 Anonymous (2003) Outbreak of severe acute respiratory syndrome--worldwide, 2003. *MMWR Morb Mortal Wkly Rep* 52: 226–228

4 Anonymous (2003) Update: severe acute respiratory syndrome – worldwide and United States, 2003. *MMWR Morb Mortal Wkly Rep* 52: 664–665

5 Anonymous (2003) Update: Outbreak of severe acute respiratory syndrome – worldwide, 2003. *MMWR Morb Mortal Wkly Rep* 52: 241–6, 248

6 Ksiazek TG, Erdman D, Goldsmith CS, Zaki SR, Peret T, Emery S, Tong S, Urbani C, Comer JA, Lim W et al (2003) A novel coronavirus associated with severe acute respiratory syndrome. *N Engl J Med* 348: 1953–1966

7 Peiris JS, Lai ST, Poon LL, Guan Y, Yam LY, Lim W, Nicholls J, Yee WK, Yan WW, Cheung MT et al (2003) Coronavirus as a possible cause of severe acute respiratory syndrome. *Lancet* 361: 1319–1325

8 Drosten C, Gunther S, Preiser W, van der WS, Brodt HR, Becker S, Rabenau H, Panning M, Kolesnikova L, Fouchier RA et al (2003) Identification of a

novel coronavirus in patients with severe acute respiratory syndrome. *N Engl J Med* 348: 1967–1976

9 Marra MA, Jones SJ, Astell CR, Holt RA, Brooks-Wilson A, Butterfield YS, Khattra J, Asano JK, Barber SA, Chan SY et al (2003) The genome sequence of the SARS-associated coronavirus. *Science* 300: 1399–1404

10 Rota PA, Oberste MS, Monroe SS, Nix WA, Campagnoli R, Icenogle JP, Penaranda S, Bankamp B, Maher K, Chen MH et al (2003) Characterization of a novel coronavirus associated with severe acute respiratory syndrome. *Science* 300: 1394–1399

11 Kuiken T, Fouchier RA, Schutten M, Rimmelzwaan GF, van Amerongen G, van Riel D, Laman JD, de Jong T, van Doornum G, Lim W et al (2003) Newly discovered coronavirus as the primary cause of severe acute respiratory syndrome. *Lancet* 362: 263–270

12 Chong PY, Chui P, Ling AE, Franks TJ, Tai DY, Leo YS, Kaw GJ, Wansaicheong G, Chan KP, Ean Oon LL et al (2004) Analysis of deaths during the severe acute respiratory syndrome (SARS) epidemic in Singapore: challenges in determining a SARS diagnosis. *Arch Pathol Lab Med* 128: 195–204

13 Ding Y, Wang H, Shen H, Li Z, Geng J, Han H, Cai J, Li X, Kang W, Weng D et al (2003) The clinical pathology of severe acute respiratory syndrome (SARS): a report from China. *J Pathol* 200: 282–289

14 Franks TJ, Chong PY, Chui P, Galvin JR, Lourens RM, Reid AH, Selbs E, McEvoy CP, Hayden CD, Fukuoka J et al (2003) Lung pathology of severe acute respiratory syndrome (SARS): a study of 8 autopsy cases from Singapore. *Hum Pathol* 34: 743–748

15 Lang ZW, Zhang LJ, Zhang SJ, Meng X, Li JQ, Song CZ, Sun L, Zhou YS, Dwyer DE (2003) A clinicopathological study of three cases of severe acute respiratory syndrome (SARS). *Pathology* 35: 526–531

16 Leung WK, To KF, Chan PKS, Chan HLY, Wu AKL, Lee N, Yuen KY, Sung JJY (2003) Enteric involvement of Severe Acute Respiratory Syndrome-associated coronavirus infection. *Gastroenterology* 125: 1011–1017

17 Nicholls JM, Poon LL, Lee KC, Ng WF, Lai ST, Leung CY, Chu CM, Hui PK, Mak KL, Lim W et al (2003) Lung pathology of fatal severe acute respiratory syndrome. *Lancet* 361: 1773–1778

18 Goldsmith CS, Tatti KM, Ksiazek TG, Rollin PE, Comer JA, Lee WW, Rota PA, Bankamp B, Bellini WJ, Zaki SR (2004) Ultrastructural characterization of SARS coronavirus. *Emerg Infect Dis* 10: 320–326

19 Ng ML, Tan SH, See EE, Ooi EE, Ling AE (2003) Proliferative growth of SARS coronavirus in Vero E6 cells. *J Gen Virol* 84: 3291–3303

20 Becker WB, McIntosh K, Dees JH, Chanock RM (1967) Morphogenesis of avian infectious bronchitis virus and a related human virus (strain 229E). *J Virol* 1: 1019–1027

21 Dubois-Dalcq M, Holmes KV, Rentier B (1984) Assembly of *Coronaviradae*, in: *Assembly of Enveloped RNA Viruses*, Springer-Verlag, Wien, 100–119

22 Oshiro LS, Schieble JH, Lennette EH (1971) Electron microscopic studies of coronavirus. *J Gen Virol* 12: 161–168

23 Pedersen KW, van der Meer Y, Roos N, Snijder EJ (1999) Open reading frame 1a-encoded subunits of the arterivirus replicase induce endoplasmic reticulum-derived double-membrane vesicles which carry the viral replication complex. *J Virol* 73: 2016–2026

24 Gosert R, Kanjanahaluethai A, Egger D, Bienz K, Baker SC (2002) RNA replication of mouse hepatitis virus takes place at double-membrane vesicles. *J Virol* 76: 3697–3708

25 Nakajima N, Asahi-Ozaki Y, Nagata N, Sato Y, Dizon F, Paladin FJ, Olveda RM, Odagiri T, Tashio M, Sata T (2003) SARS coronavirus-infected cells in lung detected by new in situ hybridization technique. *Jpn J Infect Dis* 56: 139–141

26 Shieh WJ, Huang S, Paddock CD, Guarner J, Muller S, Goldsmith CS, Tatti K, Packard M, Subbarao K, Zaki SR. Immunohistochemical, *in situ* hybridization, and ultrastructural localization of SARS-associated coronavirus in a fatal case of severe acute respiratory syndrome in Taiwan. *Hum Pathol; in press*

27 To KF, Tong JH, Chan PK, Au FW, Chim SS, Chan KC, Cheung JL, Liu EY, Tse GM, Lo AW et al (2004) Tissue and cellular tropism of the coronavirus associated with severe acute respiratory syndrome: an in-situ hybridization study of fatal cases. *J Pathol* 202: 157–163

28 Anonymous (1997) Acute lung injury patterns: Diffuse alveolar damage and bronchiolitis obliterans-organizing pneumonia. In: AA Katzenstein (ed): *Katzenstein and Askin's Surgical Pathology of Non-Neoplastic Lung Disease*, 3rd ed., WB Saunders, Philadelphia, 14–47

29 Zaki SR, Bellini WJ (1997) Measles, in: Connor DH, Chandler FW, Schwartz DA, Manz HJ, Lack EE (eds): *Pathology of Infectious Diseases*, Appleton and Lange, Stamford, CT, 233–244

30 Wong KT, Shieh WJ, Kumar S, Norain K, Abdullah W, Guarner J, Goldsmith CS, Chua KB, Lam SK, Tan CT et al (2002) Nipah virus infection: pathology and pathogenesis of an emerging paramyxoviral zoonosis. *Am J Pathol* 161: 2153–2167

31 Guarner J, Shieh WJ, Dawson J, Subbarao K, Shaw M, Ferebee T, Morken T, Nolte KB, Freifeld A, Cox N, Zaki SR (2000) Immunohistochemical and in situ hybridization studies of influenza A virus infection in human lungs. *Am J Clin Pathol* 114: 227–233

32 Shieh WJ, Guarner J, Paddock C, Greer P, Tatti K, Fischer M, Layton M, Philips M, Bresnitz E, Quinn CP et al (2003) The critical role of pathology in the investigation of bioterrorism-related cutaneous anthrax. *Am J Pathol* 163: 1901–1910

33 Haagmans BL, Kuiken T, Martina BE, Fouchier RA, Rimmelzwaan GF, van Amerongen G, van Riel D, de Jong T, Itamura S, Chan KH et al (2004) Pegylated interferon-alpha protects type 1 pneumocytes against SARS coronavirus infection in macaques. *Nat Med* 10: 290–293

34 McAuliffe J, Vogel L, Roberts A, Fahle G, Fischer S, Shieh WJ, Butler E, Zaki S, St.Claire M, Murphy B, Subbarao K (2004) Replication of SARS coron-

avirus administered into the respiratory tract of African Green, rhesus and cynomolgus monkeys. *J Virol* 330: 8–15

35 Subbarao K, McAuliffe J, Vogel L, Fahle G, Fischer S, Tatti K, Packard M, Shieh WJ, Zaki S, Murphy B (2004) Prior infection and passive transfer of neutralizing antibody prevent replication of severe acute respiratory syndrome coronavirus in the respiratory tract of mice. *J Virol* 78: 3572–3577

36 Roberts A, Vogel L, Guarner J, Hayes N, Murphy B, Zaki S, Subbarao K. SARS coronavirus infection of golden Syrian hamsters. *J Virol; in press*

Coronaviruses with Special Emphasis on First Insights Concerning SARS
ed. by A. Schmidt, M.H. Wolff and O. Weber

Genome organization and structural aspects of the SARS-related virus

Caroline R. Astell, Robert A. Holt, Steven J. M. Jones and Marco A. Marra

Genome Sciences Centre, British Columbia Cancer Agency, Suite 100–570 West 7th Ave., Vancouver, B.C., Canada V5Z 4S6

Background

The first appearance of severe acute respiratory syndrome (SARS) occurred in Guangdong province in southern China with the earliest cases dating from November 16, 2002. By February 14, 2003 the WHO reported a total of 305 cases of acute respiratory syndrome of unknown etiology in Guangdong province (WHO WER 7/2003). At the time of writing this review, scientists in the Guangdong province of China believe that the SARS virus may have shifted to human hosts by at least five independent events, however sequence information to support this conclusion on these five isolates is still incomplete. The SARS virus was spread to Hong Kong by a physician from Guangdong when he traveled to Hong Kong and stayed at the Metropole Hotel on Feb 21. From there, world-wide dissemination of the virus to Vietnam, Singapore, Taiwan and Canada plus other locations occurred.

The SARS agent was initially believed to be an influenza virus, possibly an avian influenza virus, parainfluenza virus (metapneumovirus) or a bacterium, *Chlamydia pneumoniae* However, by March 19, the WHO reported that these agents were unlikely to be the cause and hence suggested that a new agent was responsible. Within a few days four groups obtained evidence that a coronavirus-like agent might be the causative agent using PCR primers for known coronaviruses to amplify short fragments of DNA which were sequenced ([1–3]; R. Tellier, personal communication). In addition de Risi's group at UCSF used a DNA microarray-based assay to detect viral sequences from samples cultured in Vero6 cells. These results were made available over the internet and have now appeared in print [4]. This group also recovered a ~ 1kb fragment of viral cDNA which was purified from contaminating cellular cDNAs by selecting the fragment on a DNA microarray and sent the DNA to the Washington University Genome Sequence Centre. The sequence was determined and the results indicated that it was most closely related to coronaviruses.

Hence all of these results suggested a novel coronavirus-like agent might be the cause of SARS.

With the world-wide scientific community uncertain of the causative agent of SARS and the fact that SARS had now been transported to Canada by travelers from Asia, the Genome Sciences Centre (GSC) at the BC Cancer Agency decided on March 27 to apply it's high-throughput DNA sequencing capabilities to fully characterize the genome of the "new" virus. Colleagues at the British Columbia Centre for Disease Control (BC CDC) as well as the National Microbiology Laboratory (NML) were contacted. The NML in Winnipeg, Canada's National Reference Laboratory which has a level 4 biosafety facility, had already received patient samples from Toronto and Vancouver and had succeeded in growing the virus in Vero6 cells. The NML purified the virus and were able to send to the GSC a sample of highly purified viral RNA (150 ng) which simplified considerably our ability to rapidly sequence the genome. This sample was obtained from the second victim of SARS in Toronto and was termed Tor2. As soon as the virus sample arrived at the BC CDC (approximately 5 PM on April 6) our rapid sequencing effort began.

The initial strategy for sequencing the genome was to use primers designed from homologous regions of all known coronaviruses to amplify overlapping fragments from the genome and then sequence these fragments. However, we repeated experiments to amplify a small region of the replicase gene using pancoronavirus primers, sequenced this fragment and confirmed that the sequence was related about 80 % at the protein level but only 50% at the nucleic acid level. This relatively low level of homology at the nucleic acid level caused us to shift our initial strategy to that of using combined oligo-dT and random primers to create a library of cDNA clones in two different vectors that could be submitted to our high-throughput sequencing pipeline.

RT-PCR of SARS-CoV genome and construction of genomic libraries

The manipulation of full-length viral RNA was carried out in a level 2 biosafety laboratory. The strategy used to sequence the SARS genome was to construct a library of DNA fragments spanning the ~30,000 base genome. Purified viral RNA (55 ng) was used in an oligo-dT and random primers RT-PCR reaction using the SuperScript Choice System for cDNA synthesis (Invitrogen Canada Inc., Burlington, Ontario, Canada). At this stage, the samples were handled in a level 1 laboratory. EcoR I linkers were added to the DNA fragments and the products analyzed on an agarose gel. As expected, the products were barely visible and showed a range of sizes from ~ 400 bp–3000 bp. The fragments were resolved on a low melting point agarose gel and fragments of 1000–4000 bp were recovered. These frag-

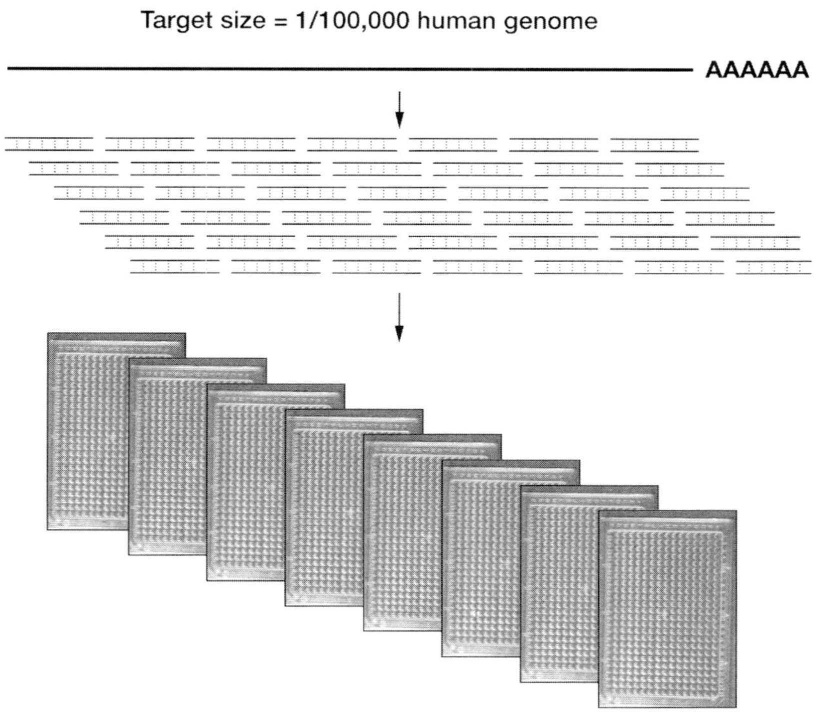

Figure 1. Whole genome shotgun approach used to sequence the SARS coronavirus genome. The SARS genome is approximately 1/100,000 the size of the human genome. A library of fragments (~2,000 bp in length) was generated and arrayed into ten 384-well plates. The clones were sequenced from either end and the data assembled into the full length 29,751 nucleotide sequence [11] (see text for details).

ments were amplified using the EcoR I linker as primers and ligated with the plasmid pCR4-TOPO TA cloning vector (Invitrogen) at the EcoR I site or with pBR194 [5] using the Not I site. Each library was transformed into DH10B T1 cells (Invitrogen) and plated on 22 cm^2 agar plates and transformants obtained using ampicillin selection. After 16 hours, colonies were picked and grown in 2X YT and plasmid DNAs purified using our standard high-throughput alkaline lysis procedure.

DNA sequencing, assembly of reads and analysis of data

The fragments generated by the cloning procedure are illustrated schematically in Figure 1. Each fragment was sequenced from both ends with appropriate primers using BigDye terminator reagent (version 3, Applied Biosystems, Foster City, CA, USA). The fragments were resolved by electrophoresis on either an AB 3700 or AB 3730XL automated sequencing instrument and the data was collected automatically and transferred electronically to the Bioinformatics team for analysis. DNA sequence chromatograms were processed and trimmed for sequence quality using PHRED software [6]. Sequence reads were subsequently screened for non-viral contaminating sequences (almost exclusively plasmid vector sequences allowing us to infer that the virus RNA sample provided by the NML had been highly purified. The assembly of the sequence reads was carried out using the PHRAP sequence assembly software [7]. The sequences were also analyzed using BLAST [8] and FASTA [9] to search the viral and non-redundant protein datasets derived from the National Centre for Biotechnology Information (NCBI). This revealed that the sequences were coronavirus related, but quite unlike any previously characterized coronavirus. Sequence data was accumulated until it was apparent that additional reads increased the depth of coverage but not the length of the sequence. Of the first 3,080 sequence reads, 2,634 assembled into one large contig.

Once the full-length genome was assembled (minus the extreme few bases at the 5' end) a manual annotation of the genome was carried out using a series of computational resources. Annotation of the SARS virus sequence was carried out using the ACEDB genome database system [10]. Release 1 of the draft sequence was made public on the BCCA GSC website on April 12, 2003 in addition to being submitted to the NCBI Genbank sequence database. On April 14, the CDC (Atlanta) released their independently derived sequence for the Urbani strain of the SARS virus obtained using an RT-PCR method and direct sequencing of fragments. On comparison of these two sequences 12 nucleotides differed between the two strains. On further analysis four of these differences were resolved, leaving a total of only 8 differences between these strains [11]. Version 2 of our sequence was posted to our website on April 14, 2003 and this update was simultaneously submitted to the Genbank database. Release 2 of the genome sequence had an average PHRED consensus quality score of 89.96 with the lowest quality bases at the 5' and 3'ends of the viral genome. This average score corresponds to an expected error rate in sequence determination of 1 error in $10^{8.96}$ base pairs. However, such an error rate corresponds only to the sequencing technology itself and does not account for other sources of potential error, e.g. reverse transcriptase errors during early phases of library construction. Each base in the sequence was determined on average 60 times (30 times in a forward direction and 30 times in a reverse direction). A subsequent release included the 5' most nucleotides which were determined by the RACE procedure using the RLM-RACE kit (Ambion Inc., Woodward, Austin, TX, USA). Release 3, the complete genome sequence, was deposited in Genbank (accession AY274119). We also immediately made available our clones via our website www.bcgsc.ca.

We subsequently validated all the clones and have also made these validated clones available to qualified researchers.

In addition to the sequencing efforts at the BC GSC [11] and the CDC Atlanta [12] groups, the Washington University Genome Sequence Centre in collaboration with the de Risi group in San Francisco used a method very similar to the one used at the GSC to generate a library of cDNA clones which were sequenced by the shotgun method [4]. These scientists assembled about 25,000 bases of sequence data which was freely sent to the SARS group at the CDC in Atlanta by J. deRisi on April 12, 2003. Shortly after the publication of the Tor2 and Urbani sequences, another group reported determining the sequence of several related isolates by the whole genome shotgun approach [13]; however of the more than 100 sequences now deposited at GenBank, most have been generated by sequencing of RT-PCR fragments using the Tor2 or Urbani sequences to design primers.

Relatedness of the SARS-CoV with other coronaviruses

Coronaviruses are members of the order *Nidovirales*, family *Coronaviridae*, genus *Coronavirus* [14]. Comparison of the Tor2 [11] (Genbank AY274119) and the Urbani sequence [12] (Genbank AY 278741) data showed that the sequences were essentially identical with only 8 bases difference out of ~29,700 bases. The analysis of the sequences by both groups was also very similar. The nomenclature used by each group differed slightly and in this review we maintain the naming system used for the Tor2 sequence [11]. For the convenience of the reader, Table 1 summarizes the nomenclature used by both groups as well as that used by Thiel et al. [15].

Preliminary analysis of the SARS genome sequence using BLAST and FASTA identified a total of 14 putative open reading frames (ORFs) possessing initiating codons (Fig. 2). For completeness, all detected ORFs were annotated in the initial genome analyses. Marra et al. [11] annotated ORFs that did not match database sequences but were identified if they were larger than 40 amino acids and had a strong match to the TRS consensus upstream of the potential initiating methionine residue. In contrast, Rota et al. did not identify potential proteins of less than 50 amino acids [12]. It is important to note that for some of these predicted ORFs no experimental evidence or sequence similarity information currently exists to support the notion that they actually do produce proteins *in vivo*.

All five major ORFs found in all known coronavirus genomes were identified: the replicase proteins (ORFs 1a and 1b), the spike or S protein ORF, the M or membrane glycoprotein ORF, the E or small membrane protein ORF and the N or nucleocapsid ORF. Coronaviruses were originally divided into three serotypes, groups 1 and 2 (predominantly mammalian viruses) and 3 (predominantly avian viruses) based on antigenic cross-reactivity. This grouping of the viruses also agrees fairly well with the

Table 1. Summary of terninology used for SARS-CoV Open Reading Frames

Marra et al.[11]	Rota et al. [12]	Thiel et al. [15]	Protein encoded
1a	1a	1a	Replicase
1b	1b	1b	Replicase
2	S	2	Spike
3	X1	3a	Unknown
4	X2	3b	Unknown
5	E	4	E small membrane
6	M	5	Membrane glycoprotein
7	X3	6	Unknown
8	X4	7a	Unknown
9	N/R	7b	Unknown
10	N/R	8a	Unknown
11	X5	8b	Unknown
12	N/R	9a	Nucleocapsid
13	N/R	9b	Unknown
14	N/R	N/R	Unknown

NB. In animal isolates of the SARS-CoV, ORFs 10 and 11 are replaced by a 122 aa of unknown function. This is the result of an additional 29 nt in the animal genome that are apparently deleted in almost all human isolates. In this paper that protein is referred to as ORF 10'.
N/R, not recognized. Rota et al. did not recognize these ORFs because their minimal length cutoff was greater that 50 amino acids.

phylogenetic similarity of the viral genomes; however, some genomes have diverged sufficiently that the viruses are no longer antigenically cross-reactive. Phylogenetic analysis of four of the SARS ORFs (Rep, S, M, and N) by both the Vancouver and CDC Atlanta groups using unrooted analyses provided evidence (for all four comparisons) that the SARS virus represents a fourth group within the coronavirus family [11, 12]. Figures 3A and B illustrate the comparison for ORF 1a [11] and ORF1b [12], respectively. However, others have now constructed a rooted phylogenetic tree, using the ORF1b gene of equine torovirus. This analysis suggests that the SARS-CoV is more related, albeit distantly, to group 2 coronaviruses than to any other group and shares a common ancestor early in coronavirus evolution (Fig. 3C) [16].

Analysis by both Marra et al. [11] and Rota et al. [12] also suggested that the SARS-CoV is not a *recent* recombinant between two (or more) other known coronaviruses, which may have explained its sudden appearance in humans and its pathogenicity. However, Rest and Mindell [17] have completed a more in-depth analysis of the RNA-dependent RNA polymerase (RdRp) coding sequence and found evidence that during evolution of the SARS-CoV the 3' region of the RdRp gene may have been derived from avian coronaviruses possibly due to a recombination event. Yet another study by Stavrinides and Guttman suggests that the left portion of the SARS genome is derived from mammalian-like viruses while the right portion is derived from avian sources [18]. The position of recombination appears to be within the 3' end of the S protein gene. Stavrinides and

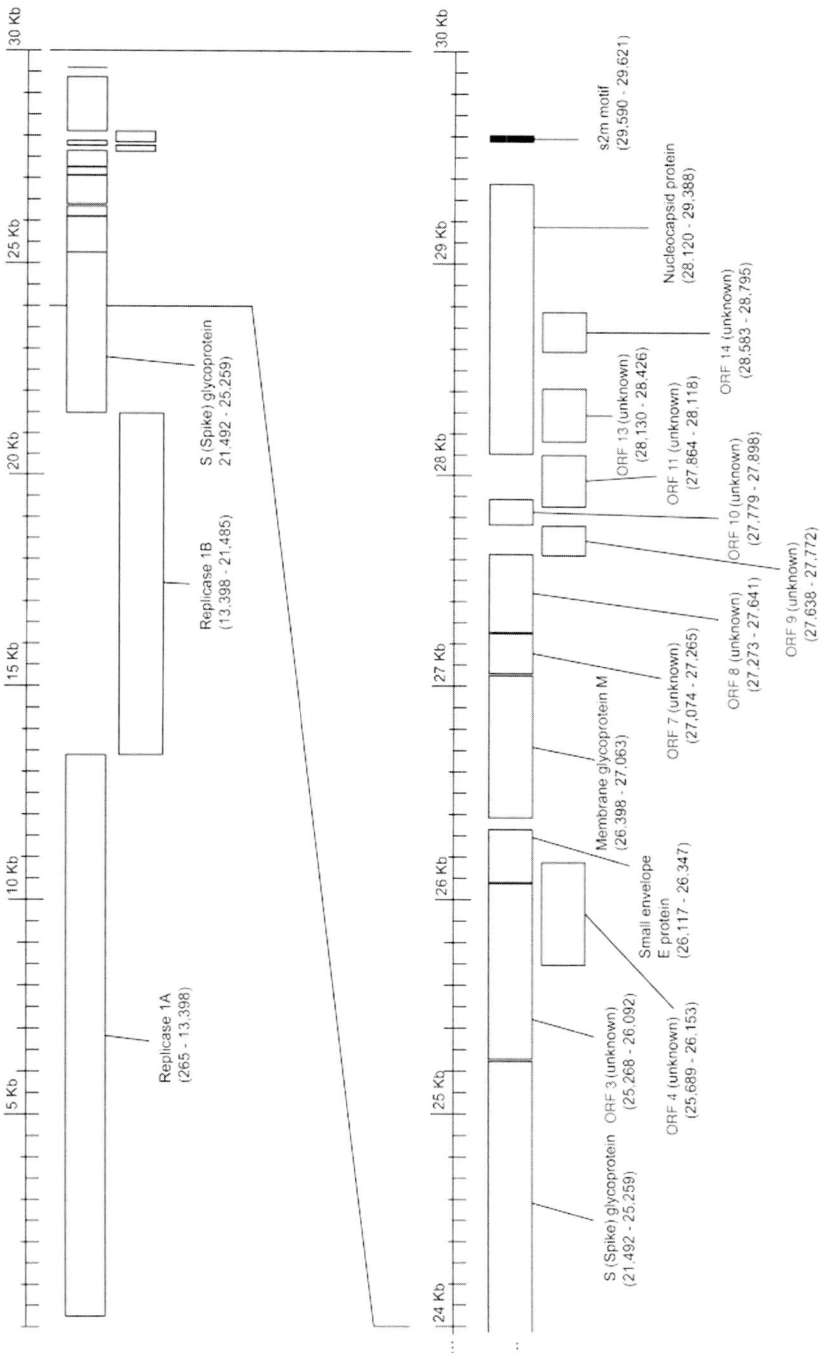

Figure 2. Map of the predicted ORFs and s2m motif in the Tor2 SARS virus genome sequence (reprinted with permission from [11]).

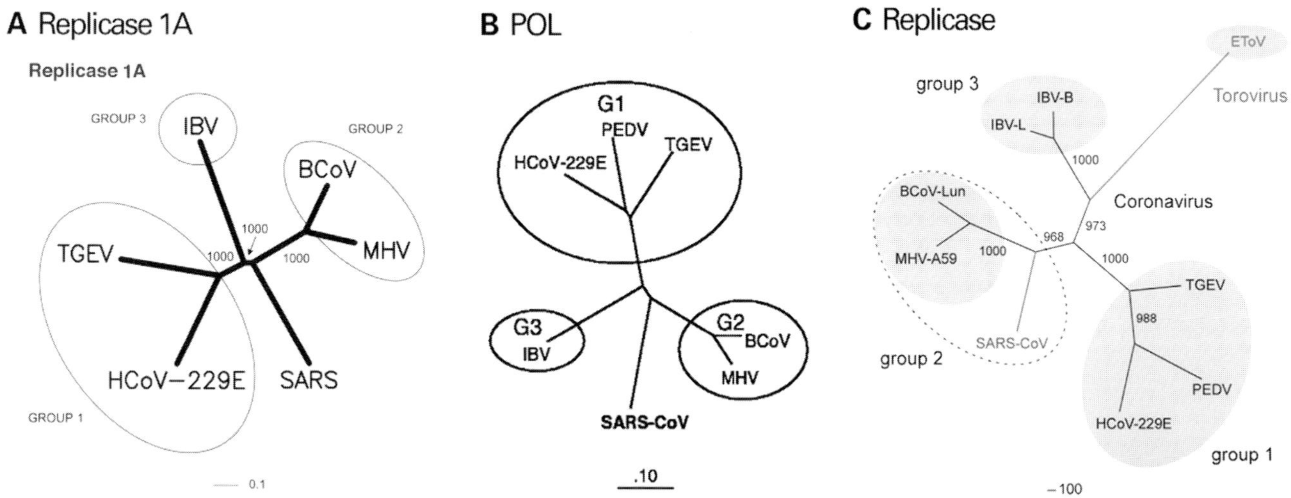

Figure 3. Phylogenetic analysis of SARS coronavirus open reading frames. (A) is ORF1a [11] and (B) is the POL gene from ORF 1b [12] obtained using an unrooted phylogenetic analysis methods, (C) is ORF 1b obtained using a rooted phylogenetic analysis method [16]. (Fig. 3A reprinted with permission from [11], Fig. 3B reprinted from [12], Fig. 3C reprinted from [16], with permission from Elsevier.)

Guttman proposed that this recombination within the S protein gene may have been the event that allowed the SARS virus to spread to human hosts [18]. However, the lack of evidence for a mammalian virus that is closely related to SARS to the left of the recombination point and an avian virus closely related to sequences to the right, leaves room for an alternative interpretation. The SARS-CoV may have arisen by an ancient recombination occurring a long time ago in the natural history of the SARS coronavirus and that subsequently this recombinant virus has been evolving over a long time period would seem like a more rational interpretation of these data. There are currently over 100 SARS-CoV complete or partial sequences in GenBank http://www.ncbi.nlm.nih.gov/query.fcgi?db=nucleotide&cmd=search&term=%22SARS+coronavirus%22, including several isolates from civet cats, one of several possible animal hosts responsible for transmitting the virus to humans [19]. While it is unclear if civet cats are the natural reservoir for this novel coronavirus, there does appear to have been another transfer event (maybe from civet cats or rats) in Guangdong, reported in December 2003. Analysis of this sequence will hopefully shed more light on the origin of the human SARS virus, however at this point, most hypotheses are based on a very limited amount of data. Future characterization of many additional animal SARS virus isolates will help to elucidate the true origin of the human SARS-CoV.

Mechanism of transcript expression by coronaviruses including identification of TRS sequences in the SARS-CoV

The expression of coronavirus genes is thought to occur by discontinuous transcription of the plus sense genomic RNA to generate a series of subgenomic RNAs which are subsequently transcribed into opposite sense mRNA [20, 21] (Fig. 4). Sequences referred to as TRS (transcription regulatory sequences) occur within the genomic RNA upstream of the major ORFs. These TRS sequences which have a common core sequence (5'-UAAACGAAC-3') are believed to facilitate the dissociation of the replicase complex from the genomic RNA and reassociation with similar sequences within the template RNA near the 5' end of the genome referred to as the leader sequence, generating a nested set of minus strand subgenomics RNAs. The mRNAs are then transcribed in a continuous fashion from these subgenomics negative strands, generating a nested set of mRNAs. Hence each of the mRNAs contains a leader sequence of ~ 72 nt (corresponding with the 5' end of the viral genome) attached to one of the downstream viral ORFs and all sequence 3' to that region.

In the bioinformatic analysis of the SARS genome by Marra et al. [11] candidate TRS sequences upstream of 10 of 13 "internal" ORFs and within the 72 nt leader sequence upstream of ORFs 1a and 1b were identified. Putative TRS sequences containing the central nucleotides of the core

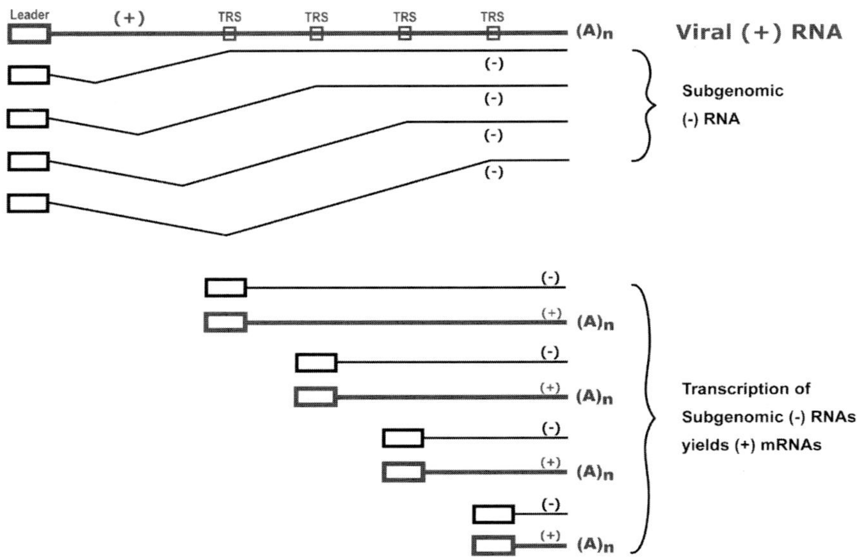

Figure 4. Preferred transcription model for coronaviruses. The mechanism illustrated is believed to be responsible for generating the nested set of mRNAs used to express coronavirus proteins. The coronavirus plus strand genome is transcribed into subgenomic minus strand RNAs. During the transcription process the RdRp encounters one of several TRS (transcription regulatory sequences) located upstream of the viral ORFs. The RdRp then jumps to the 5' leader sequence and finishes synthesis of the transcripts. The family of subgenomics minus strands are then copied into a family of subgenomic plus strands, the mRNAs used for translation of the viral proteins. The mRNA for ORF1a and ORF1b is synthesized from a full length minus strand transcript [22, 23] and during translation can undergo a –1 ribosomal frameshift (see text and Fig. 7 below).

sequence, 5'-ACGAAC-3', were identified upstream of 11 of the 14 ORFs in the SARS-CoV. Some were identified as strong (good matches to the consensus sequence) while others were classed as weak while still other upstream regions appeared not to contain an obvious TRS core sequence. Those lacking obvious TRS core sequences include ORFs 4, 13 and 14. It was speculated that possibly the three putative ORFs without an upstream TRS are translated from a longer transcript (containing an upstream ORF) by a process of internal ribosomal initiation [11]. Functional bicistronic mRNAs have been observed for other coronavirus subgenomic mRNAs [22, 23]. The ORFs 1a and 1b are expected to be translated from full length mRNAs copied from full-length negative sense RNA.

Two groups of investigators have used Northern blotting to identify the subgenomic species of RNA expressed in Vero6 cells infected by the SARS virus. Rota et al. [12] detected 5 subgenomic RNAs while Snijder et al. [16] and Thiel et al. [15] identified a total of 8 subgenomic RNAs (1.8, 2.1, 2.6,

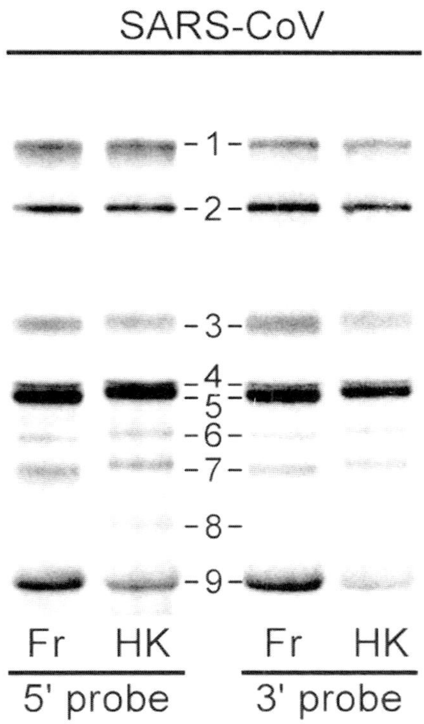

Figure 5. Transcripts generated in cultured cells infected with either the Frankfurt-1 (Fr) or HKU-39849 (HK) isolates of the SARS-CoV [16]. The transcripts were detected using 5' or 3' probe genomic probes. There are 8 subgenomic transcripts ranging from 1.8 to 8.4 kb plus the full-length transcript (reprinted from [16] with permission from Elsevier).

3.0, 3.5, 3.8, 4.6 and 8.4 kb) (Fig. 5) plus the full-length mRNA (29.7 kb) from which ORFs 1a and 1b are expected to be translated. The molar ratio of the fragments indicates that some transcripts are clearly more abundant than others, with the most abundant transcripts the ones that likely are translated into the E and M proteins. If the inability to detect additional subgenomic transcripts is not simply due to their low level of expression, it would appear that the use of bicistronic mRNA is likely the method used to express at least half of the putative proteins encoded by the ORFs in the right one third of the SARS genome. Thiel et al. [15] have also confirmed the leader to body fusion sites on the subgenomic mRNAs using RT-PCR to transcribe the mRNAs expressed in SARS-CoV-infected Vero6 cells. Subsequent PCR amplification using a second "body" primer plus a primer specific for the leader sequence generated fragments that were sequenced to determine the junction of the leader to the body of the mRNA.

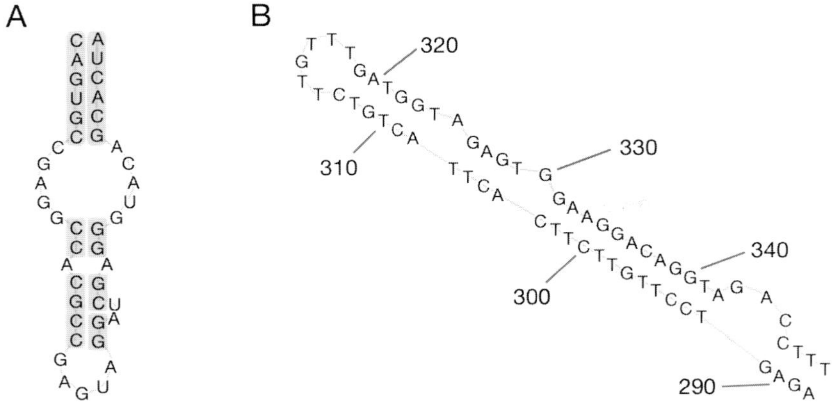

Figure 6. Secondary structural motifs within the SARS-CoV genome. (A) illustrates the conserved s2m motif found near the 3' end of many coronavirus genomes [24], (B) illustrates the putative SARS RNA packaging signal within the 3' end of ORF 1b [26] (reprinted with permission).

Other non-coding features of the SARS-CoV genome

Coronavirus genomes are single-stranded plus sense RNAs which are both capped at the 5' end and polyadenylated at the 3' end. There is a putative 2'-O-methyl transferase and putative mRNA cap 1-methyl transferase within the large replicase gene (see below, section "Coding potential of the SARS CoV, ORFs 1a and 1b-replicase) of the SARS-CoV suggesting that these proteins have a role in synthesizing the cap structure. However, so far there is no putative guanyl transferase gene identified, nor is there a polyA polymerase gene identified. However since the incoming viral genome is polyadenylated and the replication mechanism described above would provide an explanation for the presence of a polyA tract, this is the likely mechanism by which the mRNAs are polyadenylated.

In addition there is a 32 nt region corresponding to the conserved s2m motif [24]. This imperfect hairpin structure (Fig. 6A) is a feature of all astroviruses and has also been found in avian infectious bronchitis virus (avian IBV) and the ERV-2 equine rhinovirus. Due to their high degree of sequence similarity and occurrence in viruses that are evolutionarily distant, Jonassen et al. [24] proposed that this motif is indicative of multiple horizontal transfer events.

A recent bioinformatic analysis of the SARS-CoV genome has identified a putative genome packaging signal. The packaging signal for two laboratory coronavirus models systems, murine hepatitis virus (MHV) and bovine coronavirus (B-CoV) has been identified an ~ 69 nt region near the

3' end of ORF 1b, the second half of the large ORF encoding the replicase gene. This sequence is capable of driving the packaging of foreign RNA into MHV particles [25]. Qin et al. [26] have characterized the secondary structure of this packaging signals using alignment of the sequences and a RNA secondary structure program, RNA Structure 3.71 [27]. The structural motif for the packaging signals of several coronaviruses appears to be a long stem-loop structure of which the top of loops are similar. Analysis of the SARS genome showed that a similar structure (Fig. 6B) is found in a hypervariable region of ORF1b displaced slightly upstream relative to the packaging signals for MHV and BCoV. This packaging signal needs to be tested experimentally and may prove to be a useful target for development of an antiviral agent.

Coding potential of the SARS-CoV

In this section we summarize the coding potential of each of the 14 ORFs identified by Marra et al. [11] and Rota et al. [12] (see Tab. 2). We also include information about the proteins that has become available during the past 9 months since the genome sequences were published. A search on the plus sense strand identified a number of ORFs (Fig. 2). There are a number of smaller ORFs on the minus strand but to date no coronavirus has been shown to encode genes on the minus sense strand.

ORFs 1a and 1b-replicase

The left two thirds (21.2 kb) of the genome was found to contain two large ORFs corresponding to the replicase 1a and 1b regions. ORF 1a is translated into a large polypeptide of ~4,000 aa while a fused ORF1ab can be translated into a polyprotein of ~7,000 aa. As is the case with other coronaviruses, ORFs 1a and 1b can be fused together into one large ORF by a –1 frameshift event which is believed to occur by a process of slippage on the ribosome [28]. In the case of the SARS virus the C-terminal end of the ORF 1a polypeptide is .... L-N-G-F-A-V-STOP (Fig. 7). At least part of the time a –1 frameshift occurs, yielding a read-through polypeptide with the sequence ....L-N-R-V-C-G-V – etc. A pseudoknot, a specialized region of secondary structure within the mRNA, immediately downstream from the position of the frameshift, is believed to cause the ribosome to pause during translation. Upstream of the pseudoknot is a consensus "slippery sequence" NNNAAAN.. or ..NNNTTTN.. where the first three Ns can be any nucleotide but they must be the same nucleotide [29]. In the case of the SARS genome the sequence is ...TTTAAACGGG.... When the ribosome encounters the pseudoknot, there is a pause in reading of the mRNA and the mRNA is shifted back one nucleotide, allowing only partial yet stable

Table 2. Predicted SARS-CoV replicase cleavage products and their mode of expression (see text for details). Modified from [16].

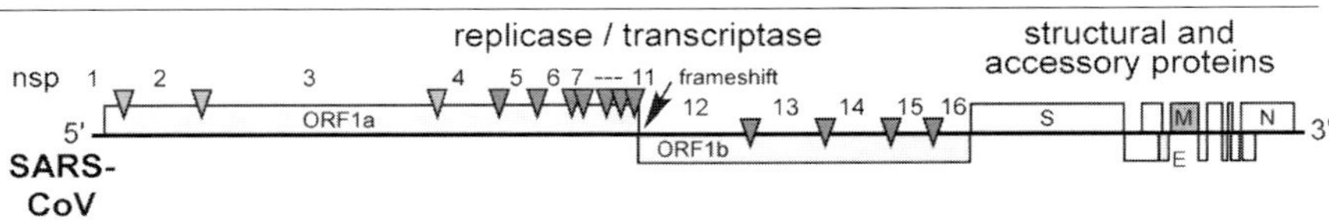

Protein order[a] in polyproteins pp1a/pp1ab	Position in polyproteins pp1a/pp1ab (amino acid residues)[b]	Protein size (amino acid residues)	Associated putative functional domain(s)[c]	Predicted mode of expression and release from polyproteins[d]
nsp1-pp1a/pp1ab	1Met-Gly180	180	?	TI + PL2^{pro}
nsp2-pp1a/pp1ab	181Ala-Gly818	638	?	PL2^{pro}
nsp3[*]-pp1a//pp1ab	819Ala-Gly2740	1922	Ac, X, PL2^{pro}, Y (TM1), ADRP	PL2^{pro}
nsp4-pp1a/pp1ab	2741Lys-Gln3240	500	TM2	PL2 + 3CL^{pro}
nsp5-pp1a/pp1ab	3241Ser-Gln3546	306	3CL^{pro}	3CL^{pro}
nsp6-pp1a/pp1ab	3547Gly-Gln3836	290	TM3	3CL^{pro}
nsp7-pp1a/pp1ab	3837Ser-Gln3919	83	?	3CL^{pro}
nsp8-pp1a/pp1ab	3920Ala-Gln4117	198	?	3CL^{pro}
nsp9-pp1a/pp1ab	4118Asn-Gln4230	113	?	3CL^{pro}
nsp10-pp1a/pp1ab	4231Ala-Gln4369	139	GFL	3CL^{pro}
nsp11-pp1a	4370Ser-Val4382	13	?	3CL^{pro} + TT
nsp12-pp1ab	4370Ser-Gln5301	932	RdRp	RFS + 3CL^{pro}
nsp13-pp1ab	5302Ala-Gln5902	601	ZD, NTPase, HEL1, mRNA CAP 1-mt	RFS + 3CL^{pro}
nsp14-pp1ab	5903Ala-Gln6429	527	Exonuclease (ExoN homolog)	RFS + 3CL^{pro}
nsp15-pp1ab	6430Ser-Gln6775	346	NTD, endoRNase (XendoU homolog)	RFS + 3CL^{pro}
nsp16-pp1ab	6776Ala-Asn7073	298	2′-O-MT	RFS + 3CL^{pro} + TT

Predictions are based on the SARS-CoV sequences published by Michael Smith Genome Sciences Centre (Vancouver, Canada; Entrez Genomes accession number NC_004718 (AY274119)[4]) and the Centers for Disease Control and Prevention (Atlanta, USA; GenBank accession number AY278741[5]) and an alignment of SARS-CoV with previously characterized coronavirus sequences as summarized in Refs. [32-34].

[a] For convenience, replicase cleavage products were provisionally numbered non-structural protein (nsp) 1–16 according to their position in the polyproteins.

[b] Amino acids of replicase proteins pp1a and pp1ab were numbered assuming that, as in other coronaviruses, a −1 ribosomal frameshift occurs; use of the slippery sequence UUUAAAC[10] is predicted to yield a peptide bond between Asn4378 and Arg4379 in pp1ab.

[c] Abbreviations: PL2^{pro}, papain-like proteinase 2; ADRP, adenosine diphosphate-ribose 1″-phosphatase; TM, transmembrane domain; 3CL^{pro}, 3C-like cysteine proteinase; GFL, growth factor-like domain; RdRp, RNA-dependent RNA polymerase; ZD, putative Zinc-binding domain; HEL1, superfamily 1 helicase; NTD, nidovirus conserved domain; ExoN, 3′-to-5′ exonuclease; 2′-O-MT, S-adenosylmethionine-dependent ribose 2′-O-methyltransferase. Domains Ac, X, and Y are described in Refs [33, 35]. The mRNA cap-1 methyltransferase (in nsp 13) has been described [37].

[d] Indicated are the SARS-CoV proteinases predicted to be involved in cleavage of the N- and/or C-termini of the cleavage products; TI, translation initiation; TT, translation termination; RFS, ORF1a/ORF1b ribosomal frameshift.

interactions with the peptidyl-tRNA and aminoacyl-tRNA on the ribosome. Figure 7A illustrates the SARS virus mRNA sequence with the codons lined up opposite the anticodons for leucine (L) and asparagine (N) when the normal reading frame is used, while Figure 7B illustrates the position when a –1 frameshift occurs. In Figure 7C the ribosome continues translation in the –1 reading frame, generating a polypeptide ~ 7,000 nt in length.

Initial annotation of this large ORF identified the RdRp (POL) gene, a putative RNA helicase and two proteases, a chymotrypsin-like protease 3CL^{pro} and a papain-like protease PL^{pro} [11, 12]. Gorbalenya and coworkers have been studying the coronavirus replicase ORFs for several years [30–32] and have recently provided an extensive analysis of the SARS-CoV 1a and 1b ORFs [16] (Tab. 2).

These very large "replicase" proteins are processed autocatalytically by two or three viral proteinases encoded within ORF 1a [33]. In all other

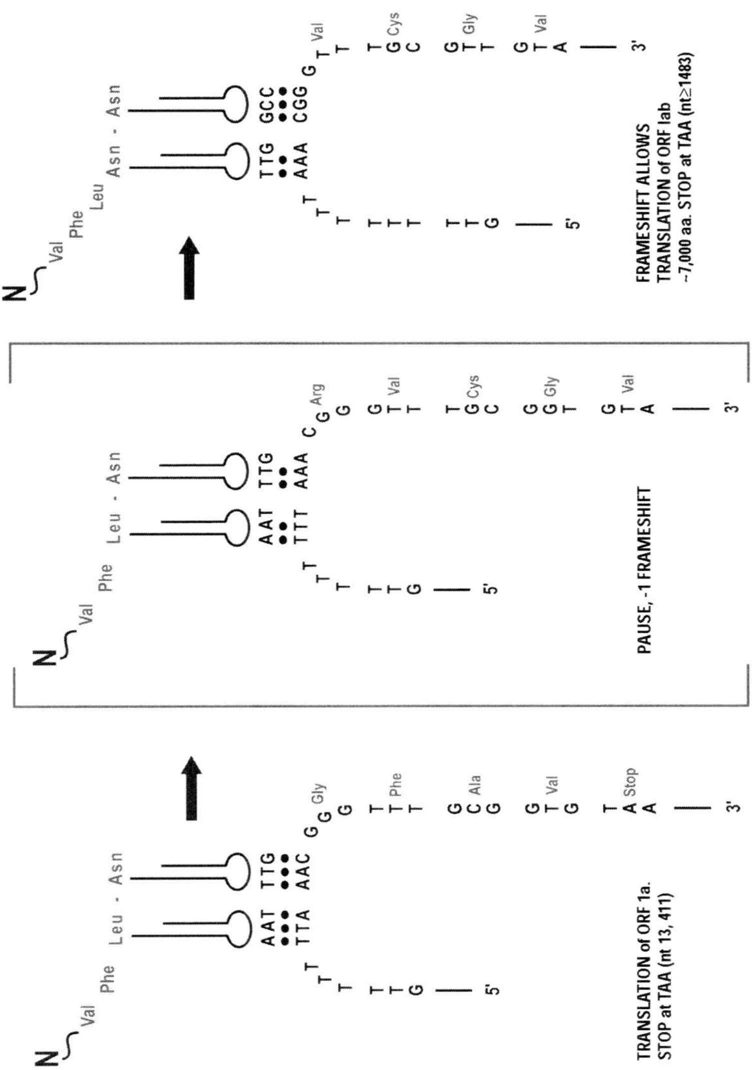

Figure 7. Ribosomal frameshifting within ORF1a and b of the SARS-CoV. Orf1a and ORF1b are large open reading frames encoding as many as 16 non-structural proteins. Translation of the ORF1b proteins is believed to occur due to a –1 frameshift which occurs on the ribosome. There is a pseudoknot within the RNA immediately downstream of the frameshift site. Translation of the RNA is believed to pause near the end of ORF1a and the RNA is shifted back one nucleotide, shifting to a different reading frame (see text for details).

coronaviruses three proteinases, a $3CL^{pro}$, $PL1^{pro}$ and $PL2^{pro}$ function in cleaving these polyproteins [34, 35]. However, Rota et al. [12] and more recently Snijder et al. [16] proposed that the $PL1^{pro}$ has been lost during evolution such that only the $3CL^{pro}$ and $PL2^{pro}$ virally encoded proteinases function in processing of the SARS-CoV replicase polyprotein. The putative recognition sites within the 1a and 1b regions are summarized in Table 2. The $PL2^{pro}$ is predicted to autocatalytically cut at the first three arrowheads near the N-terminal end of the polyprotein, while the $3CL^{pro}$ is predicted to cut at all other sites. If all consensus sites are recognized by these enzymes then the 1a and 1ab polyproteins will generate 16 proteins ranging in size from 18 amino acids up to 1922 amino acids. The sizes and putative function of these proteins is summarized in Table 2 (modified from Snijder et al. [16]). Also, each of these proteins is assigned a number, in order, designated as nsp (nonstructural protein) 1 to 16. Some of these proteins would be translated from both the 1a and the 1ab polypeptides, while others would be translated exclusively from the 1b region on the full-length frame-shifted transcript.

The replicase subunits are thought to exist as a large membrane-associated complex including at least the RdRp, RNA helicase, and several putative RNA processing enzymes such as Poly(U) specific endoribonuclease (XendoU,nsp 15), a 3' to 5' exonuclease (ExoN,nsp 14), S-adenosylmethionine-dependent ribose 2'O-methyltransferase (2'-O-MT,nsp 16,), adenosine diphosphate-ribose 1''-phosphatase (ADRP, nsp3) (Tab. 2). Several other proteins are predicted to be membrane associated and may facilitate formation of the membrane-associate replicase complex. One can imagine a large complex that synthesizes discontinuously the subgenomic minus strands and then transcribes these into the functional mRNAs.

Two functions that seem not to have been identified are a polyA polymerase activity and 5' capping activity. Coronavirus RNAs are known to be both 5' capped and 3' polyadenylated. It is probable that the genomic plus strands that have a polyA tail are transcribed into subgenomic minus strands and when these are converted to mRNAs, the polyA tail is added by copying the template strand. Presumably loss of the polyA tract would destine that genome to be lost from the gene pool. How the 5' cap structure is formed is unclear. There is a consensus sequence for a mRNA cap-1 methyltransferase [36] and a 2'-O-MT [16] which may play some role in 5' cap formation but so far a nucleotidyl transferase activity has not been identified in the viral genome.

Since the large ORF 1 polyproteins must be cleaved to generate the functional enzymes needed for virus replication, there is much interest in the viral protease as targets for the development of antivirals. A crystal structure of human coronavirus 229E $3CL^{pro}$ [37] was published about the same time the SARS-CoV genome sequence became available. Based on the 229E 3-D structure for the $3CL^{pro}$, Anand et al. [37] were able to model the SARS-CoV $3CL^{pro}$ and a few months later a 3D structure for this protease (both the free protein and complexed with a peptide inhibitor) appeared [38], providing the basis for drug design. The active protease is believed to be a dimer. Also, Fan et al. [39] have expressed the $3CL^{pro}$ in bacterial cells and provided evidence that the active protease is a dimer. Substrate specificity was analyzed using a series of 11 oligopeptides corresponding to the 11 predicted cleavage sites within the ORF1a and 1b regions (Tab. 2).

Another ORF 1a/1b polypeptide of unknown function, nsp9, has also been expressed, purified and crystallized [40].

ORF 2 – spike

The next largest ORF is ORF2 encoding the spike or S protein. The S protein is predicted to be 1255 amino acids in length and like other coronavirus S proteins it is likely heavily glycosylated. Mutations in this gene have previously correlated with altered pathogenesis and virulence in other coronaviruses [14]. Bioinformatic analysis of the SARS S protein using SignalP [41] showed a likely signal peptide at the N terminus (13–14 amino acids) and TMHMM [42] identified a strong transmembrane domain near the C-terminus, consistent with this protein being a type I membrane protein embedded in the viral envelope with most of the protein exposed on the surface. Proteomic analysis by Krokhin et al. [43] has also confirmed twelve glycosylation sites on this protein and the attached sugars for 4 of these sites have already been identified. Many of the SARS structural proteins appear to be membrane-associated proteins. A model of the predicted membrane-associated nature and orientation of these proteins is shown in Figure 8 (modified from http://athena.bioc.uvic.ca/sars/map/diagram-main.html/). It is believed that three molecules of the coronavirus S proteins form the characteristic peplomers or corona-like structure of this viral family. For some coronaviruses, specific regions of the S protein that bind to cellular receptors have been identified. Also it is known that various coronaviruses use different cellular receptors to mediate entry of the virus into host cells, hence it will be important to establish both the cellular receptor for the SARS-CoV and the viral attachment site on the S protein as possible antiviral targets for this new pathogen.

In several coronaviruses it is known that the S protein is cleaved into an N-terminal S1 subunit and C-terminal S2 subunit either by a viral or host protease [33], however it is not expected that the SARS-CoV S protein is similarly cleaved. Rota et al. [12] noted that the basic amino acid cleavage sites found in group 2 and group 3 coronaviruses (RRFRR, RRSRR, RSRR, RARS, and RARR) are not present in the SARS S protein. The S glycoprotein for the Sars-CoV shows a remarkably low sequence homology with other coronavirus S proteins. This low homology is especially notable in the N-terminal 700 amino acids of the protein. Spiga et al. [44] have presented a molecular modeling analysis of the S1 and S2 regions of

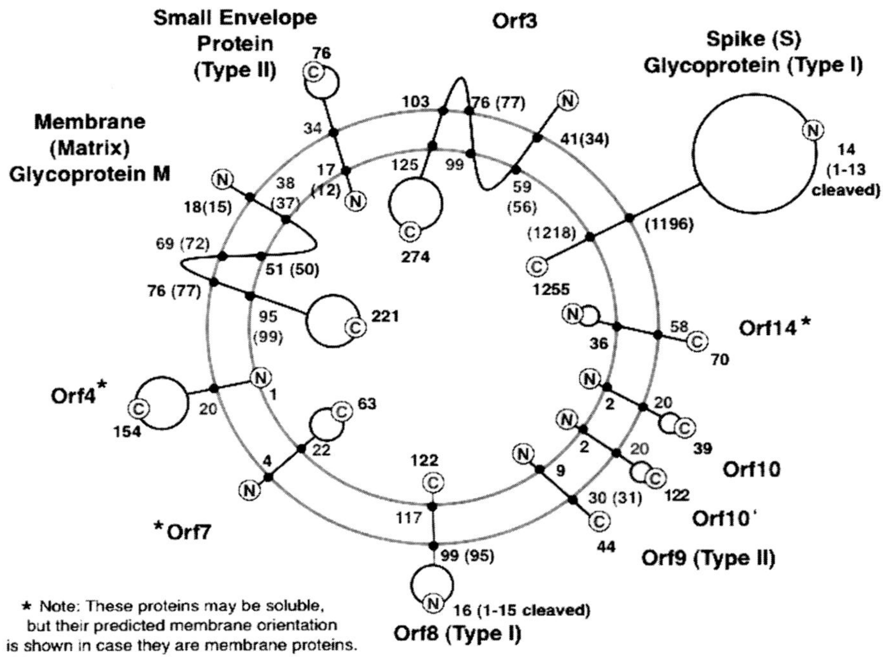

Figure 8. Predicted membrane association and orientation of "structural" proteins encoded by the SARS-CoV. Major coronavirus proteins such the spike (S), membrane glycoprotein (M) and small membrane (E) proteins are known to be part of the viral envelope. The remainder of the proteins may be associated with the viral envelope or may be associated with cellular membranes. For simplicity all the proteins are illustrated as being associated with a hypothetical circular membrane structure. Modified from http://athena.bioc.uvic.ca/sars/ (with permission of R. Roper and C. Upton).

the SARS-CoV S protein using the crystal structure of *Clostridium botulinum* neurotoxin B protein. These molecular models predict the overall shape and surface hydrophobicity of the S1 and S2 subunits and until a crystal structure is available, these will be a good starting point for design of antiviral drugs.

ORF3 – unknown function

ORF3 encodes a 274 aa protein that lacks significant similarities to any known proteins (BLAST, FASTA, or PFAM [45]). SignalP analysis [41] suggests that there may be a signal peptide at the N-terminus and internally, TMPred [46] and TMHMM predict three trans-membrane domains with a

149 aa C-terminal domain inside the viral or cellular membrane (Fig. 8). This region may also contain an ATP-binding domain.

It is important to note that many of the ORFs in the right two thirds of the SARS-CoV genome are predicted to code for membrane-associated proteins. In Figure 8, for convenience, a circular membrane envelope is used to illustrate the predicted orientation of these putative proteins in a membrane. Certainly the E, M and S proteins are embedded in the viral envelope, however there is no evidence that the other proteins are associated with the viral envelope or embedded in host cell membranes.

ORF4 – unknown protein

ORF4 has the potential to encode a 154 aa protein which overlaps completely with ORF 3 and ORF 5, but in a different reading frame. There is no obvious upstream TRS for this ORF, however it may be translated from the mRNA for ORF 3 using internal initiation [11]. This suggestion is supported by the data of Thiel et al. [15] in which the 4.6 kb mRNA transcript for ORF 3 is predicted to be bicistronic (capable of expressing Thiel's 3a and 3b polypeptides). This putative protein appears to encode a single transmembrane helix suggesting that if it is expressed, the product may be a membrane-associated protein (Fig. 8).

ORF 5 – E protein

ORF 5 encodes the small membrane E protein. It is 76 amino acids in length and BLAST and FASTA analyses show significant matches to other coronavirus small membrane E proteins. Both SignalP and TMPred analyses reveal a single transmembrane helix, again suggesting that this is a membrane-associated protein. TMHMM predicts the protein is a type II membrane protein with the majority of the hydrophilic domain and C terminus on the surface of the viral envelope (Fig. 8).

ORF 6 – M protein

The membrane glycoprotein or M protein is encoded by ORF6. This 221 aa protein is related to other coronavirus membrane or matrix glycoproteins. It is believed that during assembly of progeny virions the RNA-nucleocapsid complex associates non-covalently with the M protein embedded in the membranes of the ER, resulting in viral particles budding into the lumen of the ER. The virus then migrates through the Golgi complex and exits the cell, likely by exocytosis [14]. Signal P predicts that the M protein has a signal peptide that is likely not cleaved, while TMHMM and TMpred analyses suggest that there are three transmembrane domains (aa 15–37, 50–72, and 77–00). The 121 aa hydrophilic domain at the C-teminus of the protein is predicted to be inside the viral particles (Fig. 8) where it is expected to interact with the nucleocapsid protein.

ORF 7 – unknown protein

ORF 7 likely encodes yet another putative membrane protein. Although TMHMM and SignalP do not predict a transmembrane helix, TMPred does. The transmembrane helix is predicted to be between residues 3 and 22, with the N-terminus on the outside of the viral membrane (Fig. 8). The possible function of this 63 aa putative polypeptide is unknown as there are no significant matches using BLAST and FASTA analyses.

ORF 8 – unknown protein

ORF 8 is another ORF that may code for a protein of 122 amino acids. Again BLAST and FASTA searches failed to find significant homology with known proteins and again TMPred and TMHMM analyses predict that there is a single transmembrane domain near the C-terminus. SignalP indicates a signal sequence at the N-terminus that is likely cleaved between residues 15 and 16. However, there is no evidence yet to indicate that this protein is expressed in infected cells.

ORF 9 – unknown protein

The putative protein encoded by ORF 9 is only 44 amino acids in length (Rota et al. [12] used a cutoff of 50 aa, hence they did not include this protein in their analysis) (Tab. 1). Using FASTA there are some weak similarities with a putative sterol-C5 desaturase and a *Clostridium perfringens* protein (SWISS-PROT Q9M883 and CPE2366, respectively). Again TMPred predicts a strong transmembrane helix with no real preference for the orientation of the protein in the membrane. In Figure 8 this protein has been drawn it with the N terminus inside the particle and the C terminus outside.

ORF 10 – unknown protein

ORF 10 is interesting as it is only a 39 aa protein, yet there is a strong TRS sequence upstream of this ORF [11]. From studies on animal SARS viruses, ORF 10 and 11 proteins would actually be fused due to an additional 29 nt in these genomes. Hence in these animal SARS virus isolates as well as one human isolate (GZ01) these additional 29 nts result in an ORF that would encode a 122 aa protein (see ORF 10' below) [19]. The small ORF 10 protein is predicted to be another putative transmembrane protein with the N terminus located on the inside of the membrane and the C terminus outside (Fig. 8).

ORF 11 – unknown protein

ORF11 is predicted to encode an 84 aa protein. It contains limited homology to the human E2 glycoprotein precursor. SignalP and TMHMM predict that this protein, if expressed, is likely soluble.

ORF 10' – unknown protein

As discussed above all animal isolates contain an additional 29 nt [19] which predict that the ORF 10 and ORF 11 protein would not be expressed, but rather a fusion protein of 122 amino acid, ORF 10' would be expressed. This protein is also likely a transmembrane protein (see Fig. 8) with the N terminus inside the membrane.

ORF 12 – Nucleocapsid protein

The nucleocapsid gene encodes a 422 aa protein that has significant homology to other coronavirus N proteins. It does however have a short basic region (KTFPPTEPKKDKKKKTDEAQ) that appears to be unique to the SARS-CoV. Further analysis suggested that this region is part of a bipartite nuclear localization signal [11]. This motif may indicate that the SARS-CoV N protein is capable of being transported to the nucleus where it may play some novel role in pathogenesis of the virus. The nucleocapsid protein is known to associate with the viral RNA to form the RNA-protein complex that interacts with the M protein initiating encapsidation of the particle as it passes into the lumen of the ER [14]. Of interest is that a protein (~46 kDa) found in serum from convalescent SARS patients has been characterized by MALDI_TOF MS to be the SARS N protein [43]. Mass spectrometry has also been applied to the S protein allowing confirmation of 12 glycosylation sites in the protein [43].

The final two ORFs (13 and 14) do not have a TRS upstream so if they are expressed, they would likely be translated from the mRNA encoding the N protein.

ORF 13 – unknown protein

This ORF has the potential to encode a protein of 98 aa. There are no transmembrane helices detected and BLAST shows no homology to known proteins.

ORF 14 – unknown protein

The ORF 14 protein also has no known homologies using BLAST and TMPred predicts a single transmembrane helix, hence this protein, if expressed, is likely a membrane associated protein. However like the ORF4 protein the prediction of the membrane location is not strong. If embedded in the membrane it is expected that the N-terminus would be oriented toward the inside of the membrane.

The role of these minor proteins (ORFs 3, 4, 7, 8, 9, 10, 11, 13, and 14) will need further study to evaluate their role, if any, in the SARS-CoV replication cycle. Unpublished preliminary data indicates that at least one of these proteins is expressed.

Future direction for SARS-CoV research

It is quite remarkable that, in the one year since the first clinical reports of a new emerging virus, so much has been learned about the SARS-CoV. In late March 2003 the virus was identified as probably a new coronavirus and within two weeks its entire genome was sequenced [11, 12]. The speed with which this was accomplished is unprecedented. It is also remarkable that more than 1300 papers have been published on SARS in the past year (PubMed). In comparison, it took several years before the human immunodeficiency virus (HIV) was identified in 1983-4 as the agent responsible for a newly described immunodeficiency disease, AIDS [14]. Characterization of HIV has led to the development of a number of drugs that slow the progression of AIDS and multi-drug therapies ("highly active antiretroviral therapy" or HAART) have changed HIV infection from a terminal disease to a chronic one. However, 20 years after the discovery of HIV, no vaccine is available, a reflection of the remarkably intractable task of developing an HIV vaccine.

In contrast, development of improved tests for the SARS-CoV RNA as well as serological test to detect antibodies to viral proteins were well underway very shortly after this viral genome sequence became available [47]. Amazingly, a SARS chip was available by June 2003 [48]. Also, structural information about the main protease $3CL^{pro}$ [38], nsp9 protein [40], E protein [49] and S protein [44] (in the first two cases crystallographic determination of the structures and in the latter two cases, molecular models) is allowing preliminary, directed development of anti-SARS drugs to begin. In addition, small inhibitory RNA (siRNA) therapy may prove to be effective in treating this viral infection and again preliminary studies have begun to evaluate potential siRNAs [50].

Another area that will be a focus during the next few years is the development of a SARS vaccine. The success of vaccines for avian, bovine, feline, and porcine coronaviruses bodes well for the development of a vaccine against the SARS-CoV [51] and a report of a recent conference in Switzerland indicates preliminary progress from a number of laboratories towards developing a vaccine directed against the S, E and N proteins using a variety of inactivated virus, recombinant vectors, recombinant antigens, as well as DNA-based vaccines (http://www.who.int/vaccine_research/diseases/sars/events/2003/11/en/).

Yet further reason for optimism is the very recent discovery by Li et al. [52] that unlike other coronaviruses, the SARS-CoV uses a receptor on cells – the angiotensin-converting enzyme 2 or ACE2 – and drugs that block this receptor already have been developed for other conditions. The ACE2 inhibitors have been tested in humans, and some appear to be safe, but they have not yet been commercialized [52, 53]. In addition, the other half of the interaction, the receptor binding domain on the S protein, has been localized to residues 303 to 537 of the S protein [53]. Also learning from the experience with HIV virus in which soluble receptor protein (sCD4) proved ineffective in blocking HIV infection while a multivalent CD4-IgG fusion protein does seem to be effective, it has been speculated that soluble ACE2-IgG fusions may prove useful in treating SARS infections [53].

One aspect of the SARS viral genome lends itself to speculation about the origin of the SARS-CoV. While the natural host has not been identified, if appears that the virus spread from civet cats into humans. Since the civet cat virus and only one human isolate of the SARS-CoV contains the additional 29 nt in the ORF 10/11 region, it is tempting to speculate that transfer of the virus to humans was accompanied by a deletion of 29 nt. If this is the case, the characterization and function of ORF 10, ORF11 and ORF 10' may provide considerable insight into why the SARS-CoV is so pathogenic in humans.

Acknowledgements

This work was supported by funds from Genome British Columbia and Genome Canada.

The GSC high throughput large scale sequencing and bioinformatics pipelines are also supported by the BC Cancer Foundation of the BCCA, GBC/GC, NSERC, CIHR, NHGRI, NCI, and Western Diversification.

MAM and SJMJ are Scholars of the Michael Smith Foundation for Health Research.

We wish to acknowledge all those who contributed to the rapid sequencing of the Tor2 SARS genome. At the GSC these include A. Brooks-Wilson, Y. Butterfield, J. Khattra, J. Asano, S. Barber, S. Chan, A. Cloutier, S. Coughlin, D. Freeman, N. Girn, O. Griffiths, S. Leach, M. Mayo, H. McDonald, S. Montgomery, P. Pandoh, A. Petrescu, G. Robertson, J. Schein, A. Siddiqui, D. Smailus, J. Stott, and G. Yang. Our collaborators at the NML were F. Plummer, A. Antonov, H. Artsob, N. Bastien, K. Bernard, T. Booth, D. Bowness, M. Czub, M. Drebot, L. Fernando, R. Flick, M. Garbutt, M. Gray, A. Grolla, S. Jones, H. Feldmann, A. Meyers, A. Kabani, Y. Lio, S. Normand, U. Stoher, G. Tipples, S. Tyler, R. Vogrig, D. Ward and B. Watson. Our collaborators at the BC CDC were R. Brunham, M. Krajden, D. Skowronski, and M. Petric and a the U. Victoria they were C. Upton and R. Roper.

This review summarizes research published to Dec 31, 2003. Due to space limitations not all papers could be cited. Two accidental laboratory derived infections (Senior, K.) [55, 56] and only one new confirmed case of SARS have occurred since June 2003. The new community acquired case occurred in Guangdong province in December 2003. It appears that surveillance and quarantine procedures in place helped to identify and isolate this case preventing further transmission to the patient's contacts.

References

1 Peiris JS, Lai ST, Poon LL, Guan Y, Yam LY, Lim W, Nicholls J, Yee WK, Yan WW, Cheung MT (2003) Coronavirus as a possible cause of severe acute respiratory syndrome. *Lancet* 361: 1319–1325

2 Ksiazek TG, Erdman D, Goldsmith CS, Zaki SR, Peret T, Emery S, Tong S, Urbani C, Comer JA, Lim XX et al (2003) A novel coronavirus associated with severe acute respiratory syndrome. *N Engl J Med* 348: 1848–1951

3 Drosten C, Gunther S, Preiser W, van der Werf S, Brodt HR, Becker S, Rabenau H, Panning M, Kolesnikova L, Fouchier RA et al (2003) Identification of a novel coronavirus in patients with severe acute respiratory syndrome. *N Engl J Med* 348(20): 1967–1976

4 Wang D, Urisman A, Lui Y-T, Springer M, Ksiazek TG, Erdman DD, Mardis ER, Hickenbotham M et al (2003) Viral discovery and sequence recovery using DNA microarrays. *PLoS Biol* 1: e2 (2003)

5 Venter JC, Adams MD, Myers EW, Li PW, Mural RJ, Sutton GG, Smith HO, Yandell M, Evans CA, Holt RA, (2001) The sequence of the human genome. *Science* 291: 1304–1351

6 Ewing B, Green P (1998) Base-calling of automated sequencer traces using phred. II. Error probabilities. *Genome Res* 8: 186–194

7 Gordon D, Abajian C, Green P (1998) Consed: a graphical tool for sequence finishing. *Genome Res* 8: 195–202
8 Altschul SF, Gish W, Miller W, Myers EW, Lipman DJ (1990) Basic local alignment search tool. *J Mol Biol* 215: 403–410
9 Lipman DJ, Pearson WR (1985) Rapid and sensitive protein similarity searches. *Science* 227: 1435–1441
10 Durbin R,Thierry J Mieg (1991) A *C. elegans* database documentation, code and data available from anonymous FTP servers at lirmm.lirmm.fr, cele.mrc-lmb.cam.ac.uk and ncbi.nlm.nih.gov
11 Marra MA, Jones SJ, Astell CR, Holt RA, Brooks-Wilson A, Butterfield YS, Khattra J, Asano JK, Barber SA, Chan SY et al (2003) The genome sequence of the SARS-associated coronavirus. *Science* 300: 1399–1404 (published online 1 May, 2003)
12 Rota PA, Oberste MS, Monroe SS, Nix WA, Campagnoli R, Icenogle JP, Penaranda S, Bankamp B, Maher K, Chen MH et al (2003) Characterization of a novel coronavirus associated with severe acute respiratory syndrome. *Science* 300: 1394–1399 (published online, 1 May, 2003)
13 Ruan YJ, Wei CL, Ee AL, Vega VB, Thoreau H, Su ST, Chia JM, Ng P, Chiu KP, Lim L et al (2003) Comparative full-length genome sequence analysis of 14 SARS coronavirus isolates and common mutations associated with putative origins of infection. *Lancet* 361: 1779–1785
14 Fields BN, Knipe DM, Howley PM, Griffin DE (eds) (2001) *Fields Virology*. Lippincott Williams and Wilkins, Philadelphia
15 Thiel V, Ivanov KA, Putics A, Hertzig T, Schelle B, Bayer S, Weissbrich B, Snijder EJ, Rabenau H, Doerr HW et al (2003) Mechanisms and enzymes involved in SARS coronavirus genome expression. *J Gen Virol* 84: 2305–2315
16 Snijder, EJ, Bredenbeek PJ, Dobbe JC, Thiel V, Ziebuhr J, Poon LL, Guan Y, Rozanov M, Spaan WJM, Gorbalenya AE (2003) Unique and conserved features of genome and proteome of SARS-coronavirus, an early split-off from the coronavirus group 2 lineage. *J Mol Biol* 331: 991–1004
17 Rest JS, Mindell DP (2003) SARS associated coronavirus has a recombinant polymerase and coronaviruses have a history of host-shifting. Infect. Genet. and Evol. 3: 219–225
18 Stavrinides J, Guttman DS (2004) Mosaic evolution of the severe acute respiratory syndrome coronavirus. *J Virol* 78: 76–82
19 Guan Y, Zheng BJ, He YQ, Liu ZX, Zhuang CL, Cheung CL, Luo SW, Li PH, Zhang LJ, Guan YJ et al (2003) Isolation and characterization of viruses related to the SARS coronavirus from Southern China. *Science* 5643: 276–278
20 Lai MMC, Cavanagh D (1997) The molecular biology of coronaviruses. *Adv Virus Res* 48: 1–100
21 Sawicki SG, Sawicki DL (1998) A new model for coronavirus transcription. *Adv Exp Med Biol* 440: 215–220
22 Lai MMC, Holmes KV (2001) *Coronaviridae*: the viruses and their replication. In: Fields BN, Knipe DM, Howley PM, Griffin DE (eds) (2001) *Fields Virology*. Lippincott Williams and Wilkins, Philadelphia, 1163–1185

23 Siddell SG (1995) The *Coronaviridae*. Plenum Press, New York
24 Jonassen CM, Jonassen TO, Grinde BJ (1998) A common RNA motif in the 3' end of the genomes of astroviruses, avian infectious bronchitis virus and an equine rhinovirus. *Gen Virol* 79: 715–718
25 Woo K, Joo M, Narayanan K, Kim KH, Makino S (1997) Identification and characterization of a coronavirus packaging signal. *J Virol* 71: 824–827
26 Qin L, Xiong B, Luo C, Guo Z-M, Hao P, Su J, Nan P, Feng Y, Shi Y-X, Yu X-J et al (2003) Identification of probable genomic packaging signal sequence from SARS-CoV genome by bioinformatics analysis. *Acta Pharmacologica Sinica* 24: 489–496
27 Matthews DH, Sabina J, Zuker M, Turner DH (1999) Expanded sequence dependence of thermodynamic parameters improves prediction of RNA secondary structure. *J Mol Biol* 288: 911–940
28 Brierley I, Digard P, Inglis SC (1989) Characterization of an efficient coronavirus ribosomal frameshifting signal: requirement for an RNA pseudoknot. *Cell* 57: 537–547 (1989)
29 Geidroc DP, Theimer CA, Nixon PL (2000) Structure, stability and function of RNA pseudoknots involved in stimulating ribosomal frameshifting. *J Mol Biol* 298: 167–185
30 Gorbalenya AE, Koonin EV, Donchenko AP, Blinov VM (1989) Coronavirus genome: prediction of putative functional domains in the non-structural polyprotein by comparative amino acid sequence analysis. *Nucl Acids Res* 17: 4847–4861
31 Gorbalenya AE (2001) Big nidovirus genome. When count and order of domains matter. *Adv Exp Biol Med* 494: 1–17
32 Ziebuhr J, Thiel V, Gorbalenya AE (2001) The autocatalytic release of a putative RNA virus transcription factor from its polyprotein precursor involves two paralogous papain-like proteases that cleave the same peptide bond. *J Biol Chem* 276: 33220–33232
33 Zeibuhr J, Snijder EJ, Gorbalenya AE (2000) Virus-encoded proteinases and proteolytic processing in the *Nidovirales*. *J Gen Virol* 82: 853–879
34 Gorbalenya AE, Koonin EV, Lai MM (1991) Putative papain-related thiol proteases of positive-strand RNA viruses. Identification of rubi- and aphthovirus proteases and delineation of a novel conserved domain associated with proteases of rubi-, alpha- and coronaviruses. *FEBS Letts* 288: 201–205
35 Baker SC, Yokomori K, Dong S, Carlisle R, Gorbalenya AE, Koonin EV, Lai MM (1993) Identification of the catalytic sites of a papain-like custeine proteinase of murione coronaviruses. *J Virol* 67: 6056–6063
36 von Grotthuss M, Wyrwicz LS, Rychlewski L (2003) mRNA cap-1 methytransferase in the SARS genome. *Cell* 113: 701–702
37 Anand K, Ziebuhr J, Wadhwani P, Mesters JR, Hilgenfeld R (2003) Coronovirus main proteinase (3CLpro) structure: basis for design of anti-SARS drugs. *Science* 300: 1763–7
38 Yang H, Yang M, Ding Y, Liu Y, Lou Z, Zhou Z, Sun L, Mo L, Ye S, Pang H (2003) The crystal structure of severe acute respiratory syndrome virus main

protease and its complex with an inhibitor. *Proc Natl Acad Sci USA* 100: 13190–13195

39 Fan K, Wei, P, Feng, Q, Chen S, Huang C, Ma L, Lai B, Pei J, Liu Y, Chen J et al (2004) Biosynthesis, purification and substrate specificity of SARS coronavirus 3C-like proteinase. *J Biol Chem* 279: 1637–1642

40 Campanacci V, Egloff MP, Longhi S, Ferron F, Rancurel C, Salomoni A, Durousseau C, Tocque F, Bremond N, Dobbe JC et al (2003) Structural genomics of the SARS coronavirus: cloning, expression, crystallization and preliminary crystallographic study of the Nsp9 protein. *Acta Crystallogr D Biol Crystallogr* 59: 1628–1631

41 Nielson H, Engelbrecht S, Brunak, von Heijne G (1997) Identification of prokaryotic and eukaryotic signal peptides and prediction of their cleavage sites. *Protein Eng* 10: 1–6

42 Sonnhammer EL, von Heijne G, Krogh A (1998) A hidden Markov model for predicting transmembrane helices in protein sequences. *Proc Int Conf Intell Syst Mol Biol* 6: 175–182

43 Krokhin O, Li Y, Andonov AQ, Feldman H, Flick R, Jones S, Stroeher U, Bastien U, Dasuri KV, Cheng K et al (2003) Mass spectrometric characterization of proteins from the SARS Virus: A preliminary report. *Mol Cell Proteomics* 2: 346–356

44 Spiga O, Bernini A, Ciutti A, Chiellini S, Menciassi N, Finetti F, Caurarono V, Anselmi F, Prisch F, Niccolai N (2003) Molecular modelling of S1 and S2 subunits of SARS coronavirus spike glycoprotein. *Biochem Biophys Res Commun* 310: 78–83

45 Bateman A, Birney E, Cerruti L, Durbin R, Etwiller L, Eddy SR, Griffiths-Jones S, Howe KL, Marshall M, Sonnhammer EL (2002) The Pfam protein families database. *Nucl Acids Res* 30: 276–280

46 Hoffman K, Stoffel W (1993) *Biol Chem Hoppe-Seyler* 374: 166

47 Basu P (2003) Biotech firms jump on SARS bandwagon. *Nat Biotech* 21: 720

48 Frankish H (2003) SARS genome chip available to scientists: the NIAID hopes that widespread access to the SARS genome chip will catalyse research into effective treatments for the virus. *Lancet* 361: 2212

49 Shen X, Xue JH, Yu CY, Luo HB, Qin L, Yu XJ, Chen J, Chen LL, Xiong B, Yue LD et al (2003) Small envelope protein E of SARS: cloning, expression, purification, CD determination, and bioinformatics analysis. *Acta Pharmacol Sin* 24: 505–511

50 Zhang R, Guo Z, Lu J, Meng J, Zhou C, Zhan X, Huang B, Yu X, Huang M, Pan X et al (2003) Inhibiting severe acute respiratory syndrome-associated coronavirus by small interfering RNAs (siRNAs). *Chin Med J* 116: 1262–1265

51 Cavanagh D (2003) Several acute respiratory syndrome vaccine development: experiences of vaccination against avian infectious bronchitis coronavirus. Avian Pathol. 32: 567–582

52 Li W, Moore MJ, Vasilieva N, Sui J, Wong SK, Berne MA, Somasundaran M, Sullivan JL, Luzuriaga K, Greenough TC et al (2003) Angiotensin-converting

enzyme 2 is a functional receptor for the SARS coronavirus. *Nature* 426: 450–454

53 Dimitrov DS (2003) The secret life of ACE2 as a receptor for the SARS virus. *Cell* 652–653

54 Xiao X, Chakraboti S, Dimitrov AS, Gramatikoff K, Dimitrov DS (2003) *Biochem Biophys Res Commun* 312: 1394–1399

55 Senior K (2003) Recent Singapore SARS case a laboratory accident. *Lancet Infec Dis* 3: 679

56 Lim PL, Kurup A, Gopalakrishna G, Chang KP, Wong CW, Ng LC, Se-Thoe SY, Oon L, Bai X, Stanton LW et al (2004) Laboratory-acquired severe acute respiratory syndrome. *New Engl J Med* 350: 1740–1745

Coronaviruses with Special Emphasis on First Insights Concerning SARS
ed. by A. Schmidt, M.H. Wolff and O. Weber

Virological laboratory diagnosis of SARS

Wolfgang Preiser[1], Christian Drosten[2], Hans Wilhelm Doerr[1]

[1] *Institute for Medical Virology, Johann Wolfgang von Goethe University Hospital, Paul Ehrlich-Str. 40, 60596 Frankfurt/Main, Germany;*
[2] *Bernhard Nocht Institute for Tropical Medicine, Hamburg, Germany*

Introduction

The enormous speed with which, through unprecedented international collaboration coordinated by WHO, the novel coronavirus causing SARS, termed SARS-CoV, was isolated and characterized [1], allowed the development of diagnostic tests when the first SARS epidemic was still in full swing (Severe Acute Respiratory Syndrome (SARS): Laboratory diagnostic tests – 29 April 2003: http://www.who.int/csr/sars/diagnostictests/en/). As early as mid-April 2003, sequences of polymerase chain reaction (PCR) primers were made publicly available on the WHO SARS website (PCR primers for SARS developed by WHO Network Laboratories – 17 April 2003: http://www.who.int/csr/sars/primers/en/) to facilitate the introduction of laboratory testing in affected countries.

Soon afterwards the first commercial assays became available, and numerous laboratories all over the world started preparing for SARS diagnosis using these or various in-house assays. Important research efforts were - and still are, as of April 2004 - directed towards improving SARS laboratory testing, including the development of novel genome targets for nucleic acid detection and of recombinant antigens for serological diagnosis.

Nevertheless, despite these efforts, it has to be recognized that the laboratory diagnosis of SARS so far remains problematic. Problems with test specificity have led to false-positive results for SARS-CoV on occasions, which created enormous public concern and confusion. In addition, some of the results of newly developed antibody tests have yielded results that are difficult to reconcile with epidemiological and other information and may be related to insufficient test sensitivities or specificities.

In this chapter, we will endeavour to briefly list and describe the currently available laboratory test methods for SARS-CoV, including their performance as far as has been published. We will then outline the current WHO-endorsed strategy for the laboratory diagnosis of suspected SARS

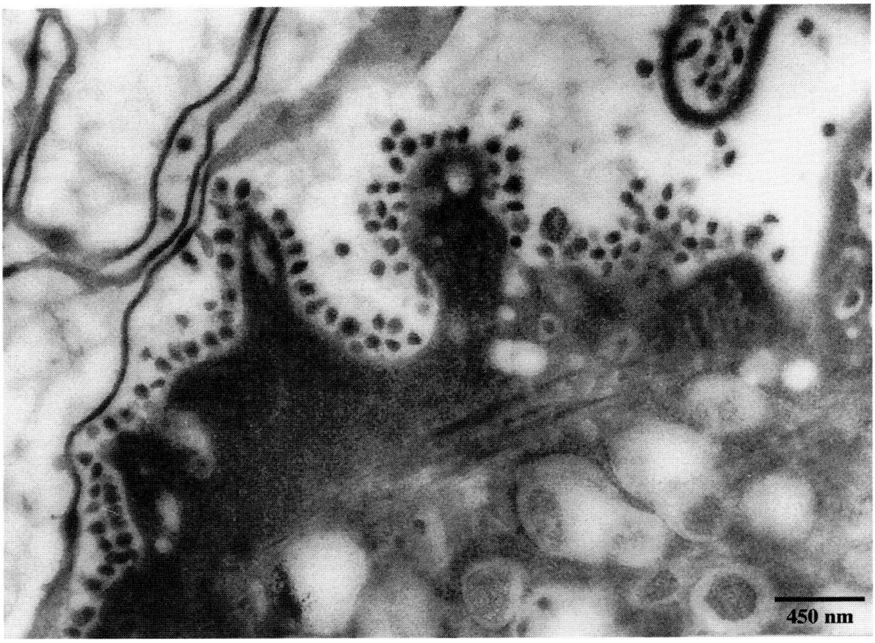

Figure 1. SARS-CoV particles in Caco-2 cell culture.

cases, including recommendations for dealing with such cases, and provide an outlook regarding future developments.

Available virological laboratory tests for SARS-CoV

Virus detection

Virus isolation

In contrast to the previously known human-pathogenic coronaviruses, HCoV-229E and HCoV-OC43, SARS-CoV is relatively easily propagated in cell culture. The most commonly used cell lines are Vero (African green monkey kidney) cells, but fetal rhesus kidney (FRhK-4) cells and – interesting in the light of possible gastrointestinal pathology caused by SARS-CoV – the human colonic carcinoma cell line Caco-2 (HTB-37) may also be used (Fig. 1). Cells commonly used for the isolation of human respiratory viruses are however unsuitable. The authors were able to isolate SARS-CoV on Vero cells from lower respiratory tract specimens (sputum, bronchoalveolar lavage) from the two Frankfurt/Main SARS cases; a marked

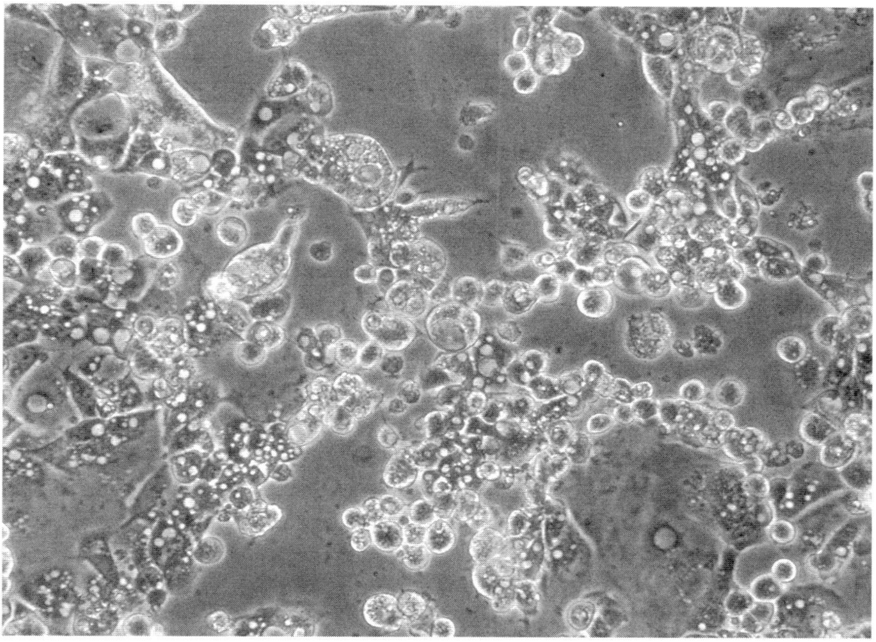

Figure 2. Cytopathic effect (CPE) in Caco-2 cell culture caused by SARS-CoV infection 72 hours after infection.

cytopathic effect (CPE) became visible only a few days after inoculation ([2]; Fig. 2).

To confirm the presence of SARS-CoV, further tests are required. Human SARS-CoV immune (convalescent) serum may be used for immunostaining of infected cells (Fig. 3). Alternatively, viral nucleic acid testing (see below) may be performed on cell culture supernatant. The latter is recommended by WHO (Use of laboratory methods for SARS diagnosis – 1 May 2003: http://www.who.int/csr/sars/labmethods/en/).

Relatively few isolations of SARS-CoV were made during the SARS outbreak which caused more than 8,000 "probable" SARS cases. This may be due to the fact that many laboratories refrained from virus isolation due to biosafety concerns, and if it was attempted, long transport times and the use of patient sample types with a low viral load, such as those from the upper respiratory tract, may have affected its success rate, despite the agent's relatively high degree of resistance to various environmental conditions [3].

The advantage of virus isolation is that it demonstrates the presence of infectious virus and thus proves active – and potentially infectious – SARS-CoV infection in the patient. Of course, negative cell culture results do not exclude a diagnosis of SARS (see below). Virus isolation furthermore allows further studies to characterize the virus strain implicated, which will

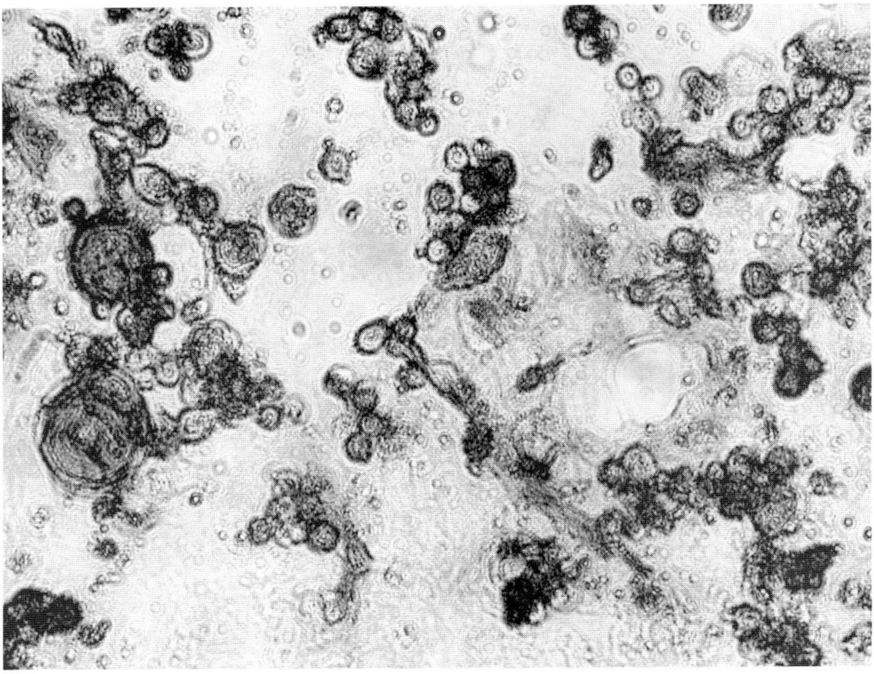

Figure 3. Immunostaining of SARS-CoV infected cells using human immune serum.

be of enormous importance should SARS re-emerge. Such information might not only shed light on the transmissibility and virulence of different strains of SARS-CoV but also on its presumed animal reservoir [4].

While it is internationally agreed that virus isolation from suspect SARS cases has to be performed under at least biosafety safety level (BSL) 3 conditions (WHO post-outbreak biosafety guidelines for handling of SARS-CoV specimens and cultures – 18 December 2003: http://www.who.int/csr/sars/biosafety2003_12_18/en/), it has to be stressed that during the outbreak that ended in July 2003, not a single laboratory infection seems to have occurred. In contrast, there have been several such incidents since; two without further human-to-human spread (Singapore, September 2003, and Taiwan, December 2003), and with spread beyond the laboratory workers themselves (Beijing, April 2004). Therefore, it is obviously not so much the routine diagnostic work-up of suspect SARS specimens that poses a risk to laboratory workers but the neglect of well-known precautions during scientific work which involves much higher volumes and concentrations of infectious materials. If possible, isolation of the causative agent should therefore always be attempted from suspect and probable SARS cases if suitable facilities are available.

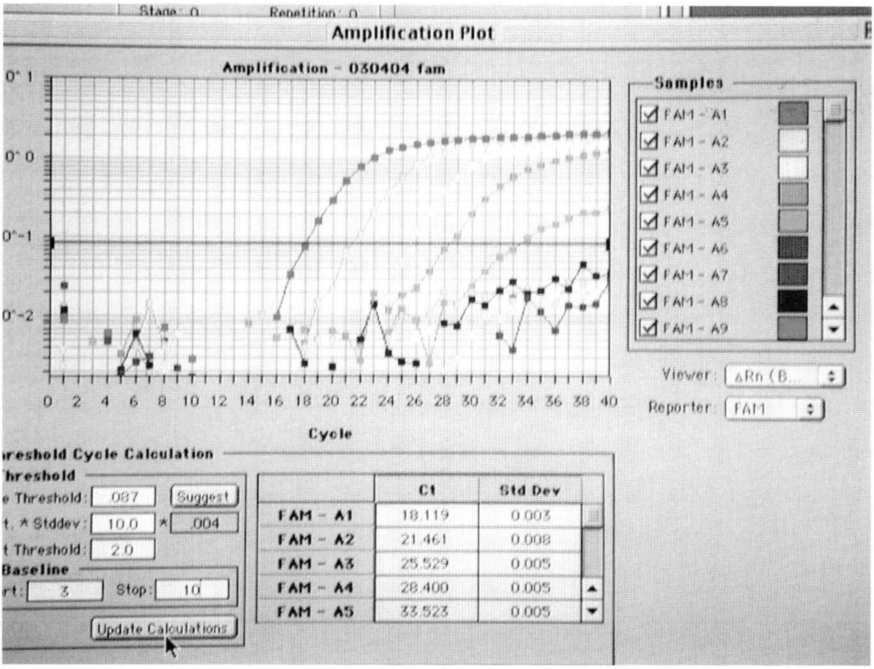

Figure 4. "TaqMan" real-time PCR amplification plot.

Viral nucleic acid detection

All three groups that simultaneously but independently succeeded in isolating and characterizing SARS-CoV published methods for the detection of the agent's RNA [5–7]. These first-generation reverse transcription (RT)-polymerase chain reactions (PCR) all target the viral replicase gene, and detection of PCR products is *via* agarose gel electrophoresis.

SARS-CoV RNA has since been found in various clinical materials. Published papers describe its detection in respiratory secretions both from the lower and the upper respiratory tract, in stool, in urine, and in the blood, as well as in different tissues and organs. Subsequently developed PCR methods employ real-time formats and allow quantification of SARS-CoV RNA (Fig. 4). Using such a method, Drosten et al. [5] were able to demonstrate high concentrations of viral RNA of up to 10^8 molecules per ml in sputum samples; on the other hand, only low concentrations were detected in specimens from the upper respiratory tract, such as throat swabs, and in plasma during the acute phase of the illness. However, faecal specimens obtained late during convalescence, beyond the time period for which strict isolation of patients is usually recommended, tested positive. In patients from Hong Kong, Peiris et al. [8] found the amount of nasopharyngeal

SARS-CoV to peak around 10 days after onset of symptoms, at which time 19 of 20 patients were PCR positive in nasopharyngeal aspirates, all 20 in stool and 10 in urine samples.

Currently, two real-time RT-PCR test kits, both targeting the viral replicase gene, are commercially available, the RealArt HPA coronavirus LC kit (Artus, Hamburg, Germany) and the LightCycler SARS-CoV quantification kit (Roche, Penzberg, Germany). A recently conducted international external quality assurance study for SARS-CoV nucleic acid testing (NAT) distributed 10 coded, inactivated samples to 58 laboratories in 38 different countries [9]. The seven positive samples contained between 94 and 940,000 RNA copies of SARS-CoV strains Frankfurt 1 or HKU-1 per ml when reconstituted. Almost 90% of laboratories reported correct results for all samples containing more than 9,400 viral RNA copies/ml while not producing false-positive results in the three negative ones. The use of commercial test kits was found to positively influence diagnostic performance. The encouraging outcome of this exercise confirms the success of the considerable efforts undertaken by WHO to support laboratories in establishing SARS-CoV diagnostic tests rapidly as a means to effectively respond to the SARS outbreak. Through the European Network for Imported Viral Infections (ENIVD; http://www.enivd.de), an inactivated standard preparation of SARS-CoV is available for diagnostic purposes.

To improve the insufficient negative predictive value of PCR-based methods to rule out SARS in suspect cases, efforts were made to increase their methodological sensitivity. Besides increasing the volume of patient sample material from which RNA is extracted [10], an attractive approach seemed to target the viral nucleocapsid gene of which, due to the unique transcription strategy of coronaviruses, more than one mRNA copy is present in infected cells [11]. However, in a recent study a technically optimized nucleocapsid in-house assay failed to consistently detect SARS-CoV RNA in 66 clinical samples from confirmed SARS patients with an overall positivity rate around 70% [12]. This is in agreement with results obtained by other groups [13].

The same study, however, found viral RNA detectable in all lower respiratory tract samples by all test methods. It therefore concluded that, rather than further optimizing PCR methods and protocols, efforts should be directed towards developing safe and convenient methods for obtaining specimens from the lower respiratory tract of suspect SARS patients. In the very early phase of clinical illness, prior to the onset of respiratory symptoms, plasma may provide a convenient and safe alternative sample material; Grant et al. [14] were able to detect SARS-CoV RNA in 19 of 24 patients (79%) tested within three days after onset of fever. The same study confirmed the brief duration of viraemia in SARS cases and thus offers reassurance for blood transfusion services. However, should SARS re-emerge on a large scale, methods have already been developed and evaluated that would allow screening of donated blood for SARS-CoV RNA [15].

While it is clear from the studies cited above – and numerous others – that PCR cannot rule out the presence of SARS-CoV in patients with certainty, there is also a risk of false-positive results being caused by contamination of samples in laboratories performing PCR, or of true-positive results caused by related viruses when methods of low specificity for SARS-CoV are employed. In August 2003, there was considerable confusion when mild respiratory infections in an institution for the elderly in Canada were initially reported to be positive by SARS-CoV tests; these later turned out to be infections with a different human coronavirus, OC43. When a small number of SARS cases occurred in the southern Chinese province of Guangdong in January 2004, there was some uncertainty for several weeks as to the true diagnosis in some of the cases, as independent confirmation could not be obtained for some patients tested positive locally. For these reasons, WHO has issued clear guidance on how such samples should be handled and tested [16].

For the interpretation of laboratory results, WHO recommends that PCR results for SARS-CoV should only be regarded as confirmed positive if (1) at least two different clinical specimens (e.g. nasopharyngeal and stool) or (2) the same type of clinical specimen collected on two or more days during the course of the illness (e.g. two or more nasopharyngeal aspirates) were tested or (3) if two different assays or repeat PCR using the original clinical sample on each occasion of testing yielded positive results on one specimen (Use of laboratory methods for SARS diagnosis – 1 May 2003: http://www.who.int/csr/sars/labmethods/en/). Besides including appropriate negative and positive controls in each PCR run, possible PCR inhibition should be controlled for by spiking the patient sample with a weak positive control and testing it in parallel with the unspiked sample. In the post-outbreak period – when each truly positive SARS-CoV result will have massive implications for public health etc. –, a second aliquot of the original sample should be sent unopened to the national SARS reference laboratory for re-testing, and a third aliquot retained for use by an international SARS reference and verification laboratory nominated by WHO, if necessary.

In summary, PCR is able to detect viral RNA in between 50 and 85% of stool, blood and upper respiratory tract samples from acutely ill SARS patients. While the use of commercial kits may increase the reliability of results, the sensitivity and thus the negative predictive value of PCR require further improvement. While this is unlikely to come from changing the PCR target gene region, increasing the volume of sample from which RNA is extracted [10], testing lower respiratory tract specimens [12], or testing several samples from each patient [17] may be useful approaches. Nevertheless, a diagnosis of SARS cannot currently be ruled out by a negative PCR result.

Antibody detection

Neutralisation test (NT)

This assay became available as soon as SARS-CoV had been isolated and propagated *in vitro*. It is the only antibody test that allows to assess and quantify, by means of serial titrations of patient sera, their ability to neutralize the infectivity of SARS-CoV. Although this has yet to be demonstrated in humans, the NT titer may therefore be correlated to clinical immunity and is used to assess humoral immunity in animal studies [18]. Furthermore, NT is recommended as a means to rule out non-specific antibody reactivity that might occur in other tests, e.g. through cross-reactivity with antibodies directed against other, non-SARS human coronaviruses. One disadvantage of NT is that it is limited to institutions with BSL-3 cell culture facilities as it involves the propagation of SARS-CoV.

Immunofluorescence test (IFT, IFA)

IFT was the first type of solid-phase antibody assay to be used for SARS and remains the widely employed "gold standard", together with NT (see above). Even before the exact nature of the newly isolated agent was known, specific seroconversion and thus, primary infection, were demonstrated in the Frankfurt SARS patients by means of indirect IFT, using infected cells (and non-infected cells as control), serum samples obtained from the patients at different points of time and anti-human IgG conjugate antibody labelled with a fluorescent dye [5] (Fig. 5). Peiris et al. found seroconversion in 93% of 75 patients by day 30 after onset of symptoms. None had antibodies prior to day 10, and the mean time period to seroconversion was 20 days [18].

An IFT assay is now commercially available (Euroimmun, Lübeck, Germany). As it employs gamma-irradiated infected cells that have been demonstrated to be non-infectious and includes both negative (uninfected) cell controls and appropriate positive and negative control sera, it is suitable for use under BSL-2 conditions; ideally, patient samples should be heat inactivated prior to testing to exclude infectivity. Positive samples should also be tested in serial dilutions to provide a titer which may be helpful to demonstrate acute or very recent infection (see below).

Other serological methods

A number of other serological test methods such as enzyme immunoassay (EIA), Western blot and rapid antibody tests have been developed. They employ infected cell lysates or recombinant proteins as antigens, and some

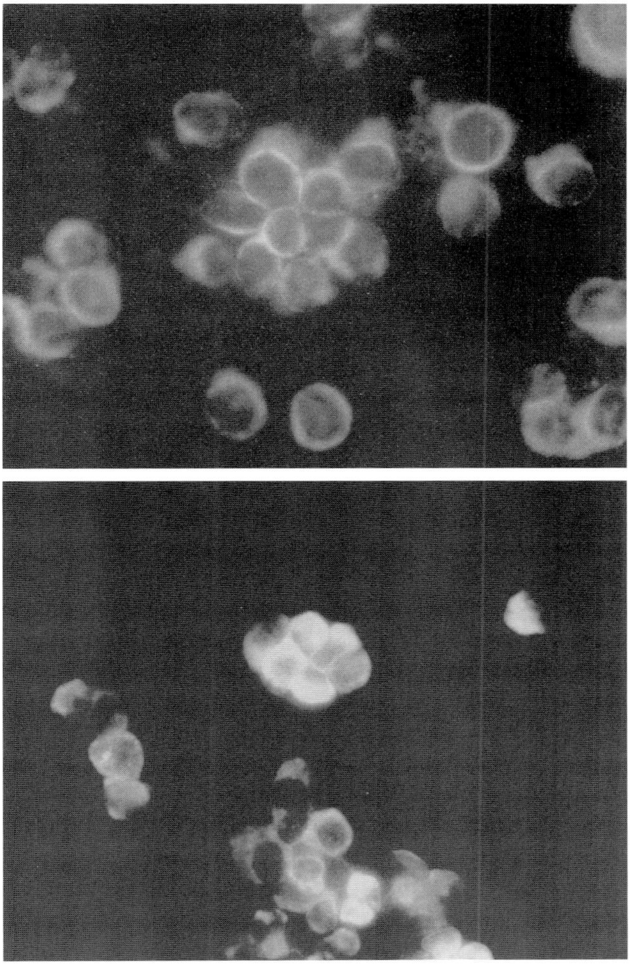

Figure 5. Seroconversion against SARS-CoV demonstrated in Frankfurt SARS patient by IFT. Serum sample obtained 8 days (top) and 14 days (bottom) after onset of illness.

are even commercially available. However, none of these assays has been thoroughly evaluated yet, by means of comparison with either IFT or NT. It is therefore currently impossible to give well-founded recommendations regarding their use. Particularly some well advertised "rapid tests" have caused much excitement in the lay press, as they seemed to offer a quick answer; the speed with which an antibody test result is available, however, does not help at all with the commonest and most urgent practical problem, i.e. to reliably establish a diagnosis in suspect cases, for which antibody testing is unsuitable due to the appearance of antibodies only later in the course of disease (see above). However, from about three weeks after a possible contact with a SARS patient, e.g. during travel or in a health care setting, antibody testing is a useful tool to exclude that SARS-CoV infection has taken place.

According to WHO recommendations, serodiagnosis may be used for (normally retrospective) confirmation of a diagnosis of SARS if either seroconversion is demonstrated by IFT or EIA (i.e. a negative antibody test on an acute serum followed by a positive antibody test on a convalescent serum) or if an at least four-fold rise in antibody titer is demonstrated between such paired sera tested in parallel. Reassuringly, most studies so far showed seroconversion six and more weeks after the beginning of the illness in almost 100% of SARS patients [19].

Results demonstrating SARS-CoV antibodies in a small proportion of sera obtained from individuals prior to the emergence of SARS remain to be confirmed and may reflect a lack of specificity of the assays used rather than pre-existing circulation of the virus. On the other hand, the finding of SARS-CoV antibodies in animal handlers without a history of clinical disease compatible with SARS and presumably exposed to closely related but possibly non-human-pathogenic coronaviruses isolated from different species of animals in southern China [20, 21] may point to a possible explanation for such phenomena. However, most studies found no background seroprevalence against SARS-CoV in the control populations screened so far.

Therefore, antibody testing is suited to retrospectively confirm the diagnosis of SARS and may help to further elucidate the epidemiology of this novel disease. While of course unsuitable during the acute phase of illness when a reliable diagnosis is needed most urgently, it has the advantage of requiring only a blood specimen and probably being little time-sensitive once patients are beyond the first few weeks of their illness.

It needs to be borne in mind that the international case definition for SARS was based on a combination of clinical and epidemiological factors and did not require specific virological or serological testing (although evidence of SARS-CoV infection was added from May 1st, 2003, as a facultative criterion to upgrade a suspect to a probable case). Since the clinical manifestation rate of SARS-CoV infection appears to be high (>80%), the epidemiology of SARS does not need to be revised. However, much remains to be done to define the optimal antigens for use in EIA and other assays, including large-scale comparative evaluations on panels of well-defined sera. WHO has called for countries in which large numbers of SARS cases occurred to make such panels available to the scientific community.

Current status of virological laboratory diagnosis of SARS

In the light of currently available information, it is regarded as unlikely that SARS-CoV continues to circulate in the human population of previously affected areas. Nevertheless, the cases in Guangdong at the beginning of 2004 have demonstrated that a re-introduction from the still unknown animal reservoir is possible, and repeated laboratory accidents have underlined the need for stringent infection control procedures and their strict application in laboratories working with the agent, as these are the only places of which it is known for sure that infectious SARS-CoV still exists [22].

It is therefore imperative that vigilance for SARS be maintained. WHO has defined three geographical zones according to their presumed risk for potential SARS recurrence and issued recommendations for SARS surveillance for each of them [23].

In the "potential zone of re-emergence", comprising Guangdong and other, adjacent areas where animal-to-human transmission of SARS-CoV might again occur, "SARS alert" plus enhanced SARS surveillance should be in place and special studies for SARS-CoV infections in animal and human populations conducted. In "nodal areas", comprising Hong Kong, Vietnam, Singapore, Canada, and Taiwan, that experienced sustained local transmission in spring 2003 or the entry of numerous persons from the potential zone of re-emergence, only "SARS alert" plus enhanced SARS surveillance are deemed necessary. In "low risk areas", i.e. the rest of the world, surveillance should be directed to clusters of "alert" cases among health care workers, other hospital staff, patients and visitors in the same health care unit.

A "SARS alert" is defined as at least two health care workers developing clinical illness, or at least three individuals – health care workers and/or other hospital staff and/or patients and/or visitors – in the same health care unit developing hospital-acquired illness, within the same 10-day period, that fulfills the clinical case definition of SARS. Fulfilling the clinical case definition also means that "no alternative diagnosis can fully explain the illness", i.e. it requires certain other laboratory tests for infectious agents – such as influenza and other viruses – to be conducted if appropriate.

For such cases, and in those recognized through "enhanced SARS surveillance", such as otherwise causally undiagnosed cases of atypical pneumonia, a laboratory case definition was developed based on PCR, antibody tests or virus isolation to be undertaken in a national or regional reference laboratory. Only clinically compatible and laboratory-confirmed cases should be reported to WHO.

At the SARS Laboratory Workshop held in October 2003 in Geneva, experts from the enlarged international laboratory network made several recommendations [24]. These included

(1) the establishment of a quality assurance programme and the standardisation of laboratory tests and protocols;
(2) the establishment of a WHO SARS reference and verification laboratory network to undertake verification of suspected cases of SARS-CoV

infection, with terms of reference requiring such laboratories to be active members of the quality assurance programme;

(3) to require all sporadic (non-epidemic) cases of suspected SARS-CoV infection to be verified by a WHO reference and verification laboratory external to the country in which the case occurred;

(4) to acquire and assist in the development of a panel of positive SARS-CoV control sera;

(5) to develop algorithms for assessing the need to test patients for SARS-CoV infection based on an epidemiologic and geographic risk assessment;

(6) to endorse the guidelines for biosafety in laboratories handling diagnostic specimens potentially containing SARS-CoV or culturing SARS-CoV, which should be done in biocontainment level 3 facilities where tests involve virus propagation, or in biocontainment level 2 facilities with level 3 work practices where tests involve manipulations of live virus without propagation;

(7) to strongly recommend that countries maintain an inventory of laboratories working with SARS-CoV, and an inventory of cultures of SARS-CoV in those laboratories.

Because of the risks of inappropriate use of scarce resources and of overwhelming the health system unnecessarily by false alarms, the low pre-test probability for SARS has to be taken into account in low risk settings during the post-epidemic period.

If a case is to be investigated, respiratory samples – ideally including nasopharyngeal aspirates, provided full infection control procedures are in place to protect staff and other patients – and stool specimens should be routinely collected for virus isolation and/or detection by RT-PCR during the first and second weeks of illness, as well as plasma or serum specimens early on and in the second or third week to demonstrate seroconversion or a significant rise in antibody titer by testing acute and convalescent sera in parallel.

Laboratory testing is to be conducted through a three-tier system. Therefore, all clinical samples have to be separated into three aliquots at the time of collection or in a secure laboratory in which there is no ongoing work on SARS-CoV. One aliquot is for use by the local diagnostic laboratory, and the second has to remain unopened for use by the national reference laboratory. The third aliquot should be retained in case verification by a WHO SARS reference and verification laboratory becomes necessary. This happens if a positive clinical specimens is reported by either the local diagnostic laboratory or the national reference laboratory.

Regarding the interpretation of laboratory results, specimens found positive by PCR or virus isolation require confirmation on the second, previously unopened aliquot of the same specimen in a second laboratory, and on a second, independently collected specimen, too. The genome region amplified by PCR should be specific for SARS-CoV and not conserved amongst other known coronaviruses, and PCR products should be sequenced to verify the presence of SARS-CoV.

A four-fold or greater rise in antibody titer on parallel testing by IFT, EIA – using a well-characterised antigen – or another serological test between acute and convalescent phase sera are collected at least 8-10 days apart indicates a suspect case but confirmation by NT is mandatory, because of the possibility of antibodies cross-reacting with other human coronaviruses.

The purpose of these guidelines is clearly to ensure a maximum specificity of laboratory results in order to avoid false alarms which would put unnecessary stress on health systems and might – in the long run – lead to lowered vigilance. Should SARS re-emerge on a larger scale, some of the confirmatory requirements might have to be modified again.

Outlook

Despite the rapid discovery of the causative agent and the early development of diagnostic tests, further progress on the laboratory diagnosis of SARS has been somewhat slower than might have been expected. Although numerous PCR-based assays have been developed, some of which are technically superb, there is still no test that could be used to rule out the diagnosis of SARS in a suspect case, due to the comparatively low virus excretion during the early course of SARS.

In the current post-outbreak phase, thorough evaluation of suspect cases for other agents known to cause atypical pneumonia, such as influenza and parainfluenza viruses, *Legionella pneumophila*, *Mycoplasma pneumoniae* etc. is even more important. Furthermore, if a decision is made to also include SARS in the differential diagnosis – which necessitates thorough and up-to-date information about the patient's personal, work and travel history as well as about the current epidemiological situation worldwide – the recommendations made by WHO (see [23] above; but check for updates!) should be followed meticulously.

The two laboratory-acquired SARS cases in Singapore and in Taiwan in the second half of 2003, and the sporadic SARS cases reported from Guangdong at the beginning of 2004, demonstrate that through a functioning surveillance and alert system, as recommended by WHO, newly emerging cases may be detected in a timely fashion, confirmed by laboratory testing including independent confirmation, and further spread thus prevented. The most recent laboratory-associated cases in Beijing (April 2004), however, cast some doubt on the quality of the local surveillance system.

In little more than one year, a lot has been learned about this novel virus and the disease it causes, but undoubtedly much remains to be understood. The availability and prudent application of SARS-CoV laboratory tests has allowed to address several important questions, but it has also become clear that much more remains to be done. Given how little attention the previously known human coronaviruses had received in human virological laboratory diagnosis, SARS even offers a chance to improve our understanding of their epidemiology and clinical relevance by developing and applying suitable tests.

For the time being, however, great care has to be exercised when using SARS-CoV tests in clinical settings. It is a prerequisite to stay up-to-date on current recommendations issued by WHO, relevant national organizations, and scientific bodies. A recent meeting of the WHO Scientific Research Advisory Committee on SARS [25] has identified several priority issues for laboratory research, including the evaluation and standardization of current and future diagnostic tests for SARS, the improvement of serological tests with respect to specificity and sensitivity, studying the nature of cross-reactions between different coronaviruses, determining the importance of virus strain variation for diagnostic tests, and finding new technologies that can be applied to develop inexpensive, sensitive and specific laboratory tests that are reliable in the first few days of illness.

References

1 Drosten C, Preiser W, Gunther S, Schmitz H, Doerr HW (2003) Severe acute respiratory syndrome: identification of the etiological agent. *Trends Mol Med* 9(8): 325–327

2 Rickerts V, Wolf T, Rottmann C, Preiser W, Drosten C, Jakobi V, Leong HN, Brodt HR (2003) Clinical presentation and management of the severe acute respiratory syndrome (SARS) [Klinik und Behandlung des schweren akuten respiratorischen Syndroms]. *Dtsch Med Wochenschr* 128(20): 1109–1114

3 Rabenau HF, Cinatl J, Morgenstern B, Bauer G, Preiser W, Doerr HW (2004) Stability and inactivation of SARS-associated coronavirus. *Med Microbiol Immunol (Berl)* 194: 1–6

4 Breiman RF, Evans MR, Preiser W, Maguire J, Schnur A, Bekedam H, MacKenzie JS (2003) Role of China in the quest to define and control severe acute respiratory syndrome. *Emerg Infect Dis* 9(9): 1037–1041

5 Drosten C, Günther S, Preiser W, van der Werf S, Brodt HR, Becker S, Rabenau H, Panning M, Kolesnikova L, Fouchier RA et al (2003) Identification of a novel coronavirus in patients with severe acute respiratory syndrome. *N Engl J Med* 348(20): 1967–1976

6 Peiris JS, Lai ST, Poon LL, Guan Y, Yam LY, Lim W, Nicholls J, Yee WK, Yan WW, Cheung MT et al (2003) Coronavirus as a possible cause of severe acute respiratory syndrome. *Lancet* 361: 1319–1325

7 Ksiazek TG, Erdman D, Goldsmith CS, Zaki SR, Peret T, Emery S, Tong S, Urbani C, Comer JA, Lim W et al (2003) A novel coronavirus associated with severe acute respiratory syndrome. *N Engl J Med* 348: 1953–1966

8 Peiris JS, Chu CM, Cheng VC, Chan KS, Hung IF, Poon LL, Law KI, Tang BS, Hon TY, Chan CS et al (2003) Clinical progression and viral load in a community outbreak of coronavirus-associated SARS pneumonia: a prospective study. *Lancet* 361: 1767–1772

9 Drosten C, Doerr HW, Lim W, Stöhr K, Niedrig M (2004) SARS molecular detection external quality assurance. *Emerg Infect Dis* 10: 2200–2203

10 Poon LLM, Chan KH, Wong OK, Yam WC, Yuen KY, Guan Y, Lo YMD, Peiris JSM (2003) Early diagnosis of SARS Coronavirus infection. *J Clin Virol* 28: 233–238

11 Lai MM, Cavanagh D (1997) The molecular biology of coronaviruses. *Adv Virus Res* 48: 1–100

12 Drosten C, Chiu LL, Panning M, Leong HN, Preiser W, Tam JS, Gunther S, Kramme S, Emmerich P, Ng WL, Schmitz H, Koay ESC (2004) Evalution of advanced reverse transcription-PCR assays and an alternative PCR target region for detection of severe acute respiratory syndrome-associated coronavirus. *J Clin Microbiol* 42: 2043–2047

13 Poon LL, Chan KH, Wong OK, Cheung TK, Ng I, Zheng B, Seto WH, Yuen KY, Guan Y, Peiris JS (2004) Detection of SARS coronavirus in patients with severe acute respiratory syndrome by conventional and real-time quantitative reverse transcription-PCR assays. *Clin Chem* 50(1): 67–72

14 Grant PR, Garson JA, Tedder RS, Chan PK, Tam JS, Sung JJ (2003) Detection of SARS coronavirus in plasma by real-time RT-PCR. *N Engl J Med* 349(25): 2468–2469

15 Schmidt M, Brixner V, Ruster B, Hourfar MK, Drosten C, Preiser W, Seifried E, Roth WK (2004) NAT screening of blood donors for severe acute respiratory syndrome coronavirus can potentially prevent transfusion associated transmissions. *Transfusion* 44(4): 470–475

16 World Health Organization (WHO). WHO SARS International Reference and Verification Laboratory Network: Policy and Procedures in the Inter-Epidemic Period – 23 January 2004. WHO website at http://www.who.int/csr/resources/publications/en/SARSReferenceLab.pdf (accessed 4 May 2004)

17 Yam WC, Chan KH, Poon LL, Guan Y, Yuen KY, Seto WH, Peiris JS (2003) Evaluation of reverse transcription-PCR assays for rapid diagnosis of severe acute respiratory syndrome associated with a novel coronavirus. *J Clin Microbiol* 41(10): 4521–4524

18 Gao W, Tamin A, Soloff A, D'Aiuto L, Nwanegbo E, Robbins PD, Bellini WJ, Barratt-Boyes S, Gambotto A (2003) Effects of a SARS-associated coronavirus vaccine in monkeys. *Lancet* 362(9399): 1895–1896

19 Li G, Chen X, Xu A (2003) Profile of specific antibodies to the SARS-associated coronavirus. *N Engl J Med* 349: 508–509

20 Centers for Disease Control and Prevention (2003) Prevalence of IgG Antibody to SARS-Associated Coronavirus in Animal Traders — Guangdong Province, China, 2003. MMWR Morb Mortal Wkly Rep 52(41): 986–987

21 Guan Y, Zheng BJ, He YQ, Liu XL, Zhuang ZX, Cheung CL, Luo SW, Li PH, Zhang LJ, Guan YJ et al (2003) Isolation and characterization of viruses relat-

ed to the SARS coronavirus from animals in southern China. *Science* 302(5643): 276–288

22 Berger A, Drosten Ch, Doerr HW, Sturmer M, Preiser W (2004) Severe acute respiratory syndrome (SARS)--paradigm of an emerging viral infection. *J Clin Virol* 29(1): 13–22

23 World Health Organization (WHO). Alert, verification and public health management of SARS in the post-outbreak period – 14 August 2003. WHO website at http://www.who.int/csr/sars/postoutbreak/en/ (accessed 4 May 2004)

24 World Health Organization (WHO). Summary of the discussion and recommendations of the SARS laboratory workshop, 22 October 2003 – 5 November 2003. WHO website at: http://www.who.int/csr/sars/guidelines/en/SARSLab meeting.pdf (accessed 4 May 2004)

25 World Health Organization Department of Communicable Disease Surveillance and Response. WHO Scientific Research Advisory Committee on Severe Acute Respiratory Syndrome (SARS). Report of the first meeting. Geneva, Switzerland, 20–21 October 2003. WHO website at: http://www.who.int/csr/resources/publications/WHO_CDS_CSR_GAR_2004_16/en/ (accessed 4 May 2004)

ed. by A. Schmidt, M.H. Wolff and O. Weber

Performance evaluation of a Bayer Healthcare Diagnostics research-based SARS coronavirus assay

Charlene E. Bush-Donovan[1], Tony Mazzulli[2], Jill J. Detmer[1] and Johan Surtihadi[1]

[1] *Bayer Healthcare Diagnostics, 725 Potter Street, Aquatic Park Center 4, Berkeley, CA 94710-2722, USA*
[2] *Department of Microbiology, Mount Sinai Hospital, 600 University Avenue, Toronto, Ontario M5G 1X5, Canada*

Introduction

Severe acute respiratory syndrome (SARS) is an emerging infectious disease caused by a highly contagious coronavirus (SARS-CoV) that is transmitted through direct or indirect contact with secretions from mucous membranes [1, 2]. The disease first appeared in southern China in late 2002, and rapidly spread to 31 countries within the first 6 months of 2003 [3–5]. At the end of this epidemic, the World Health Organization (WHO) estimated the number of probable SARS cases at 8,098 with 774 deaths [6]. Since the initial epidemic was declared over by the WHO in July 2003, there have been several new laboratory confirmed cases of SARS in late 2003 and 2004 resulting from accidental research laboratory exposure (in Singapore, Taiwan and China) and animal or environmental exposure (in China) [7–10].

A recent Centers for Disease Control and Prevention (CDC) guideline for clinical specimen collection, diagnostic testing and an interpretation algorithm for SARS-CoV infection has been developed [11]. According to these guidelines, respiratory tract, blood and stool are the preferred specimens for serological and molecular diagnostic testing through the clinical course of the disease. Several enzyme immunoassays and immunofluorescent assays for serological diagnosis and reverse-transcriptase PCR (RT-PCR) assays for detection of SARS-CoV RNA in clinical specimens have been described [12–15].

Bayer Healthcare Diagnostics developed a research based RT-PCR assay for detection and quantification of SARS-CoV in clinical specimens during the 2002–2003 outbreak of SARS. (This assay is for research use only, not for use in diagnostic procedures.) This article describes this assay, together with the assay's validation and performance and compares it with the

RealArt™ HPA-Coronavirus LC RT PCR Kit (Artus GmbH, Hamburg, Germany) for detection of SARS-CoV RNA in clinical specimens.

SARS coronavirus detection assays

In an astounding research accomplishment, the full-length genome sequence of the SARS-CoV was available within weeks after the identification of the pathogen and the initial global WHO alert [16, 17]. The availability of the nucleotide sequence allowed for the development of specific molecular diagnostic assays to detect SARS-CoV RNA in clinical specimens.

Bayer Healthcare Diagnostics developed a one-step, real-time quantitative RT-PCR assay for SARS-CoV RNA quantification. Full genomic sequences of SARS-CoV were used to design homologous forward and reverse primers and fluorescent labeled TaqMan probe targeting a 67-base pair nucleocapsid genomic region. Primer and probe design included a BLAST search with other human coronaviruses and human genomic DNA to exclude sequence cross reactivity [18]. A second heterologous amplification system including forward and reverse primers, fluorescent labeled TaqMan probe and target was included as an internal control for the assay process including sample preparation and PCR amplification.

One-step amplification reactions were performed using the Qiagen® OneStep RT-PCR kit (Qiagen, Valencia, CA, USA) in a reaction volume of 25 μl containing 5 μl of target (extracted patient tissue RNA and heterologous internal control RNA). Reactions were first incubated at 55°C for 30 min to complete the reverse transcriptase step followed by incubation at 95°C for 15 min to inactivate the RT enzyme. Reactions were then thermocycled with the following parameters: denaturation at 95°C for 30 sec followed by 40 cycles of 60°C for 60 sec and 72°C for 30 sec. The Stratagene MX3000P™ Real-Time PCR System (Stratagene, La Jolla, CA, USA) was used to analyze the emitted fluorescence during amplification. Positive and negative controls, containing standardized SARS viral culture RNA extract from cell culture supernatants of VeroE6 cells (National Center for Infectious Diseases, CDC, Atlanta, GA, USA) and nuclease-free RNA diluent, respectively, were included in each run. External standards for SARS-CoV RNA quantification were prepared with serial dilutions of quantified SARS-CoV RNA culture extract, with concentrations ranging from 10 to 10^6 copies/5 μl reaction. The quantification standards were value assigned in comparison with three lots of purified RNA transcripts generated from the nucleocapsid region cloned into a plasmid (pCR-N9). The plasmid was provided through a material transfer agreement with the CDC. The RNA transcripts were prepared from the T7 promoter using the MEGAscript™ In Vitro Transcription Kit (Ambion, Austin, TX, USA). The concentration of the transcripts was determined by measuring the absorbance at 260 and

280 nm. These quantified viral RNA standards were treated as purified samples, tested in 5 µl volumes in an amplification reaction and used to calculate SARS-CoV viral load in clinical specimens.

The RealArt™ HPA-Coronavirus LightCycler® RT Reagents Assay (Artus GmbH, Hamburg, Germany) with a LightCycler® real-time PCR instrument (Roche Diagnostics, Laval, Canada) was performed according to the manufacturer's instructions. Viral load was calculated from a standard curve based on four external positive controls, ranging from 10 to 10^4 copies/µl, included in the assay kit. Assay performance was defined in the User Manual provided with the RealArt™ HPA-Coronavirus LC RT PCR Kit (Artus).

The performance of the Bayer Healthcare Diagnostics research-based SARS-associated coronavirus assay (Bayer Assay) and the Artus RealArt™ HPA-Coronavirus LC RT PCR assay (Artus Assay) were compared for detection of SARS-CoV RNA in clinical specimens. Identical parallel RNA extracts from clinical specimens were used in this performance evaluation.

Bayer Healthcare research-based SARS-associated coronavirus assay performance

Assay sensitivity is defined as the lowest concentration of SARS virus that can be detected 95% of the time, and is expressed in terms of the limit of detection (LoD). Assay sensitivity was determined by testing a serial dilution panel of SARS viral culture RNA extract, consisting of 9 levels ranging from 0.5 copies/5 µl to 20 copies/5 µl and analyzed with the Stratagene MX3000P™ Real-Time PCR System (Stratagene). Each level of the dilution panel was tested in a total of 27 replicates (9 replicates per run over 3 runs).

In a real-time PCR assay, the threshold cycle is defined as the cycle at which the system begins to detect the increase in signal associated with an exponential growth of PCR product during the log-linear phase. The percent detected, that is the percentage of results with the threshold cycle (CT) value less than 40, at each level of the dilution panel was calculated. The percent detected was then fitted against the log concentration using a logistic regression model. The LoD was estimated by the concentration where the model predicted percent detected was 95%.

Table 1 shows the observed and predicted percent detected for each dilution level of the SARS viral culture RNA extract panel. The LoD was estimated by the concentration where the predicted % detected was 95% (Fig. 1). Based on this panel, the estimated LoD was 9.30 copies/5 µl (0.974 log copies/5 µl).

In a real-time quantitative RT-PCR assay, the mean CT value is inversely proportional to the log input concentration. In practice, one way to assess

Table 1: Observed and predicted % detected for the viral RNA culture extract panel

Concentration (copies/5 μl)	Log concentration	N	Observed % detected	Predicted % detected (from logistic regression model)
0.5	-0.301	27	7.4%	6.2%
1	0.000	27	22.2%	20.2%
2	0.301	27	44.4%	49.2%
3	0.477	27	66.7%	68.0%
4	0.602	27	81.5%	78.8%
5	0.699	27	85.2%	85.1%
7.5	0.875	27	92.6%	92.6%
10	1.000	27	92.6%	95.7%
15	1.176	27	100.0%	98.0%
20	1.301	27	100.0%	98.8%

the linearity of such an assay is to plot the mean CT value against the log input concentration and fit a simple linear regression. Assay linearity is established if the regression plot has a slope close to the theoretical value of –3.32.

Assay precision (reproducibility) is a measure of assay variability in repeated testing of replicates of an identical input under varying test conditions, such as within-run and between-run replications. Assay precision is commonly expressed in terms of the standard deviation (SD) or coefficient of variation (% CV) associated with the test condition.

To assess the linearity and precision of the Bayer Assay, a dilution panel, made of SARS viral culture RNA, was constructed and tested across multiple runs, by two operators on three instruments. The virus panel consisted of 6 levels, ranging from 10 to 10^6 copies. The dilution levels of 10 to 10^4 copies were each tested for a total of 32 replicates (8 replicates per run over 4 runs); the dilution levels of 10^5 and 10^6 copies were each tested for a total of 20 replicates (5 replicates per run over 4 runs). The heterologous amplification system that serves as an internal control was added to each well of all dilution levels. Signal generated from the internal control increased confidence in the real-time PCR result and helped to eliminate the occurrence of false negatives.

The following analyses were performed on the data from the dilution panel:

- The percent detected (percentage of results with CT value less than 40) was calculated for each level of the dilution.
- The mean CT was calculated for each dilution level, based on all CT values that were less than 40. The mean CT was plotted against the $\log_{10}$ nominal concentration to assess linearity of the assay response. A linear regression was fitted on the plot and the regression equation and R^2 were also calculated.

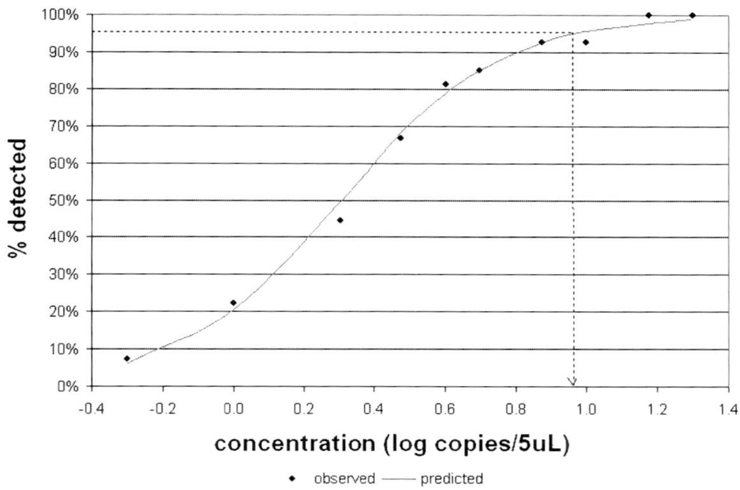

Figure 1. Assay sensitivity: percent detected (percentage of results with the threshold cycle (CT) value less than 40) fitted against the log concentration using a logistic regression model.

- A linear mixed model was used to estimate the component of variations of the CT values due to between-run and within-run variability, based on CT values that were less than 40. The assay precision was expressed in terms of SD due to between-run, within-run, and total components. The corresponding % CV was also calculated. The total SD of the CT values for the dilution panel was plotted against the nominal concentration.
- The CT values of the internal control (IC) were analyzed to assess the detection of the IC and the stability of the IC signal relative to the concentration of the panel. Additionally, the variability of the CT values of the IC, expressed in terms of the total SD was also evaluated.

Table 2 shows the percent detected, mean CT, SDs and % CV of CT, for the viral culture RNA extract panel.

Figure 2 shows the plot of the mean CT value against the $\log_{10}$ nominal concentration for the viral culture RNA extract dilution panel. The regression plot has a slope of –3.535. Furthermore, the R^2 value shown on the plot indicates that the linear regression fit the data very well, thus showing the highly linear response of the assay.

Figure 3 shows the precision profile of the assay. The total SD of the CT values for the viral culture RNA extract dilution panel was plotted against $\log_{10}$ nominal concentration. The plot shows that the precision was fairly constant from 10^2 copies to the upper limit of the dynamic range (10^6 copies). The highest SD was observed at 10 copies, with a total SD of 1.21, however, this corresponds to only about 3.3% CV.

Table 2. Linearity and precision of the viral culture RNA extract panel

Nominal concentration (copies/5 μl)	N	% detected	Mean CT	Between-run SD	Within-run SD	Total SD	Between-run %CV	Within-run %CV	Total %CV
10	32	96.9%	36.23	0.75	0.95	1.21	2.1%	2.6%	3.3%
10^2	32	100%	32.50	0.44	0.34	0.55	1.4%	1.0%	1.7%
10^3	32	100%	29.05	0.43	0.36	0.56	1.5%	1.2%	1.9%
10^4	32	100%	25.46	0.44	0.24	0.50	1.7%	0.9%	2.0%
10^5	20	100%	21.97	0.48	0.14	0.50	2.2%	0.6%	2.3%
10^6	20	100%	18.52	0.47	0.33	0.57	2.5%	1.8%	3.1%

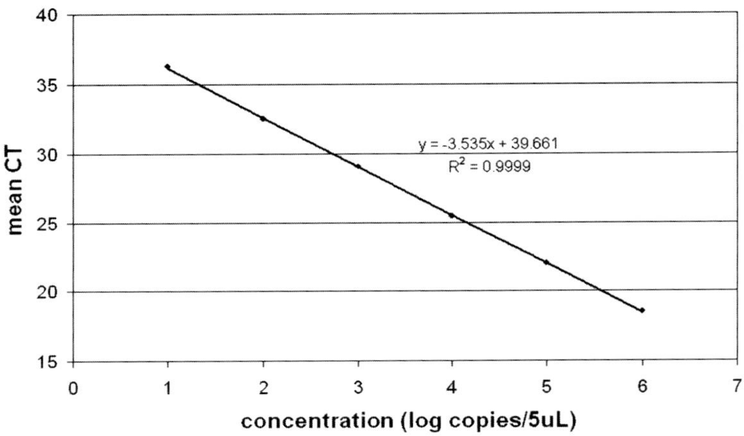

Figure 2. Assay viral culture RNA extract linearity panel: mean CT *versus* concentration. The assay response is highly linear ($R^2 = 0.9999$).

Table 3 shows the summary statistics of the internal control CT value. For the viral culture panel runs, the internal control was detected in all wells up to a target concentration of 10^6 copies. Furthermore, the variability of the CT values, expressed in terms of the total SD, was very small and stable across the dynamic range of the assay. Thus the internal control provides a reliable signal for the assay process as well as for detecting amplification inhibition.

Figure 4 shows the plot of the mean CT of the IC against the nominal concentration of the viral RNA extract panel.

Analytical specificity was assessed by testing nucleic acid extracts from a control panel of common viral and bacterial respiratory pathogens acquired from the American Type Culture Collection (ATCC, Manassas, Va, USA.). Clinical specificity was assessed by testing nucleic acid extracts

Table 3. Summary statistics of the CT values of the internal control (IC)

Panel	Panel nominal concentration (copies/5 μl)	Total N of IC	N detected	% detected	IC CT mean	Total SD
virus	10	32	32	100%	35.3	0.33
virus	10^2	32	32	100%	35.1	0.29
virus	10^3	32	32	100%	34.9	0.34
virus	10^4	32	32	100%	34.8	0.36
virus	10^5	20	20	100%	35.2	0.49
virus	10^6	20	20	100%	35.3	0.43

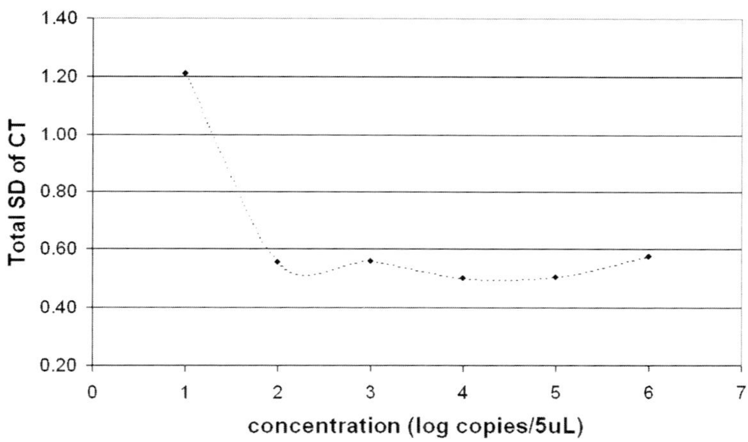

Figure 3. Assay precision profile: total standard deviation (SD) *versus* concentration. The precision was fairly constant form 10^2 copies to the upper limit of the dynamic range (10^6 copies).

from lung tissue, nasopharyngeal swabs (NPS) and whole blood. Lung was derived from patients who died during the SARS outbreak in Toronto, but who did not have SARS as defined by the CDC and WHO definitions. Permission to use the lung tissues was obtained by the Chief Coroner's Office of Ontario. NP swabs were from non-SARS patients with respiratory symptoms who did not meet the criteria for SARS. Permission to use these samples was from the IRBs at Mount Sinai Hospital and University Health Network. Whole blood samples were purchased from the Sacramento Blood Bank (Sacramento, CA, USA).

Table 4 shows the results of the specificity study. The Bayer Assay showed high specificity, in that there was no amplification signal from any nucleic acid target in the control panel or the SARS negative clinical specimens.

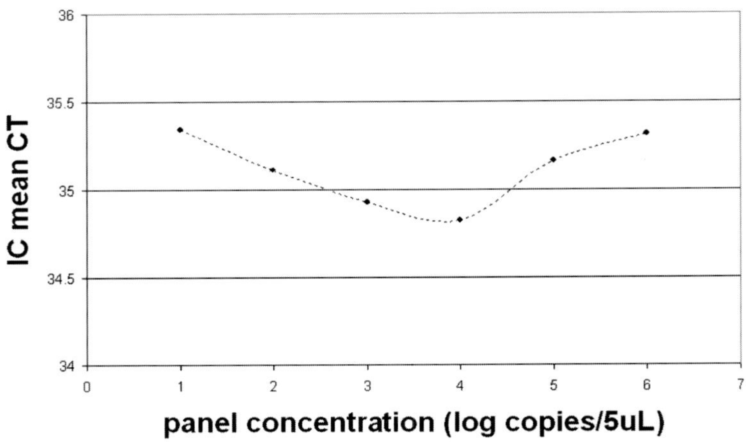

Figure 4. Mean internal control: CT *versus* concentration of the viral culture RNA extract panel. The internal control provides a reliable signal for the assay process as well as for detecting amplification inhibition.

Table 4. Summary of Bayer assay specificity

Pathogens	ATCC number	Total number of samples	SARS-CoV primer/probe set	Internal control primer/probe set
SARS coronavirus	CDC passage # 3	1	Positive	Positive
Influenza A	ATCC VR-1520	1	Negative	Positive
Influenza B	ATCC VR-101	1	Negative	Positive
Parainfluenza 1	ATCC VR-94	1	Negative	Positive
Parainfluenza 3	ATCC VR-93	1	Negative	Positive
Respiratory synocytial virus B	ATCC VR-1401	1	Negative	Positive
Adenovirus type 4	ATCC VR-1081	1	Negative	Positive
Adenovirus type 21	ATCC VR-1098	1	Negative	Positive
Mycoplasma pneumoniae	ATCC 15293	1	Negative	Positive
Human coronavirus 229E	ATCC VR740	1	Negative	Positive
SARS-CoV negative clinical samples		**Total number of samples**	**SARS-CoV primer/probe set**	**Internal control primer/probe set**
Lung tissue extracts		10	Negative	Positive
NPS extracts		10	Negative	Positive
Human genomic DNA extracts		5	Negative	Positive

Clinical performance evaluation of the Bayer Healthcare assay

Clinical specimens were collected from patients who met the CDC and WHO case definitions for probable SARS in Toronto, Canada, between March and June 2003. Permission to use the clinical samples for research purposes was obtained from the Research Ethics Boards at the Mount Sinai Hospital and University Health Network, Toronto and for the tissue samples from the Chief Coroner's Office of Ontario, Canada.

All samples were stored at –70 °C until tested. Stool and bronchoalveolar lavage (BAL) samples were collected in a clean, sterile container. NPS specimens were collected using a flexible dacron-tipped swab and placed into viral transport media (Starplex Scientific Inc., Etobicoke, Canada). Tissue samples collected during autopsies were placed into sterile containers and snap frozen immediately in a solution of absolute ethanol and dry ice.

Prior to RNA extraction, mucoid BAL specimens were mixed with an equal volume of physiological salt (0.9% NaCl) containing 1% N-acetylcysteine (Sigma-Aldrich Ltd.,Ontario, Canada) and incubated for 30 min. For non-mucoid BAL specimens and NP specimens and treated BAL specimens, RNA was extracted from 140 µl of specimen using the QIAamp Viral RNA Mini Kit (Qiagen, Mississauga, Canada).

One gram of each stool sample was mixed in 5 ml of distilled RNase-free water and vortexed. It was then allowed to settle at room temperature for 5 min before vortexing again. A volume of 140 µl of stool specimen was then mixed in 560 µl RNeasy Lysis Buffer (RLT buffer, Qiagen) and pipetted directly onto a QIAshredder spin column (Qiagen) placed in a 2 mL collection tube followed by centrifugation for 2 min. The supernatant was then transferred to a new microfuge tube and RNA was extracted using the RNeasy Mini Kit (Qiagen).

Thirty milligrams of frozen tissue derived from lung, colon, kidney, skeletal muscle and liver was homogenized in 600 µl of RLT buffer using disposable tissue grinders (Kendall Precision TM, Mansfield, MA, USA). The homogenate was then passed through QIAshredder spin columns as was done for stool specimens. RNA was extracted using the RNeasy Mini Kit (Qiagen). Extracted RNA was then frozen at –70°C prior to testing.

Postmortem lung, liver, colon, kidney, skeletal muscle and liver specimens as well as stool and NPS specimens were tested by the Bayer and/or the Artus assays to assess viral load. Table 5 shows the results comparing the two assays performed on the same RNA extract from the same tissue and Table 6 shows the results of the two assays performed on different extracts from the same tissue. The assays showed perfect qualitative agreement, with 18 specimens positive for SARS-CoV RNA by both assays and 9 specimens negative by both assays. Both assays were able to detect as few as 4 copies of SARS-CoV RNA in a microliter of clinical sample extract.

Table 5. Comparison of Bayer and Artus assays tested on clinical specimens[a]

Sample number	Sample description	Bayer assay[b] Qualitative results	Bayer assay[b] Copies of CoV per ml extract	Artus assay[c] Qualitative results	Artus assay[c] Copies of CoV per ml extract
1	Lung RL	Positive	57,525,000	Positive	25,010,000
2	Lung LUL	Positive	402	Positive	384
3	Lung LL	Negative	0	Negative	0
4	Lung RL	Positive	553,600	Positive	142,700
5	Lung LLL	Positive	1,229	Positive	838
6	Lung RUL	Positive	171	Positive	153
7	Lung LL	Positive	4	Positive	3
8	Lung LUL	Positive	7	Positive	4
9	Lung 9	Positive	21,393	Positive	4,949
10	Lung LLL	Positive	20	Positive	14
11	Lung LL	Positive	17,588,000	Positive	3,269,000
12	Lung RL	Positive	7	Positive	5
13	Small bowel	Negative	0	Negative	0
14	NPS (R)	Negative	0	Negative	0
15	NPS (S)	Negative	0	Negative	0
16	NPS (T)	Positive	7	Positive	53
17	BAL (U)	Positive	6,632	Positive	2,891
18	BAL (V)	Positive	270,400	Positive	174,900
19	BAL (W)	Negative	0	Negative	0
20	BAL (X)	Negative	0	Negative	0
21	BAL #6 right	Positive	4	Positive	27
22	Stool	Negative	0	Negative	0

[a]Quantitative results in both asseys are derived from same extract.
[b]Bayer research-based SARS-associated CoV RT-PCR assay
[c]Artus RealArt™ HPA coronavirus RT-PCR kit
RL, right lobe; RUL, right upper lobe; LUL, left upper lobe; LL, left lobe; LLL, Left lower lobe; BAL, bronchoalveolar lavage; NPS, nasopharyngeal swab

Table 6. Comparison of the Bayer and Artus assays on additional clinical tissues[a]

Sample number	Sample description	Bayer[b] Qualitative results	Bayer[b] Copies of CoV per ml extract	Artus[c] Qualitative results	Artus[c] Copies of CoV per ml extract
1	large bowel	Positive	108	Positive	365
2	kidney	Positive	496	Positive	367
3	skeletal muscle	Negative	0	Negative	0
4	small bowel	Positive	10,804,000	Positive	1,613,000
5	liver	Negative	0	Negative	0

[a]Quantitative results in both assays are derived from different extract from same patient tissue section.
[b]Bayer research-based SARS-associated CoV RT-PCR assay
[c]Artus RealArt™ HPA coronavirus RT-PCR kit

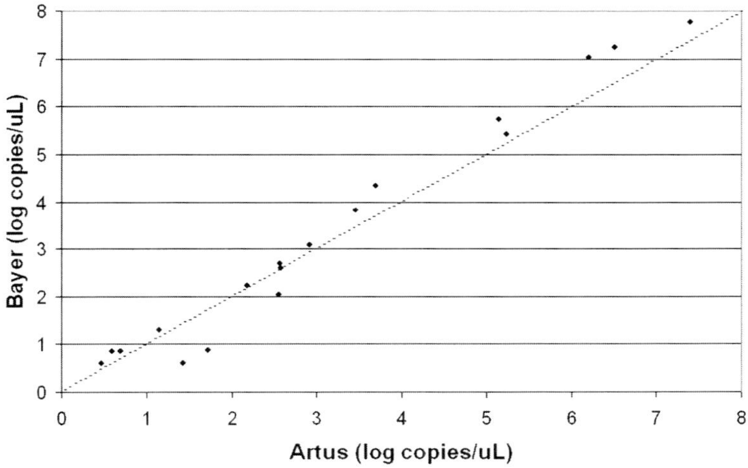

Figure 5. Comparison between Bayer and Artus assay quantification. The correlation coefficient for SARS-CoV RNA concentrations between the assays was 0.98. The Bayer results frequently quantified higher than the Artus results (about 1.4 folds).

The quantitative results of the Bayer and Artus assays given in Tables 5 and 6 were plotted in Figure 5. The correlation coefficient for SARS-CoV RNA concentrations between the Bayer and Artus assays was 0.98. As shown in the plot, the Bayer results frequently quantified higher than the Artus results. On the average, the Bayer results were 0.14 logs (about 1.4 fold) higher than the Artus assay. The higher viral loads detected by the Bayer Assay may be due to the fact that this assay targets the nucleocapsid region of the SARS RNA genome, while the Artus Assay targets the polymerase region. Other investigators have noted that PCR assays targeting the nucleocapsid region achieve higher quantitative values than assays targeting the polymerase region of the SARS-CoV genome [13, 19, 20]. It is speculated that in some tissues, subgenomic fragments that contain the nucleocapsid gene may be present and contribute to the overall signal. Further studies are needed to investigate the mechanism for the higher quantification observed between these two assays.

Discussion

Shortly after the identification of a novel coronavirus (SARS-CoV) as the etiologic agent of SARS, a number of home-brew and commercial assays were developed to aid in the laboratory diagnosis. The most widely used assays continue to be either molecular amplification assays (e.g. RT-PCR) for the detection of SARS-CoV RNA in clinical specimens or serologic assays for the detection of specific SARS-CoV antibodies in serum. However, due to the urgent need for laboratory tests during the SARS outbreak, many assays were put into clinical use worldwide without undergoing a complete assessment of their performance characteristics. This is reflected in the CDC guidelines for laboratory confirmation of SARS infection that cautions that all assays remain investigational.

The results of this study show that the newly developed RT-PCR assay by Bayer Healthcare Diagnostics performs extremely well for the detection of SARS-CoV RNA in clinical specimens. It is very sensitive, detecting as few as 10 copies of SARS-CoV RNA and has a wide dynamic range (10 to 10^6 copies). Both the analytical and clinical specificities were 100%. There was no cross reactivity with other more common respiratory viruses and testing of clinical samples from non-SARS patients were negative. It should be noted, however, that according to the CDC guidelines, one cannot rule out a diagnosis of SARS based on a negative molecular assay. Early in the course of infection, viral shedding may be too low for detection by many assays. As well, there may be differences in the performance of many assays depending upon the specimen type.

One of the first commercially available PCR assays during the outbreak was the RealArt HPA-Coronavirus LC RT-PCR assay (Artus). Both the Artus and the Bayer assays are based on real-time PCR platforms and thus provide relatively rapid results. By standardizing the specimen processing and RNA extraction methods before performing either the Artus or Bayer assays, we were able to show that both assays were highly correlated. The qualitative results (positive or negative) of the Artus and Bayer assays were identical. The quantitative results of the Bayer assay on the average were 0.14 logs (about 1.4 fold) higher than the Artus assay. The difference in viral load quantification may be due to assay design. The Bayer assay targets the nucleocapsid region while the Artus assay targets the polymerase region. Additionally, although both assays have the same input volume of 5 μl of target into the amplification reaction, the copy number of the Bayer standards ranges between 10 to 10^6 copies/5 μl while the Artus assay standards range between 50 to 5×10^4 copies/5 μl. The excellent correlation between these assays and the fact that the assays target different genomic regions suggests that each can be used to confirm a positive result obtained with the other, fulfilling the CDC requirement for a laboratory confirmed case of SARS.

At the time of writing, there are no known human cases of SARS anywhere in the world. Despite this, the potential for new cases to re-appear remains. The availability of properly validated, sensitive and specific assays is essential if new cases are to be accurately diagnosed particularly in light of the fact that the clinical definition of suspect and probable SARS remain very broad and somewhat non-specific.

References

1 World Health Organization. Consensus document on the epidemiology of severe acute respiratory syndrome (SARS). Available at: http://www.who.int/csr/sars/en/WHOconsensus.pdf. Accessed 2 December 2003

2 Peiris J, Phil D, Yuen K, Osterhaus A, Stohr K (2003) The acute respiratory syndrome. *N Engl J Med* 349: 2431–2441

3 Centers for Disease Control and Prevention. Update: outbreak of severe acute respiratory syndrome – worldwide, 2003. *MMWR Morb Mortal Wkly Rep* 52: 241–248

4 Lee N, Hui D, Wu A, Chan P, Cameron P, Joynt G, Ahuja A, Yung M, Leung C, To K et al (2003) A major outbreak of severe acute respiratory syndrome in Hong Kong. *N Engl J Med* 348: 1886–1994

5 Poutanen S, Low D, Henry B, Finkelstein S, Rose D, Green K, Tellier R, Draker R, Adachi D, Ayers M et al (2003) Identification of severe acute respiratory syndrome in Canada. *N Engl J Med* 348: 1995–2005

6 World Health Organization. Cumulative number of reported probable cases of SARS. Available at: http://www.who.int/csr/sars/country/2003_04_21/en/. Accessed 17 November 2003

7 Parry J (2004) Breaches of safety regulations are probable cause of recent SARS outbreak, WHO says. *Br Med J* 328: 1222

8 World Health Organization. (CSR): Severe acute respiratory syndrome in Singapore. Available at: http://www.who/int/csr/don/2003_09_16/en/. Accessed 16 September 2003

9 World Health Organization. Update 4: Review of probable and laboratory-confirmed SARS cases in southern China. Available at: http://www.who.int/csr/don/2004_01_27/en. Accessed 27 January 2004

10 World Health Organization. (CSR): Severe acute respiratory syndrome (SARS) in Taiwan and China. Available at: http://www.who.int/csr/don/2003_12_17/en/. Accessed 17 December 2003

11 Centers for Disease Control and Prevention. Public health guidance for community-level preparedness and response to severe acute respiratory syndrome, Supplement F: Available at: www.dhss.state.mo.us/SARS/SupF.pdf Accessed 8 January 2004.

12 Ksiazek T, Erdman D, Goldsmith C, Zaki S, Peret T, Emery S, Tong S, Urbani C, Comer J, Lim W et al (2003) A novel coronavirus associated with severe acute respiratory syndrome. *N Engl J Med* 348: 1953–1966

13 Ng E, Hui D, Chan K, Hung E, Chiu R, Lee N, Wu A, Chim S, Tong Y, Sung J et al (2003) Quantitative analysis and prognostic implication of SARS coronavirus RNA in the plasma and serum of patients with severe acute respiratory syndrome. *Clin Chem* 49: 11976–1980

14 Poon L, Chan K, Wong O, Cheung T, Ng I, Zheng B, Seto W, Yuen K, Guan Y, Peiris J (2004) Detection of SARS coronavirus in patients with severe acute respiratory syndrome by conventional and real-time quantitative reverse transcription-PCR assays. *Clin Chem* 50: 67–72

15 Mazzulli T, Farcas G, Poutanen S, Willey B, Low D, Butany J, Asa S, Kain K (2004) Severe acute respiratory syndrome-associated coronavirus in lung tissue. *Emerging Infect Dis* 10: 20–24

16 Rota P, Oberste M, Monroe S, Nix W, Campagnoli R, Icenogle J, Penaranda S, Bankamp B, Maher K, Chen M-H et al (2003) Characterization of a novel coronavirus associated with severe acute respiratory syndrome. *Science* 300 (5624): 1394–1398

17 Marra M, Jones S, Astell C, Holt R, Brooks-Wilson A, Butterfield Y, Khattra J, Asano J, Barber S, Chan S et al (2003) The genome sequence of the SARS-associated coronavirus. *Science* 300 (5624): 1399–1404

18 BLAST available from: URL: http://www.ncbi.nlm.nih.gov/BLAST/

19 Hui RK, Zeng F, Chan C, Yuen K, Peiris J, Leung F (2004) Reverse transcriptase PCR diagnostic assay for the coronavirus associated with severe acute respiratory syndrome. *J Clin Microbiol* 42: 1994–1999

20 Weidmann M, Zanotto P, Weber F, Spiegel M, Brodt H, Hufert F (2004) High-efficiency detection of severe acute respiratory syndrome virus genetic material. *J Clin Microbiol* 42: 2771–2773

Coronaviruses with Special Emphasis on First Insights Concerning SARS
ed. by A. Schmidt, M.H. Wolff and O. Weber

Current status of therapy of SARS

Arthur Chun-Wing Lau, Loletta Kit-Ying So and Loretta Yin-Chun Yam

Division of Respiratory and Critical Care Medicine, Department of Medicine, Pamela Youde Nethersole Eastern Hospital, Hong Kong SAR, PR China

Introduction

The severe acute respiratory syndrome (SARS) caused by the SARS-associated coronavirus (SARS-CoV) has caused a worldwide outbreak in 2003. This chapter will start with a description of the pathogenesis of this disease, followed by a review of the various pharmacological treatments and supportive ventilatory strategies adopted during the outbreak. The principles used to design various combinations of therapeutic agents and treatment modalities will also be described based on the present knowledge.

Pathogenesis

SARS has been postulated to cause a three-phased illness [1]. The first is the viral replication phase, which is associated with increasing viral load and the resultant host reaction in the form of fever and other systemic symptoms. While symptoms may improve or subside in some patients, the second phase of immunopathological damage occurs in the majority, and is reflected by pulmonary manifestations with varying degrees of clinical severity about 10 days after symptom onset. This phase corresponds to peaking of the viral load followed by it fall subsequent to the onset of IgG seroconversion. It is characterized by the recrudescence of fever, oxygen desaturation and radiological progression of pneumonitis, as well as intense macrophage activation in the lungs [2]. About 20% of patients may develop acute respiratory distress syndrome (ARDS) at this stage. The final phase is pulmonary destruction in a proportion of cases, especially if the over-exuberant host response in the second immunopathological phase remains uncontrolled.

Pharmacological therapy

There is no consensus on the types of pharmacological therapy which may be effective for SARS. In general, since the definitive laboratory diagnosis of SARS may only be made 3–5 days after symptom onset, empirical antibiotics are still indicated in the presence of pulmonary infiltrates. Antiviral and immunomodulatory agents have also been used empirically in the 2003 outbreak and will also be reviewed in this chapter.

Antibiotics

Although not active against SARS-CoV, antibiotics are prescribed by most physicians to SARS patients on initial presentation, before microbiological confirmation is obtained [3–5]. Antibiotics are chosen to cover both typical and atypical organisms according to published treatment guidelines for community-acquired pneumonia (CAP) [6]. Co-infection with other organisms which may or may not benefit from antibiotics was not uncommon in the last outbreak, including metapneumovirus [7], *Chlamydia*-like agents [8], influenza virus and parvovirus B19 [9]. Amoxicillin-clavulanate and clarithromycin, or levofloxacin alone are often used as initial treatment [3]. Broader spectrum antibiotics may be used in the presence of severe CAP, whereas potent anti-pseudomonal antibiotics like piperacillin-tazobactam, imipenam-cilastatin or cefoperazone-sulbactam should be reserved for potential complication by superimposed sepsis, which may be expected when corticosteroids are used or mechanical ventilation is instituted. A centre has recommended the early use of potent and broad spectrum antibiotics coverage (ceftriaxone or cefipime or levofloxacin) to treat and/or prevent possible underlying bacterial infection which may be associated with early use of pulsed doses of corticosteroid for SARS [10].

Antiviral therapy

Ribavirin

Because of its broad-spectrum antiviral activity against many DNA and RNA viruses, this nucleoside analogue was chosen as empirical treatment early in the 2003 outbreak even before the SARS-CoV was identified. Subsequent clinical experience showed that ribavirin did not appear to have significant effects on the clinical course in terms of fever subsidence, improvement in oxygen saturation and clearing up of chest radiograph shadows. The use of ribavirin was however continued in most centres because no better anti-viral agents were available, and there were reports suggesting that, despite only weak viral inhibitory activity, it appeared to possess some immunomodulatory effects. In the treatment of mouse coronavirus hepatitis these were mediated by inhibition of induction of macrophage pro-inflammatory cytokines and Th2 cytokines while preserving Th1 cytokines [11]. Monitoring of quantitative reverse transcriptase polymerase chain reaction (RT-PCR) in nasopharyngeal aspirates could not however demonstrate any antiviral effect *in vivo* [1]. Subsequently, it was also found that ribavirin has no or only slight *in vitro* activity against SARS-CoV [12], and inhibitory dosages may not be achievable clinically [13]. Because of its teratogenic effect, double contraception for up to seven months must be practised after the cessation of ribavirin therapy. Other side effects are dose related and are more common in the elderly. They include haemolytic anemia, elevated transaminase levels and bradycardia. Health Canada has stopped further use of ribavirin for SARS [14], while Hong Kong has planned to test this drug in a randomized controlled trial together with Kaletra should there be another outbreak.

Lopinavir-ritonavir (kaletra)

Among various anti-viral drugs screened, lopinavir-ritonavir co-formulation (Kaletra®, Abbott Laboratories, USA) was found to be active against the prototype SARS-CoV HKU39849 *in vitro* [15]. Only the lopinavir component has activity against SARS-CoV, while ritonavir inhibits the CYP3A-mediated metabolism of lopinavir and increases its serum concentration. Lopinavir can inhibit the coronaviral proteases and block the processing of the viral replicase polyprotein, thus preventing the replication of viral RNA. Synergism was also demonstrated with lopinavir and ribavirin when used in combination [15]. In a retrospective matched cohort study from Hong Kong, the only SARS outbreak area having experience with this drug [15], 75 patients given kaletra (lopinavir 400 mg/ritonavir 100 mg orally every 12 hours), ribavirin and corticosteroid were divided into two subgroups for analysis. Forty-four patients in whom kaletra was given as initial treatment at 5.5 days (median) after symptom onset were compared with a matched cohort who received only ribavirin and corticosteroid. The kaletra group showed reduction in the overall death rate and intubation rate, and a lower requirement for pulsed methylprednisolone rescue. In 31 patients who had received kaletra later in the course of the illness as rescue therapy following poor response to ribavirin and corticosteroid, such benefits were not seen. In another Hong Kong study [16], 41 SARS patients treated with a combination of kaletra, ribavirin and corticosteroid were compared with 111 matched historical controls given ribavirin and corticosteroid only. Lower incidences of adverse clinical outcomes in terms of ARDS or death at day 21 after symptom onset were seen in the kaletra group. The findings from these two studies suggest that kaletra when combined with ribavirin may be effective as anti-viral agent against SARS. If this is the case, then early use of kaletra may decrease initial viral load during the viral replicative phase and hence ameliorate the subsequent immunopathological lung damage. Based on these retrospective data, kaletra will be studied in combination with ribavirin in a randomized controlled trial planned for future SARS treatment in Hong Kong.

Interferons

Interferons belong to a group of cytokines controlling the cellular immune response. Their antiviral activities are mediated by direct effects on infected cells and by modulating the host's immune response [17]. *In vitro* testing of three recombinant interferons against SARS-CoV showed that interferon (IFN)-β was more potent than IFN-α or IFN-γ in prophylaxis and as antiviral agent after infection [18]. Another study reported complete inhibition of the cytopathic effects of SARS-CoV in culture by IFN subtypes, β 1b, α n1, α n3, and human leukocyte IFN-α [13]. Similar activity was also reported for IFN-β 1a in a third *in vitro* study [19], with therapeutic dosages shown to be effective and acceptable in monkeys [20]. IFN-α has been used for treatment of SARS in China and Canada [21, 22]. In an open-label uncontrolled Canadian study [22], 13 patients treated with corticosteroids alone as initial treatment were compared with nine given corticosteroids plus IFN alfacon-1 (Infergen®, InterMune Inc., Brisbane, CA, USA). The latter group showed shorter time to 50% resolution of radiographic abnormalities in the lungs, better oxygen saturation and earlier cessation of supplemental oxygen with decreased elevations in creatine kinase levels. Based on these *in vitro* and *in vivo* data, selected interferons, either alone or in combination with other antiviral drugs, appear to show promising treatment efficacy in human.

Immunomodulatory therapy

Corticosteroids

When the patient enters the immunopathological phase, intense macrophage and cytokine activation occurs in the lungs, resulting in severe pneumonitis and respiratory failure [23]. An immunomodulatory agent is usually given to control the over-exuberant host response, and corticosteroids had been most commonly used for this purpose in the 2003 outbreak.

Different series have reported different methods of corticosteroid prescription. Treatment had been started after no demonstrable response to antibiotics, as soon as epidemiologic history of contact with SARS could be established [24], or based on a set of surrogate clinical markers which may reflect over-reactive host response [3]. Because of the diversities regarding the route of administration, dosages and types (prednisolone, methylprednisolone, hydrocortisone, and dexamethasone) of corticosteroids used, as well as the duration of administration, conclusions about the efficacy of this drug are difficult to reach. Moreover, more severe disease may prompt the use of higher dosages of corticosteroid, making the relationship between efficacy and corticosteroid use obtained in retrospective analysis not straightforward.

Based on the present knowledge about the disease, it appears logical that immunomodulatory agents like corticosteroids should be avoided in the early phase of viral replication. On the other hand, they have to be considered when there are signs suggestive of an over-reactive host response, which may be reflected by clinical and radiographic deterioration. Beneficial results may depend on the administration of adequate initial corticosteroid dosages for long enough to dampen the over-active immune response while avoiding rebound or over-immunosuppression [3, 25]. Initial steroid dosages ranged from oral prednisolone 1 mg/kg/day [4] to as high as pulsed methylprednisolone 500 mg intravenous daily for 5 days [10]. Retrospective data suggest that higher doses given for two to three weeks in the more severe cases had been of benefit [3, 10, 26, 27], although some "good responders" develop recurrence of respiratory failure after initial response. For these as well as for some "poor responders" [28], pulsed corticosteroid in the form of methylprednisolone 500 mg–1 g for two days may be effective as rescue therapy [3, 9, 21, 29].

Corticosteroids must be used cautiously because side effects are common. In addition to hospital-acquired infections which are associated with comparatively more adverse outcome in patients requiring mechanical ventilation, post-SARS avascular necrosis of hips and knees are common, in the order of 10 to 30% [30]. Fibrin thrombi have been found in small pulmonary arteries in autopsy studies [2, 31, 32], together with initial swelling of pulmonary vessels [2]. Moreover, systemic vasculitis including oedema, localised fibrinoid necrosis and infiltration of lymphocytes, monocytes and plasma cells into the vessel walls of the heart, lung, liver, kidneys, adrenals and stroma of striated muscles, as well as thrombosis of small veins, were seen in three SARS cases from Guangzhou, China [33]. SARS-CoV may thus have deleterious effects on the endothelium which predispose to small vessel thrombosis. In addition, up to 74% of 31 patients diagnosed to be suffering from osteonecrosis, primarily of the hip, were found to be suffering from one or more primary coagulation disorder, including 15/18 (83%) who initially were diagnosed as "idiopathic" avascular necrosis [34]. The coagulation disorders included thrombophilia and hypofibrinolysis. Further analyses are required to clarify whether or not avascular necrosis is due to corticosteroids, to underlying coagulation abnormalities, or to the SARS-CoV infection *per se*.

Our group first developed a standard treatment protocol in mid-March 2003, very early in the SARS outbreak in Hong Kong and before the SARS-CoV was identified. The protocol allowed commencement of high (but not pulsed) dose methylprednisolone only on worsening of clinical and radiographic parameters after a trial of antibiotics, with subsequent tapering over the next three weeks should there be satisfactory response [3]. This standard protocol was eventually applied to a total of 88 consecutively admitted SARS patients (mean age 42 years), of whom 97% had laboratory-confirmed SARS [9]. An overall mortality of 3.4% was observed, with all three deaths occurring in patients above the age of 65 years. A multi-centre study [21] comparing four treatment regimens in Guangzhou, China, also found that high dosages of corticosteroids adjusted according to clinical and radiological severity produced zero mortality in 60 clinically-defined SARS patients (mean age 30.5 years). These figures compared favourably with the estimated case fatality rates of 13.2% for patients <60 years old and 43.3% for patients >60 years old [35].

Immunoglobulin

Human gamma immunoglobulins have been used to treat SARS patients with poor response to corticosteroids. Pentaglobin (Pentaglobin®, Biotest Pharma GmbH, Dreieich, Germany), an IgM-enriched immunoglobulin product, has been tried in Hong Kong and hospitals in mainland China. When pentaglobin was given at 5 mg/kg/day for three consecutive days to 12 patients who deteriorated despite ribavirin and repeated rescue methylprednisolone, some improvement in radiographic scores and oxygen requirement was noted [36]. In a Singaporean series [37], methylprednisolone in combination with high-dose intravenous immunoglobulin (0.4 g/kg) was administered once daily for three consecutive days to 15 critically ill probable SARS patients with acute lung injury or ARDS. Compared to patients not given immunoglobulin, lower mortality and a trend towards earlier recovery were found. Randomized controlled trials in larger patient groups are required to confirm the efficacy of immunoglobulins.

Convalescent plasma

Convalescent plasma was used in several centres in Hong Kong in the more severe cases not apparently responding to other treatments. Plasma was taken from SARS patients in convalescence and re-infused into these sick patients in 200 ml aliquots daily for 2–3 days. It was believed that the neutralizing immunoglobulins in convalescent plasma may be able to decrease viral load, and early infusion was reported to provide some clinical benefits [38].

Other drugs

Many other drugs have been tried or considered in desperation during the 2003 outbreak. These included thymosin alpha 1 (Zadaxin®, SciClone Pharmaceuticals Inc., San Carlos, CA, USA), tumour necrosis factor blocking agents, namely etanercept (Enbrel®, Immunex Corp., Seattle, WA, USA) and infliximab (Remicade®, Centocor Inc., Malvem, PA, USA), and some other compounds including cyclophosphamide, azathioprine, cyclosporin and thalidomide.

Traditional Chinese medicine

Traditional Chinese herbal medicine had been used with Western medicine to treat SARS with good results reported from some centres in mainland China [39–41]. Compared to using Western medicine alone, shorter time to symptom improvement and fever subsidence, shorter duration of hospitalization, and corticosteroid use were seen. Because herbal medicines are traditionally used in combination, it is difficult to dissect out the efficacy of individual agents. Glycyrrhizin, an active component derived from liquorice roots, has been found to be effective against SARS-CoV *in vitro* when administered either during or after the viral adsorption period [12]. Since it is only effective at very high concentrations, however, its clinical utility remains uncertain. Another herb called baicalin has also demonstrated some anti-SARS-CoV activity (unpublished data).

Assisted ventilation

Despite all treatment efforts, many SARS patients still developed acute hypoxemic respiratory failure. Overall, 20–30% required intensive care unit (ICU) or high dependency care, and 13–26% developed ARDS [42]. The initial management of SARS-related respiratory failure is oxygen supplementation. Assisted ventilation through non-invasive or invasive means should be considered when hypoxaemia or dyspnoea persists.

Non-invasive ventilation (NIV) delivers continuous positive airway pressure (CPAP) or bi-level pressure support through a tight-fitting facial or nasal mask. It was commonly employed in many Chinese hospitals [43] and in our own centre in Hong Kong [44]. Advantages of NIV include: (1) rapid improvement in vital signs, oxygenation and tachypnoea, especially when applied early; (2) reduction of the need for increasing dosages of corticosteroids to treat progressive respiratory failure; (3) avoidance of intubation and invasive ventilation in up to two-thirds of critically ill SARS patients; (4) reduction of infective risk for such patients through reduction in mechanical ventilation requirement and hence ventilator-associated pneumonia which may be further aggravated by the use of corticosteroids; and (5) reduction of risks to healthcare workers through obviating the need for the potentially highly infectious procedure of intubation. Since patients who respond to NIV usually do so within 24 hours, non-responders who will eventually need endotracheal intubation can be identified early [44]. CPAP of 4–10 cm H_2O, or bi-level pressure support with inspiratory positive airway pressure (IPAP) < 10 cm H_2O and expiratory positive airway pressure (EPAP) of 4–6 cm H_2O are reasonable starting pressures [42]. Lower pressures are safer to start with because of the high frequency of spontaneous pneumomediastinum and subcutaneous emphysema [1] which would naturally be aggravated by positive pressure ventilation in any form.

Our centre had applied NIV to 20 out of 88 patients with persistent SARS-related acute respiratory failure [44]. Mean age was 51.4 and coronavirus serology was positive in 95%. NIV was started 9.6 days (mean) from symptom onset and the mean duration of usage was 84.3 hours. Endotracheal intubation was avoided in 14 patients (70%), in whom ICU stay could be shortened significantly (3.1 ± 2.1 days vs. 21.3 ± 21.2 days in intubated cases) and chest radiography scores within the first 24 hours of NIV were also lower. Successful avoidance of intubation was predicted by a marked reduction in respiratory rate and supplemental oxygen requirement within 24 hours of NIV. Complications were few and reversible. No infection was documented among the 105 health care workers caring for SARS patients on NIV in a high air change (initially eight and later > 12 per hour) and uni-directional negative pressure ventilation environment.

Invasive mechanical ventilation

When patients do not improve within 1–2 days of NIV or continue to deteriorate, or if NIV is contraindicated, endotracheal intubation and mechanical ventilation should be considered. It should be emphasised that endotracheal intubation is a procedure with high infective risk, and all staff involved must adhere to stringent infection control measures must be strictly adhered to [45]. Most centres adopted a ventilatory strategy similar to that recommended for ARDS from other causes [46]. The tidal volume should be kept low at 5–6 ml/kg predicted body weight and plateau pressures maintained below 30 cm H_2O because of a higher risk of barotrauma in SARS [1].

Treatment principles in relation to clinical course

While many patients had suffered from a severe illness in the 2003 outbreak, SARS can also present with a wide spectrum of severity. A minority of patients with mild respiratory illnesses recover, either without any specific form of treatment or on antibiotic therapy alone [3]. All four sporadic cases from Guangzhou in December 2003 – January 2004 belonged to this category [47]. For the majority of patients with definite epidemiological links or microbiological confirmation, it may be prudent to administer an anti-viral agent (kaletra ± ribavirin, ± interferon) as soon as SARS is diagnosed. An effective anti-viral agent may decrease the severity of the subsequent immunopathological damage and thus the need for salvage therapy with immunosuppressants. When a patient has entered the immunopathological phase, an immunomodulatory agent will likely be indicated. The optimal choice, dosages and duration of such therapy are not known, but retrospective experience suggest that dosages may be titrated according to disease severity, and that sufficiently large dosages given for longer durations may be required for the more severe cases. Pulsed methylprednisolone may be effective as rescue therapy in case of unsatisfactory response or recurrence of respiratory failure after initial response. If response remains poor despite the above treatment, immunoglobulin or other forms of treatment may be tried. Assisted ventilation in the form of NIV should be instituted early if the clinical course is complicated with significant respiratory failure. If response remains poor after 24 hours, elective intubation should be considered early so that ample time is available for institution of infection control measures before managing the airway in this highly infectious disease. When fever recurs later in the course of SARS treatment, the clinical picture may not be easily distinguishable from superimposed bacterial or even fungal sepsis [48]. Empirical anti-pseudomonal antibiotics would usually be indicated considering that the patient would have been put on immunomodulatory agents for some time. If clinical response is still not apparent and opportunistic infection is reasonably excluded, higher dosage of methylprednisolone can be considered in pulses for SARS rescue (e.g. MP 1 g for 2 days), especially if this had not been given previously. Most patients will respond with fever subsidence, improvement in chest radiograph and oxygen saturation. Chest radiograph may slightly lag behind clinical improvement but this feature *per se* may not warrant the use of additional steroid [49]. Radiological infiltrates will usually improve gradually despite reducing dosages of corticosteroids over the next 2–3 weeks. However, in a small proportion of critical SARS patients, the course is relentless and the 28-day intensive care unit mortality could be up to 26–37% [50, 51].

Conclusion

In this chapter, we have reviewed the pathogenesis, various treatment modalities and the treatment principles of SARS. Subsequent to unprecedented collaborative efforts among medical and research communities worldwide, we have already gained a large amount of knowledge about this novel virus within the short space of just over a year. However, randomized controlled treatment trials remain to be performed to improve our understanding of the most optimal treatment for this new disease.

References

1 Peiris JS, Chu CM, Cheng VC, Chan KS, Hung IF, Poon LL, Law KI, Tang BS, Hon TY, Chan CS et al; HKU/UCH SARS Study Group (2003) Clinical progression and viral load in a community outbreak of coronavirus-associated SARS pneumonia: a prospective study. *Lancet* 361: 1767–1772

2 Nicholls JM, Poon LL, Lee KC, Ng WF, Lai ST, Leung CY, Chu CM, Hui PK, Mak KL, Lim W et al (2003) Lung pathology of fatal severe acute respiratory syndrome. *Lancet* 361: 1773–1778

3 So LK, Lau AC, Yam LY, Cheung TM, Poon E, Yung RW, Yuen KY (2003) Development of a standard treatment protocol for severe acute respiratory syndrome. *Lancet* 361: 1615–1617

4 Lee N, Hui D, Wu A, Chan P, Cameron P, Joynt GM, Ahuja A, Yung MY, Leung CB, To KF et al (2003) A major outbreak of severe acute respiratory syndrome in Hong Kong. *N Engl J Med* 348: 1986–1994

5 Booth CM, Matukas LM, Tomlinson GA, Rachlis AR, Rose DB, Dwosh HA, Walmsley SL, Mazzulli T, Avendano M, Derkach P et al (2003) Clinical features and short-term outcomes of 144 patients with SARS in the greater Toronto area. *JAMA* 289: 2801–2809

6 Niederman MS, Mandell LA, Anzueto A, Bass JB, Broughton WA, Campbell GD, Dean N, File T, Fine MJ, Gross PA et al; American Thoracic Society (2001) Guidelines for the management of adults with community-acquired pneumonia. Diagnosis, assessment of severity, antimicrobial therapy, and prevention. *Am J Respir Crit Care Med* 163: 1730–1754

7 Chan PK, Tam JS, Lam CW, Chan E, Wu A, Li CK, Buckley TA, Ng KC, Joynt GM, Cheng FW et al (2003) Human metapneumovirus detection in patients with severe acute respiratory syndrome. *Emerg Infect Dis* 9: 1058–1063

8 Hong T, Wang JW, Sun YL, Duan SM, Chen LB, Qu JG, Ni AP, Liang GD, Ren LL, Yang RQ et al (2003) *Chlamydia*-like and coronavirus-like agents found in dead cases of atypical pneumonia by electron microscopy [Article in Chinese] *Zhonghua Yi Xue Za Zhi* 83: 632–636

9 Lau ACW, So LKY, Miu FPL, Yng RWH, Poon E, Cheung TMT, Yam LYC (2004) Outcome of coronavirus-assoiciated severe acute respiratory syndrome using a standard treatment protocol. *Respirology* 9: 173–183

10 Ho JC, Ooi GC, Mok TY, Chan JW, Hung I, Lam B, Wong PC, Li PC, Ho PL, Lam WK et al (2003) High-dose pulse versus nonpulse corticosteroid regimens in severe acute respiratory syndrome. *Am J Respir Crit Care Med* 168: 1449–1456

11 Ning Q, Brown D, Parodo J, Cattral M, Gorczynski R, Cole E, Fung L, Ding JW, Liu MF, Rotstein O et al (1998) Ribavirin inhibits viral-induced

macrophage production of TNF, IL-1, the procoagulant fgl2 prothrombinase and preserves Th1 cytokine production but inhibits Th2 cytokine response. *J Immunol* 160: 3487–3493

12 Cinatl J, Morgenstern B, Bauer G, Chandra P, Rabenau H, Doerr HW (2003) Glycyrrhizin, an active component of liquorice roots, and replication of SARS-associated coronavirus. *Lancet* 361: 2045–2046

13 Tan ELC, Ooi EE, Lin CY, Tan HC, Ling AE, Lim B, Stanton LW (2004) Inhibition of SARS coronavirus infection *in vitro* with clinically approved antiviral drugs. *Emerg Infect Dis* 10: 581–586

14 Health Canada. Update #44. Severe acute respiratory syndrome. Health Canada Rescinds Routine Access to Ribavirin (2003) http://www.hc-sc.gc.ca/english/ protection/warnings/sars/update44.html (accessed 20 March 2004)

15 Chan KS, Lai ST, Chu CM, Tsui E, Tam CY, Wong MML, Tse MW, Que TL, Peiris JSM, Sung J et al (2003) Treatment of severe acute respiratory syndrome with lopinavir/ritonavir: a multicentre retrospective matched cohort study. *Hong Kong Med J* 9: 399–406

16 Chu CM, Cheng VC, Hung IF, Wong MM, Chan KH, Chan KS, Kao RY, Poon LL, Wong CL, Guan Y et al (2004) Role of lopinavir/ritonavir in the treatment of SARS: initial virological and clinical findings. *Thorax* 59: 252–256

17 Pfeffer LM, Dinarello CA, Herberman RB, Williams BR, Borden EC, Bordens R, Walter MR, Nagabhushan TL, Trotta PP, Pestka S (1998) Biological properties of recombinant alpha-interferons: 40th anniversary of the discovery of interferons. *Cancer Res* 58: 2489–2499

18 Cinatl J, Morgenstern B, Bauer G, Chandra P, Rabenau H, Doerr HW (2003) Treatment of SARS with human interferons. *Lancet* 362: 293–294

19 Hensley LE, Fritz EA, Jahrling PB, Karp CL, Huggins JW, Geisbert TW (2004) Interferon-β 1a and SARS coronavirus replication. *Emerg Infect Dis* 10: 317–319

20 Mager DE, Neuteboom B, Efthymiopoulos C, Munafo A, Jusko WJ (2003) Receptor-mediated pharmacokinetics and pharmacodynamics of interferon-β 1a following intravenous and subcutaneous dosing in monkeys. *J Pharmacol Exp Ther* 306: 262–370

21 Zhao Z, Zhang F, Xu M, Huang K, Zhong W, Cai W, Yin Z, Huang S, Deng Z, Wei M et al (2003) Description and clinical treatment of an early outbreak of severe acute respiratory syndrome (SARS) in Guangzhou, PR China. *J Med Microbiol* 52(Pt 8): 715–720

22 Loutfy MR, Blatt LM, Siminovitch KA, Ward S, Wolff B, Lho H, Pham DH, Deif H, LaMere EA, Chang M et al (2003) Interferon alfacon-1 plus corticosteroids in severe acute respiratory syndrome: a preliminary study. *JAMA* 290: 3222–3228

23 Jones BM, Ma ES, Peiris JS, Wong PC, Ho JC, Lam B, Lai KN, Tsang KW (2004) Prolonged disturbances of *in vitro* cytokine production in patients with severe acute respiratory syndrome (SARS) treated with ribavirin and steroids. *Clin Exp Immunol* 135: 467–473

24 Tsui PT, Kwok ML, Yuen H, Lai ST (2003) Severe acute respiratory syndrome: clinical outcome and prognostic correlates. *Emerg Infect Dis* 9: 1064–1069
25 Lau ACW, So LKY (2003) Severe acute respiratory syndrome treatment: present status and future strategy. *Curr Opin Investig Drugs* 4: 918–920
26 Zhao Z, Zhang F, Xu M, Huang K, Zhong W, Cai W, Yin Z, Huang S, Deng Z, Wei M et al (2003) Description and clinical treatment of an early outbreak of severe acute respiratory syndrome (SARS) in Guangzhou, PR China. *J Med Microbiol* 52: 715–720
27 Zheng ZG, Zhong NS (2003) The use of corticosteroid in management of critical SARS. *Chin Med J* 42: 676–677
28 Tsang KW,Lam WK (2003) Management of severe acute respiratory syndrome: the Hong Kong University experience. *Am J Respir Crit Care Med* 168: 417–424
29 Luo D, Qian SC (2003) SARS treatment: experience from a team in Guangdong, China. *Chin Med J* 116: 838–839
30 Chan KS, Zheng JP, Mok YW, Li YM, Liu YN, Chu CM, Ip MS (2003) SARS: prognosis, outcome and sequelae. *Respirology* 8 (Suppl): S36–S40
31 Franks TJ, Chong PY, Chui P, Galvin JR, Lourens RM, Reid AH, Selbs E, McEvoy CP, Hayden CD, Fukuoka J et al (2003) Lung pathology of severe acute respiratory syndrome (SARS): a study of 8 autopsy cases from Singapore. *Hum Pathol* 34: 743–748
32 Lang Z, Zhang L, Zhang S, Meng X, Li J, Song C, Sun L, Zhou Y (2003) Pathological study on severe acute respiratory syndrome. *Chin Med J* 116: 976–980
33 Ding Y, Wang H, Shen H, Li Z, Geng J, Han H, Cai J, Li X, Kang W, Weng D et al (2003) The clinical pathology of severe acute respiratory syndrome (SARS): a report from China. *J Pathol* 200: 282–289
34 Glueck CJ, Freiberg R, Tracy T, Stroop D, Wang P (1997) Thrombophilia and hypofibrinolysis: pathophysiologies of osteonecrosis. *Clin Orthop* 334: 43–56
35 Donnelly CA, Ghani AC, Leung GM, Hedley AJ, Fraser C, Riley S, Abu-Raddad LJ, Ho LM, Thach TQ, Chau P et al (2003) Epidemiological determinants of spread of causal agent of severe acute respiratory syndrome in Hong Kong. *Lancet* 361: 1761–1766
36 Tsang K, Zhong NS (2003) SARS: pharmacotherapy. *Respirology* 8: S25–S30
37 Lew TW, Kwek TK, Tai D, Earnest A, Loo S, Singh K, Kwan KM, Chan Y, Yim CF, Bek SL et al (2003) Acute respiratory syndrome in critically-ill patients with severe acute respiratory syndrome. *JAMA* 290: 374–380
38 Wong VW, Dai D, Wu AK, Sung JJ (2003) Treatment of severe acute respiratory syndrome with convalescent plasma. *Hong Kong Med J* 9: 199–201
39 Zhang RL, Jiao Q, Wang BG (2003) Controlled clinical study on 49 patients of SARS treated by integrative Chinese and Western medicine. *Zhongguo Zhong Xi Yi Jie He Za Zhi* 23: 654–657
40 Lin L, Han Y, Yang ZM (2003) Clinical observation on 103 patients with severe acute respiratory syndrome treated by integrative traditional Chinese and western medicine. *Zhongguo Zhong Xi Yi Jie He Za Zhi* 23: 409–413

41 Li J, Li SD, Du N. Clinical study on treatment of severe acute respiratory syndrome with integrative Chinese and Western medicine approach (2004) *Zhongguo Zhong Xi Yi Jie He Za Zhi* 24: 28–31
42 Lau ACW, Yam LYC, So LKY (2004) Management of critically ill patients with severe acute respiratory syndrome (SARS). *Int J Med Sci* 1: 1–10
43 Li H, Nie L, Wang G, Que C, Ma J, Li N, Zhao Z, Gao Z, Xv X, Lu H (2003) Clinical observation of non-invasive positive pressure ventilation (NIPPV) in the treatment of severe acute respiratory syndrome (SARS). *Beijing Da Xue Xue Bao* 35 (Suppl): 41–43
44 Cheung TMT, Yam LYC, So LKY, Lau ACW, Poon E, Kong BMH, Yung RWH (2004) Effectiveness of non-invasive positive pressure ventilation in the treatment of acute respiratory failure in severe acute respiratory syndrome. *Chest* 26: 845–850
45 Yam LYC, Chen RC, Zhong NS (2003) SARS: ventilatory and intensive care. *Respirology* 8: S31–S35
46 The Acute Respiratory Distress Syndrome Network (2000) Ventilation with lower tidal volumes as compared with traditional tidal volumes for acute lung injury and acute respiratory distress syndrome. *N Engl J Med* 342: 1301–1308
47 World Health Organisation. WHO calls for urgent investigation into sources of infection in recent SARS cases in Guangdong Province, after a fourth case is announced. 31 January 2004. http://www.wpro.who.int/sars/docs/pressreleases/pr_31012004.asp (accessed 27 March 2004)
48 Wang HJ, Ding YQ, Li X, Yang L, Zhang WL, Kang W (2003) Fatal aspergillosis in a patient with SARS who has treated with corticosteroids. *N Engl J Med* 349: 507–508
49 Yao W, Chen Y, Zhang L et al (2003) Chest X-ray changes after discontinuation of glucocorticoids treatment on severe acute respiratory syndrome (5 cases report). *Beijing Da Xue Xue Bao* 35 (Suppl): 26–28
50 Lew TW, Kwek TK, Tai D, Earnest A, Loo S, Singh K, Kwan KM, Chan Y, Yim CF, Bek SL et al (2003) Acute respiratory distress syndrome in critically ill patients with severe acute respiratory syndrome. *JAMA* 290: 374–380
51 Gomersall CD, Joynt GM, Lam P, Li T, Yap F, Lam D, Buckley TA, Sung JJ, Hui DS, Antonio GE et al (2003) Short-term outcome of critically ill patients with severe acute respiratory syndrome. *Intensive Care Med* 30: 381–387

Coronaviruses with Special Emphasis on First Insights Concerning SARS
ed. by A. Schmidt, M.H. Wolff and O. Weber

Coronavirus main proteinase: target for antiviral drug therapy

Kanchan Anand[1], Haitao Yang[2], Mark Bartlam[2], Zihe Rao[2,3] and Rolf Hilgenfeld[1]

[1] *Institute of Biochemistry, University of Lübeck, Ratzeburger Allee 160, 23538 Lübeck, Germany*
[2] *Laboratory of Structural Biology, Tsinghua University, Beijing, China*
[3] *Institute of Biophysics, Chinese Academy of Science, Beijing, China*

Introduction

During the first outbreak of severe acute respiratory syndrome (SARS) in early 2003, almost 8500 people worldwide were diagnosed with the disease, and approximately 800 died of it. The epidemic was contained by July, 2003, but since then, the disease has re-emerged in the Guangdong province in Southern China around the turn of the year 2003, although the number of cases was very limited this time. In addition, there were two cases of SARS caused by improper sample handling in research laboratories in Singapore and Taiwan. A "mini-outbreak" originated from several independent laboratory infections at a research laboratory in Beijing in March and April, 2004, and led to infection chains encompassing three generations. This time, China escaped another epidemic since fortunately, the number of diseased people was limited to nine, although there was one fatality. In any case, these isolated mini-outbreaks remind us of the global threat that SARS still represents.

In late March, 2003, a new coronavirus, SARS-CoV, was isolated from affected tissue of SARS patients and identified as the cause of the disease [1, 2]. *Coronaviridae* are RNA viruses that have been united with the families *Arteriviridae* and *Roniviridae* in the order *Nidovirales*. The phylogenetic relationship of these morphologically unrelated virus families is based on their similar polycistronic genome organization, common transcriptional and post-translational strategies, and a conserved array of homologous domains in the viral polyproteins [3–5]. Coronaviruses are responsible for a number of diseases of man and animals, some of which have major economical impacts, although the human coronaviruses have clearly been neglected before SARS emerged. Transmissible gastroenteritis virus (TGEV) infection is associated with severe and often fatal diarrhoea in young pigs [6, 7]. The human coronaviruses (HCoV) 229E and OC43 are major causes of upper respiratory tract illness in humans, in particular, common cold-like conditions [8]. To date, only the 229E strain of HCoV has been characterized in detail because until the discovery of SARS-CoV, it used to be the only isolate to grow efficiently in cell culture. In contrast to the relatively harmless disease caused by these human coronaviruses, SARS is characterized by high fever, malaise, rigor, headache, non-productive cough, or dyspnea and may progress to generalized, interstitial infiltrates in the lung, requiring intubation and mechanical ventilation [9]. The infection, however, is not restricted to the lungs. Other affected organs include the kidneys and the liver, as well as the gastrointestinal tract; hence SARS can be considered a systemic disease. Epidemiological evidence suggests that the transmission of this newly emerging pathogen occurs mainly by face-to-face contact, although other routes of transmission cannot be fully excluded.

Coronavirus main proteinase: function and overall structure

Coronaviruses are positive-stranded RNA viruses featuring a large (27–31 kB), single-stranded RNA genome. The replicase gene, encompassing more than 20,000 nucleotides, encodes two overlapping polyproteins, pp1a (replicase 1a, ~450 kDa) and pp1ab (replicase 1ab, ~750 kDa) [10] that mediate all the functions required for viral replication and transcription [11]. Expression of the 3'-proximal portion of the replicase gene requires (–1) ribosomal frameshifting [10]. The functional non-structural proteins are released from the viral polyproteins by extensive proteolytic processing. The vast majority of cleavages are mediated by the viral main proteinase, M^{pro} [12], a cysteine proteinase which is frequently also called 3C-like proteinase ($3CL^{pro}$) to indicate a similarity of its substrate specificity to that observed for picornavirus 3C proteinases ($3C^{pro}$) (see Tab. 1), although the structural similarities between the two families of proteinases are limited [13]. The M^{pro} ($3CL^{pro}$) cleaves the polyprotein at no less than 11 conserved sites involving Leu-Gln↓(Ser,Ala,Gly) sequences, a process initiated by the enzyme's own autolytic cleavage from pp1a and pp1ab [14, 15]. Importantly, this cleavage pattern appears to be conserved in the M^{pro} from SARS coronavirus (SARS-CoV), as deduced from the genomic sequence [16, 17] and shown experimentally for one cleavage site [18]. The SARS-CoV polyproteins have three non-canonical M^{pro} cleavage sites with Phe, Met or Val in the P2 position, but the same cleavage sites are unusual in other coronaviruses as well. The functional importance of M^{pro} in the viral life cycle makes this proteinase an attractive target for the development of drugs directed against SARS and other coronavirus infections.

Our laboratories have determined crystal structures for HCoV strain 229E M^{pro} at 2.54 Å resolution [18], porcine TGEV M^{pro} at 1.96 Å [13], and SARS-CoV M^{pro} (1.9 Å resolution) [19]. In addition, we have also elucidated the structures of substrate-analogous hexapeptidyl chloromethyl

Table 1: Autocleavage sites of coronavirus M^{pro} and picornavirus $3C^{pro}$

	P6	P5	P4	P3	P2	P1	P1'	P2'	P3'	P4'
HCoV M^{pro}										
N-terminal	Y	G	S	T	L	Q	A	G	L	R
C-terminal	F	G	V	N	L	Q	S	G	K	T
TGEV M^{pro}										
N-terminal	V	N	S	T	L	Q	S	G	L	R
C-terminal	Y	G	V	N	L	Q	A	G	K	V
MHV M^{pro}										
N-terminal	T	T	S	F	L	Q	S	G	I	V
C-terminal	A	G	V	K	L	Q	S	K	R	V
SARS-CoV M^{pro}										
N-terminal	T	S	A	V	L	Q	S	G	F	R
C-terminal	S	G	V	T	F	Q	G	K	F	I
HRV-2 $3C^{pro}$										
N-terminal	L	P	V	V	V	Q	G	P	N	T
C-terminal	Y	F	T	D	V	Q	G	Q	I	T
HAV $3C^{pro}$										
N-terminal	K	G	L	F	S	Q	A	K	I	S
C-terminal	M	E	L	R	T	Q	S	F	S	N
PV $3C^{pro}$										
N-terminal	E	T	A	K	V	Q	G	P	G	F
C-terminal	G	A	V	T	E	Q	G	Y	L	N
Consensus										
Coronavirus M^{pro}	–	–	small	–	L	Q	small	–	–	–
Picornavirus $3C^{pro}$	–	–	ϕ	–	small	Q	(G)	–	–	–

Cleavage site specificities of coronavirus M^{pro}s and picornavirus $3C^{pro}$s are similar but different in detail. N- and C-terminal autocleavage sites of M^{pro}s and $3C^{pro}$s are shown. HCoV, human coronavirus 229E; TGEV, porcine transmissible gastroenteritis virus; MHV, mouse hepatitis virus; SARS-CoV, SARS coronavirus; HRV 2, human rhinovirus serotype 2; HAV, hepatitis A virus; PV, poliovirus type 1 (strain Mahoney); ϕ, hydrophobic

ketone inhibitor complexes of the TGEV and SARS-CoV enzymes, at around 2.4 Å resolution [18, 19]. The structures of all three enzymes show that the coronavirus main proteinase consists of three domains, the first two of which together distantly resemble chymotrypsin while the third has a unique α-helical fold (Fig. 1). Located between domains I and II, the active site comprises a Cys-His catalytic dyad, rather than the usual triad. Domains I and II (residues 8-99 and 100-183, respectively) are six-stranded antiparallel β-barrels. A long loop (residues 184 to 199) connects domain II to the C-terminal domain (domain III, residues 200–300), which is a globular cluster of five, mostly antiparallel helices.

The interior of the β-barrel of domain I consists entirely of hydrophobic residues. A short α-helix (helix A; residues 53–58) closes the barrel like a

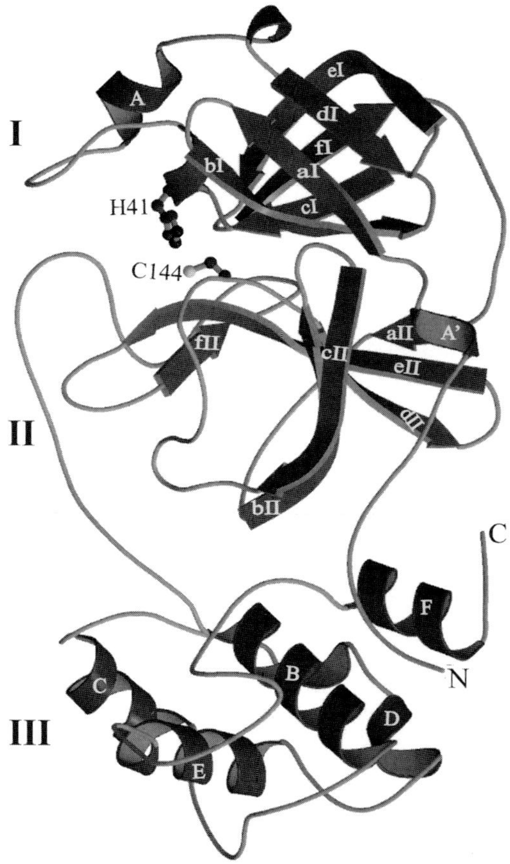

Figure 1. Domain structure of the coronavirus main proteinase monomer (shown here is TGEV M^{pro}.

lid. Domain II is smaller than domain I and also smaller than the homologous domain II of chymotrypsin and the 3C proteinase ($3C^{pro}$) of hepatitis A virus (HAV) [20–22]. Several secondary structure elements of this domain in HAV $3C^{pro}$ (strands b2II and cII and the intervening loop) are missing in the coronavirus M^{pro}. The domain II barrel of the M^{pro} is far from perfect (Fig. 1). The segment from Gly135 to Ser146 forms a part of the barrel, even though it consists mostly of consecutive loops and turns. In fact, in contrast to domain I, a structural alignment of domain II onto the picornaviral 3C proteinases has proven difficult. The superposition of domains I and II of the TGEV M^{pro} onto those of the HAV $3C^{pro}$ yields a root mean square deviation (r.m.s.d.) of 1.85 Å for 114 equivalent (out of 184 compared) C_α pairs, while domain II alone displays an r.m.s.d. of 3.25 Å for 57 (out of 85) C_α pairs.

The three M^{pro} structures determined so far are quite similar to one another. The overall r.m.s. deviations for Cα atoms between the structures is below 2 Å for all 300 Cα positions of the molecules that could be located in the electron density maps but the isolated domains exhibit significantly smaller deviations. The most variable domain appears to be the helical domain III, which shows a better spatial overlap between TGEV M^{pro} and HCoV M^{pro} than between each of these and SARS-CoV M^{pro}. To a certain extent, these numbers reflect the degree of sequence identity between the different M^{pro}s. HCoV 229E and TGEV, both being group I coronaviruses, share 61% sequence identity between their main proteinases, whereas SARS-CoV as a distant outlier of group II has 40% and 44%, respectively, of the sequence of its M^{pro} in common with HCoV 229E and TGEV [18]. Interestingly, domains I and II show a higher degree of sequence conservation (42–48% identity) than domain III (36–40%) between SARS-CoV M^{pro} and the coronavirus group I enzymes.

Dimer formation

The crystal structure of the TGEV M^{pro} provided the first indication that coronavirus main proteinases form tight dimers [13]. This has since been confirmed by the X-ray structures of the HCoV 229E and SARS-CoV M^{pro}s (Fig. 2) [18, 19]. Dimerisation also occurs in solution: we could show by dynamic light scattering that both HCoV 229E and TGEV M^{pro} exist as a mixture of monomers (~65%) and dimers (~35%) in diluted solutions (1-2 mg proteinase/ml). Lai and coworkers have demonstrated that the enzymatic activity of the SARS-CoV M^{pro} increases linearly with enzyme concentration, suggesting that the enzymatically active species is the dimer and not the monomer [23]. Crystal structures of the SARS-CoV enzyme at different pH values provided an explanation for this observation [19] (see below).

It should be noted that dimer formation as a prerequisite for enzymatic activity makes coronavirus main proteinases unique amongst the proteinases of RNA viruses, and present a clear distinction from the 3C proteinases of picornaviruses. The TGEV M^{pro} X-ray structure showed, and the other coronavirus M^{pro} structures confirmed, that the monomer-monomer contact interface comprises two regions, i.e. i) the N-terminal eight residues of molecule A and domain II of molecule B, and ii) the domains III of each protomer. Although the latter part of the interface is significantly smaller than the former, it is apparently sufficient to hold the isolated domains III together in solution, as has recently been shown for SARS-CoV M^{pro} [24]. The crystal structures show that the two molecules are oriented perpendicular to one another (Fig. 2) [13, 18, 19]. Since the architecture of the dimers including most details of intermolecular interaction are the same in TGEV M^{pro} – three independent dimers per asymmetric unit – and HCoV 229E as

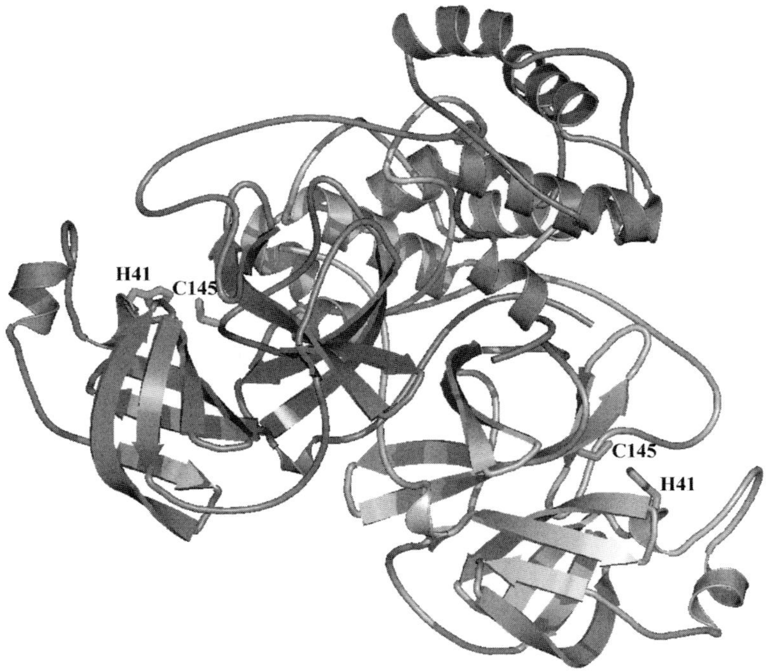

Figure 2. The SARS-CoV main protease dimer.

well as SARS-CoV M^{pro}s – both with one dimer per asymmetric unit –, i.e., in completely different crystalline environments, there can be little doubt that dimer formation is of biological relevance in these enzymes.

In the M^{pro} dimer, the N-terminal amino acid residues are squeezed in between domains II and III of the parent monomer – designated "A" in this paragraph – and domain II of the other monomer ("B"), where they make a number of very specific interactions that appear tailor-made to bind this segment with high affinity. These interactions include *intermolecular* salt bridges between the positively charged amino terminus (residue A1) and GluB165 (all residue numbers given in this section are for TGEV M^{pro}) of domain II of the neighboring molecule in the dimer, between ArgA4 and GluB286, as well as an *intramolecular* salt bridge between LysA5 and GluA291 of domain III of the parent molecule. Also, there is an important hydrophobic contact between the semiconserved LeuA3 and a hydrophobic patch on domain III which includes PheA206, AlaA209, PheA287, ValA292, the C$^{\beta}$ atom of GlnA295, and MetA296. All sequenced members of the coronavirus proteinase family have a hydrophobic residue in position 3 (SARS-CoV has Phe), while glycine is absolutely conserved in position 2.

The latter residue adopts the α_L conformation, which is easily accessible only to glycine. This conformation ensures that the N-terminal segment fits into its narrow binding canyon in the dimerization interface.

The existence of a specific binding site for the N-terminal segment of the M^{pro} could be important in the activation of the main proteinase by catalyzing its release from the viral polyprotein. The free N-terminus is created as a consequence of the first cleavage reaction performed by the proteinase, at its N-terminal autocleavage site. In the mature M^{pro} monomer, the first eight residues from the N-terminus are not a part of the globular protein structure. After the autocleavage reaction, they could easily remain bound to the substrate-binding site of the proteinase if an alternative high-affinity binding site was not provided by dimer formation. The existence of such high-affinity binding site ensures that the catalytic site is immediately liberated from the product and can act on other cleavage sites in the polyprotein. However, the exact placement of the amino terminus also has a very important structural role for the *mature* M^{pro}, and is in fact critical for its catalytic activity, as we will see below.

Catalytic site

In the active site of the M^{pro}, Cys144(145) and His41 (SARS-CoV numbering in brackets where different) form a catalytic dyad. In contrast to serine proteinases and other cysteine proteinases, which have a catalytic triad, there is no third catalytic residue present. HCoV 229E and TGEV M^{pro}s have Val84 in the corresponding sequence position (Cys in SARS-CoV M^{pro}), with its side chain pointing away from the active site. A buried water molecule is found in the place that would normally be occupied by the third member of the triad; this water is hydrogen-bonded to His41 Nδ1, Gln163 Nε2, and Asp186 Oδ1 in HCoV 229E M^{pro} (His, His, and Asp in both SARS-CoV and TGEV M^{pro}). Asp186(187) does not act on the active-site His41 through the mentioned water molecule, but rather interacts with conserved Arg40 by forming a strong inter-domain salt bridge.

There has been a long-standing debate on the exact nature of the catalytic centre in cysteine proteinases. Polgár has shown that in papain-like cysteine proteinases, the active species is a thiolate-imidazolium ion pair, with the imidazolium cation held in the correct position by an asparagine residue, the third residue of the catalytic triad [25]. However, such a mechanism does not seem to be predominant in the coronavirus main proteinases; Lai and coworkers have recently shown that if the active-site cysteine residue of SARS-CoV M^{pro} is replaced by serine, some residual enzymatic activity – decreased by a factor of 40 – can still be detected. This can be seen as an indication for the existence of a classical general base mechanism in the wild-type proteinase, involving the non-ionized Cys145 hydrogen bonded to the uncharged imidazole of His41 in the ground state of the free enzyme [26]. We note that in viral cysteine proteinases, both picornaviral 2A and 3C proteinases as well as coronaviral main proteinases, the Sγ of the active-site cysteine residue is exactly in the plane of the histidine imidazole ring, at a distance of between 3.5 and 4.0 Å, while in the papain-like cysteine proteinases, this is not the case. For hydrogen bonding to occur between the two side chains, but not for ion-pair formation, the sulfur has to be more or less in the plane of the imidazole. While this preliminary observation has to be investigated further, it seems that X-ray crystallography can contribute to this important mechanistic question by providing exact geometric details of the ground-states of the free enzymes.

Substrate binding

Comparison of the structures shows that the substrate-binding sites are well conserved among coronavirus main proteinases. This is supported by our experimental finding that recombinant SARS-CoV M^{pro} cleaves a pentadecapeptide corresponding to the N-terminal autocleavage site of the TGEV M^{pro} [18].

To allow structure-based design of drugs directed at coronavirus M^{pro}s, we sought to determine the exact binding mode of M^{pro} substrates. To this end, we synthesized the substrate analog hexapeptidyl chloromethyl ketone inhibitor, Cbz-Val-Asn-Ser-Thr-Leu-Gln-CMK (subsequently named CMK), and soaked it into crystals of TGEV and SARS-CoV M^{pro} [18, 19]. The sequence of the inhibitor was derived from the P6–P1 residues of the N-terminal autoprocessing site of TGEV M^{pro} (SARS-CoV M^{pro} and HCoV 229E M^{pro} have Thr-Ser-Ala-Val-Leu-Gln and Tyr-Gly-Ser-Thr-Leu-Gln, respectively, at the corresponding positions). At the outset, we will present here the complex between the TGEV M^{pro} and the inhibitor [18]. In the case of the SARS-CoV enzyme, some unusual binding modes were observed [19], which we will discuss later.

X-ray crystallographic analysis of the TGEV M^{pro} complex at 2.37 Å resolution revealed difference density for all residues (except the benzyloxycarbonyl (Cbz) protective group) of the inhibitor, in two (B and F) out of the six TGEV M^{pro} monomers in the asymmetric unit [18]. In these monomers, there is a covalent bond between the S_γ atom of the active-site nucleophile Cys144 and the methylene group of the chloromethyl ketone. There are no significant differences between the structures of the enzyme in the free and in the complexed state. The substrate-analogue inhibitor binds in the shallow substrate-binding site at the surface of the proteinase, between domains I and II (Fig. 3A). The residues Val-Asn-Ser-Thr-Leu-Gln occupy, and thereby define, the subsites S6 to S1 of the proteinase. Residues P5 to P3 form an antiparallel β-sheet with segment 164–167 of the long strand eII on one side, and they also interact with segment 189–191 of the loop linking domains II and III on the other. In the discussion that follows, residue numbers for TGEV M^{pro} are followed by those for the SARS-CoV enzyme in brackets.

S1 specificity site

In coronavirus M^{pro} polyprotein cleavage sites, the P1 position is invariably occupied by Gln. At the very bottom of the M^{pro} S1 subsite, the imidazole of His162(163) is suitably positioned to donate a hydrogen bond from Nε2 to the side-chain carbonyl of the P1 glutamine (Fig. 3A). In order to specifically bind glutamine and not glutamate in the S1 pocket, this histidine residue is required to be uncharged over a broad pH range. This appears to be maintained by two important interactions made by the imidazole ring: i) stacking onto the phenyl ring of Phe139(140), and ii) accepting a hydrogen bond (to Nδ1) from the hydroxyl group of the buried Tyr160(161). In agreement with this structural interpretation, any replacement of His162 completely abolishes the proteolytic activity of HCoV 229E and feline infectious peritonitis virus (FIPV) M^{pro} [27, 28]. Furthermore, FIPV M^{pro} Tyr160 mutants have their proteolytic activity reduced by a factor of >30 [27]. All of these residues are conserved in SARS-CoV M^{pro} and, in fact, in all coronavirus main proteinases. Other elements involved in the S1 pocket of the M^{pro} are the *main-chain* atoms of Ile51, Leu164(Met165), Glu165(166), and His171(172). The latter two residues form a salt bridge at the outer wall of the S1 specificity pocket in the TGEV and HCoV 229E M^{pro}s, as well as in one conformation of the SARS-CoV M^{pro}. However, the latter displays another conformation which will be discussed below.

In all structures of free coronavirus main proteinases that we determined so far, we find electron density at the bottom of the S1 pocket. We interpreted this as a water molecule or, in the case of TGEV M^{pro} where the density was more dumb-bell-shaped, as two water molecules. However, especially in the latter case, we realized that apart from a possible hydrogen bond between one of these waters and the His162 imidazole, no interactions with the proteins were made by these water molecules. Also, the positions of the two water molecules were in fact too close to one another (about 2.1–2.3 Å) [13]. When we subsequently determined the structure of the complex between the TGEV M^{pro} and the CMK inhibitor, we noted that the oxygen and the nitrogen of the side-chain amide occupied a position exactly matching that of the two water molecules in the free enzyme. It is therefore possible that the free enzyme in fact also contains some residual peptide cleavage product (perhaps from an unidentified *E. coli* protein). Having realized this possibility, we checked for residual difference electron density in other subsites but could find nothing, with the exception of a patch of relatively strong electron density at the P2 position which we had interpreted and successfully refined as a 2-methyl-2,4-pentandiol (MPD) molecule from the crystallization medium [13]. The MPD does not

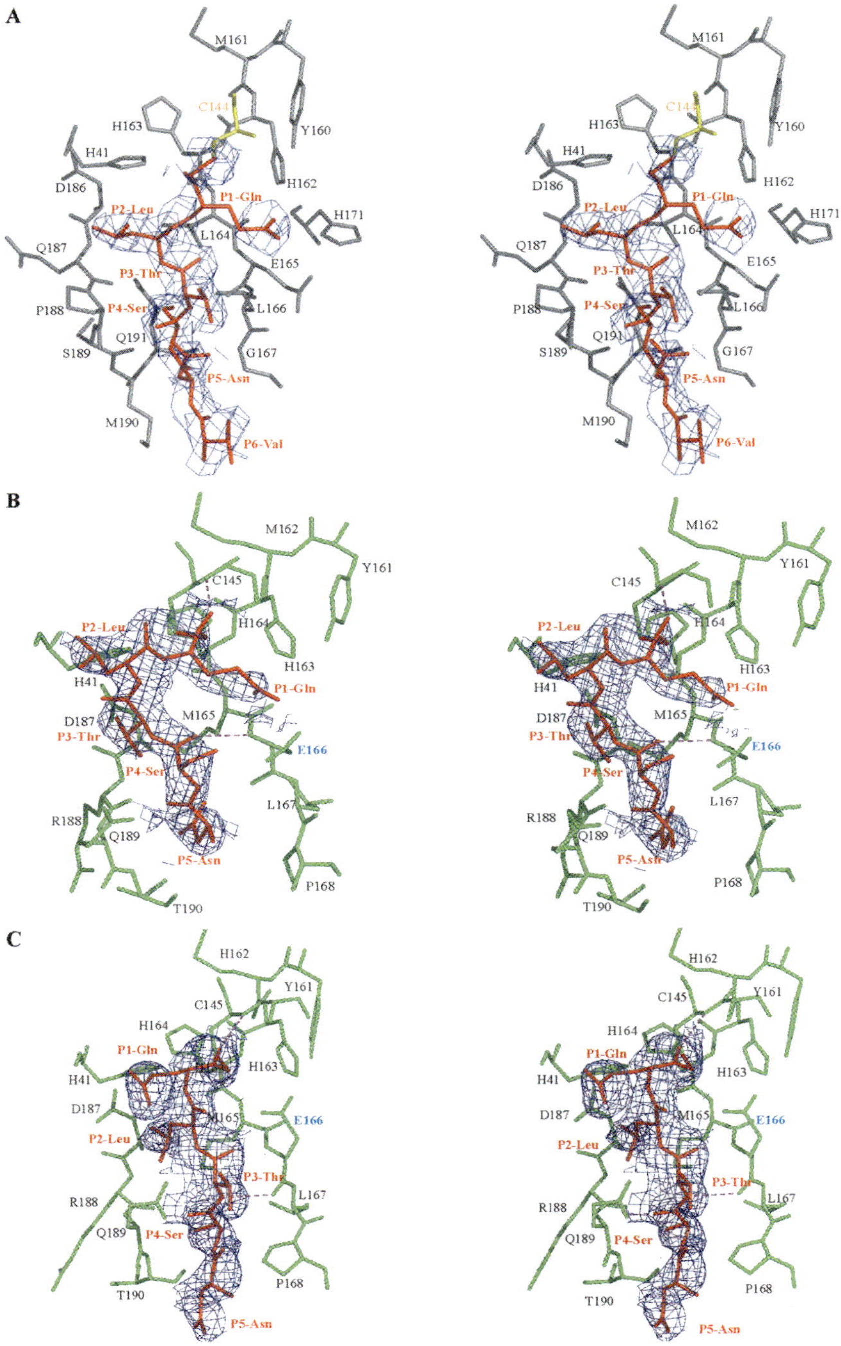
A
M161
C144
H163
Y160
H41
H162
D186
P1-Gln
P2-Leu
H171
L164
Q187
E165
P3-Thr
P4-Ser
L166
P188
Q191
S189
G167
P5-Asn
M190
P6-Val
B
M162
Y161
C145
H164
P2-Leu
H163
H41
P1-Gln
M165
D187
P3-Thr
E166
P4-Ser
L167
R188
Q189
P5-Asn
P168
T190
C
H162
Y161
C145
H164
P1-Gln
H163
H41
D187
M165
E166
P2-Leu
P3-Thr
L167
R188
Q189
P4-Ser
P168
T190
P5-Asn

fully protrude into the S2 pocket but rather occupies a position corresponding to the main chain of the peptide substrate. At this point, we still think the assignment of this density was correct, but studies on other proteinases – e.g. thermolysin – that revealed the presence of cleavage product after years of investigation taught us to be cautious.

S2 specificity site

Apart from a few exceptions, coronavirus M^{pro} cleavage sites have a Leu residue in the P2 position [28]. The hydrophobic S2 subsite of the TGEV enzyme is formed by the side chains of Leu164, Ile51, Thr47, His41, and Tyr53. In addition, residues 186–188 line the S2 subsite with some of their main-chain atoms. The P2 Leu side chain of the inhibitor is well accommodated in this pocket (Fig. 3A).

In the SARS-CoV M^{pro} [19], the S2 pocket is similar to what has been seen in HCoV M^{pro} [18] and TGEV M^{pro} [13]. One wall of the subsite is formed by methionine residues 49 and 165, which adopt positions spatially similar to TGEV and HCoV 229E M^{pro} residues Ile51 and Leu/Ile164, respectively. The longer methionine side chains restrict the S2 pocket in one direction and probably require a slight reorientation of the P2 leucine residue of the substrate, compared to TGEV M^{pro}. On the other side, the S2 pocket appears to be somewhat enlarged in SARS M^{pro}, due to the insertion of Ala46 which is not present in TGEV or HCoV 229E M^{pro}, as well as to many differences in amino acid sequence. In SARS-CoV M^{pro}, the stretch 45–50 forms a short 3_{10}-helix, whereas this region has no regular secondary structure in the other coronavirus main proteinases. The net effect of these modifications appears to be a widening of the S2 pocket on this side. This may be required for the efficient binding of a P2 phenylalanine, which is present in the C-terminal autocleavage site of the M^{pro}.

Specificity sites beyond S1 and S2

There is no specificity for any particular side chain at the P3 position of coronavirus M^{pro} cleavage sites. This agrees with the P3 side chain of our

Figure 3. X-ray crystallographic analysis of M^{pro} complexes with CMK inhibitor (stereo figures) (A) The substrate analogue inhibitor binds in the shallow substrate-binding site at the surface of the TGEV proteinase, between domains I and II. (B) In the active monomer A of the SARS-CoV M^{pro} crystallized at pH 6.0, the P1 glutamine of the inhibitor protrudes into the S1 pocket, but P2-P5 adopt an unusual binding mode. (C) In the inactive monomer B, the S1 pocket is not accessible, and the P1 glutamine points towards bulk solvent.
A: After [18], with kind permission of the American Association for the Advancement of Science (AAAS); B, C: After [19], with kind permission of The National Academy of Sciences of the USA.

substrate analog being oriented towards bulk solvent in the TGEV M^{pro} complex (Fig. 3A). At the P4 position, there has to be a small amino acid residue such as Ser, Thr, Val, or Pro because of the congested cavity formed by the side chains of Leu164, Leu166, and Gln191 as well as the main-chain atoms of Ser189. These residues are conserved or conservatively substituted (Leu164⇒Met165, Ser189⇒Thr190) in SARS-CoV M^{pro}. In the TGEV M^{pro} complex, the P5 Asn side chain interacts with the main chain at Gly167, Ser189, and Gln191 (Pro168, Thr190, Gln192 in the SARS-CoV enzyme), thus involving the loop linking domains II and III, whereas the P6 Val residue is not in contact with the protein (Fig. 3A).

Although our CMK inhibitor does not include a P1' residue, it is easily seen that the common small P1' residues (Ser, Ala, or Gly) can be easily accommodated in the S1' subsite of TGEV M^{pro} formed by Leu27, His41, and Thr47, with the latter two residues also being involved in the S2 subsite (Leu, His, and Asp in SARS-CoV M^{pro}).

Superimposition of the structures of the TGEV M^{pro}-CMK complex and the free HCoV 229E M^{pro} shows that the two substrate-binding sites are basically the same. All residues along the S4-S1 side of the cleft are identical, with the exception of the conservative M190L replacement (Ala191 in SARS-CoV M^{pro}). In the SARS pathogen, M^{pro} residues 168 and 188 - 190 show some substitutions but since these residues contribute to substrate binding with their main-chain atoms only, the identity of the side chains is less important. Indeed, the substrate-binding site of the SARS-CoV M^{pro} matches those of its TGEV and HCoV 229E counterparts quite well (Fig. 3B). And yet, the CMK inhibitor bound to the SARS-CoV M^{pro} in a remarkably different mode (Figs. 3B,C). But before we discuss substrate or inhibitor binding to the SARS-CoV main proteinase, we have to analyze the dynamical nature of the structure of the free enzyme.

pH-dependent conformational changes of the SARS-CoV M^{pro}

The SARS-CoV M^{pro} also forms a dimer in the crystal (and in solutions at concentrations of >1 mg/ml) with the two protomers oriented almost at right angles to each other [19], in an arrangement that is similar to the HCoV and TGEV M^{pro} structures [13, 18]. However, when we first determined the structure of the SARS-CoV enzyme by X-ray analysis of crystals grown at pH 6.0 [19], we were surprised to see that the substrate-binding site of one monomer (denoted "A", Fig. 4A) was in the normal, active conformation described above for the TGEV and HCoV 229E M^{pro}s, whereas the other ("B") had adopted a catalytically incompetent form (Fig. 4B). There were two major conformational changes that led to this inactivation: i) the S1 binding pocket for the glutamine residue at the cleavage site of the substrate had collapsed, and ii) so had the the oxyanion hole (Fig. 4B). We believe that these changes originate from protonation of HisB163, the con-

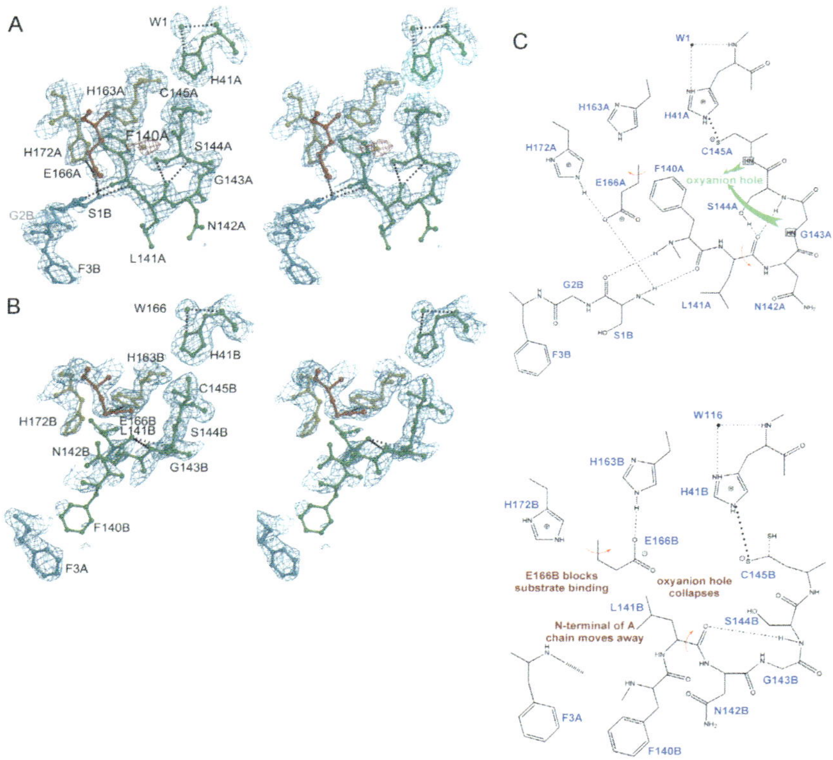

Figure 4. Conformational changes of SARS-CoV M^{pro}. (A) Substrate-binding site of one monomer in the normal, active conformation; (B) catalytically incompetent form; (C) Schematic drawing showing the S1 pocket in the active conformation (top) and the inactive conformation (bottom). After [19], with kind permission of The National Academy of Sciences of the USA.

served residue found at the bottom of the S1 pocket, in monomer B. The pH of crystallization of 6.0 is close to the pK of histidine, explaining why the residue appears to be protonated in monomer "B" but not monomer "A" of the SARS-CoV M^{pro} dimer. As a consequence of the protonation, the side chain of PheB140, which stacks onto HisB163 as long as the latter is unprotonated, moves away and reorients towards the A3 of the other monomer. In order to neutralize the positive charge of HisB163 in its relatively hydrophobic environment, GluB166 moves into the S1 pocket and forms a very strong salt bridge of 2.43 Å with HisB163. This leads to breakage of the ion pair between GluB166 and HisB172 as well as of the amino terminus, residue A1, of the other monomer in the dimer. This very amino terminus also interacts with the main chain of residue B140, the phenylalanine that moves away in response to the protonation of HisB163. This interaction,

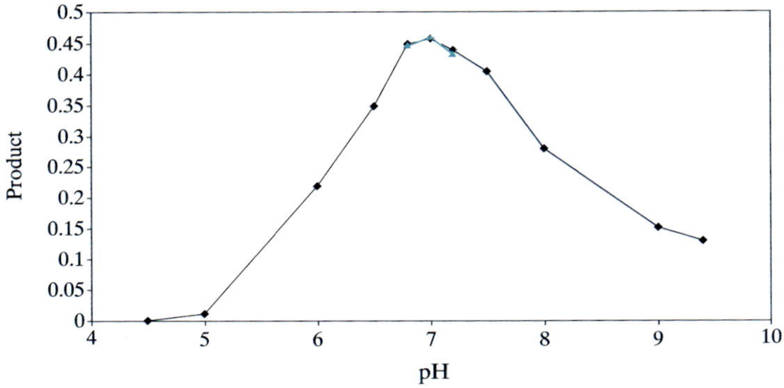

Figure 5. Activity of the SARS-CoV M^{pro} as a function of pH.

consisting of two hydrogen bonds, between the hydrogen bond with the amino group of A1 and the CO of PheB140 as well as between the CO of A1 and the NH of PheB140, is also lost as part of the conformational rearrangements. As a result, the segment around PheB140 (residues B138 - B143) is no longer fixed. It adopts a different conformation with positional differences from the A chain of up to 5.9 Å and becomes poorly ordered, although we do see continuous electron density for the main chain and for all side chains except PheB140 (Fig. 4B). In fact, the entire loop translates towards the active site. Importantly, residue 140 is part of the oxyanion loop, which stabilizes the transition state of the proteolytic reaction by donating hydrogen bonds from the main-chain amides of Gly143 and Cys145 to the negatively charged oxygen of the tetrahedral intermediate. It is essential that this loop be in the right conformation for the enzyme to exhibit full catalytic activity. However, in the inactive protomer, Gly143 moves by >3.2 Å towards the active site and leaves no space for the oxyanion to bind.

As mentioned above, the S1 binding site is partly occupied by GluB166 interacting with HisB163. In addition, CysB145 adopts two conformations, each about half occupied, one of which is filling the remainder of the collapsed S1 pocket. The other one is interacting with the catalytic HisB41 as in the active protomer. In summary, protomer "B" in the dimer is inactive because it cannot stabilize the oxyanion transition state and because it is unable to bind the P1 glutamine residue of the substrate. This agrees with the measured activity of the enzyme as dependent on pH, which displays a bell-shaped curve, with a maximum at pH 7.0 and less than 50% activity both at pH 6.0 and at pH 8.5 (Fig. 5) [29].

In a follow-up study, we equilibrated at pH 7.6 and 8.0 crystals of the SARS-CoV M^{pro} that had been grown at pH 6.0, and determined the structures by X-ray analysis [19]. At pH 7.6 (Fig. 6A), the S1 binding pocket is

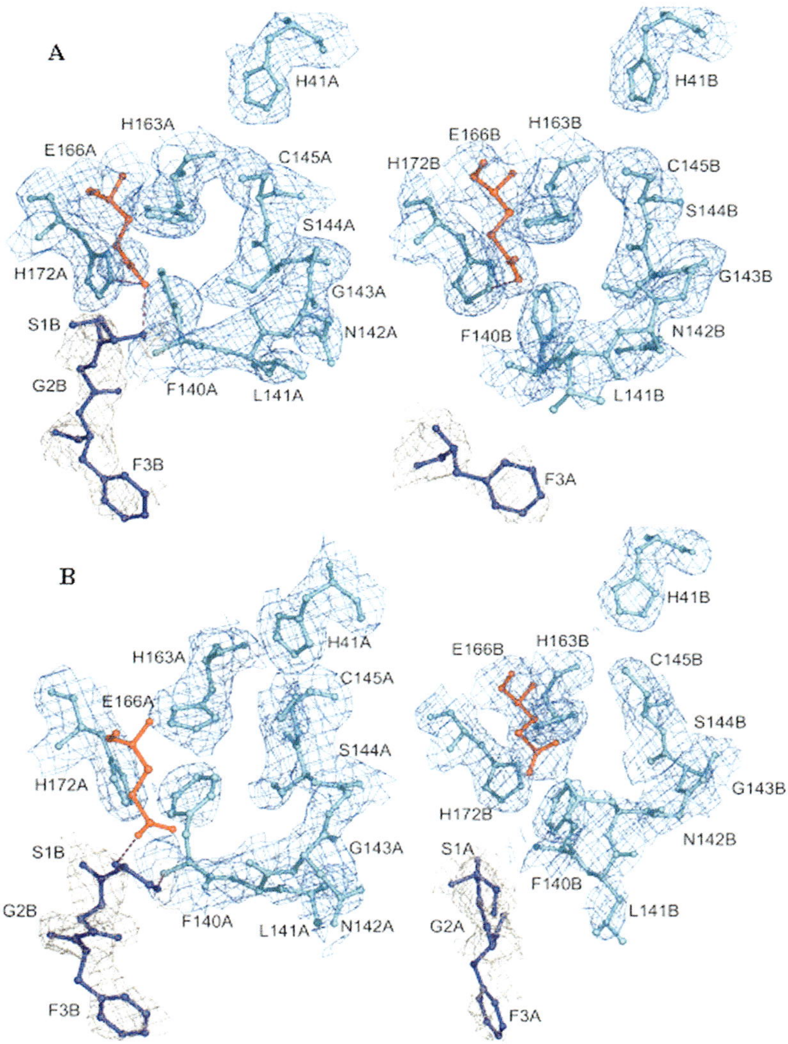

Figure 6. The S1 pocket of SARS-CoV M^{pro} equilibrated at pH 7.6 (A) and pH 8.0 (B). Left panels: molecule A, right panels: molecule B.

fully formed in both monomers and Phe140 is interacting with the now unprotonated His163. The oxyanion is correctly shaped. Glu166 forms ion pairs with His172 and the N-terminus of the other monomer in the dimer. At pH 8.0 (Fig. 6B), another interesting change takes place. The salt bridge between Glu166 and His172 breaks – but not the one between Glu166 and the amino terminus of the other protomer in the dimer –, resulting in

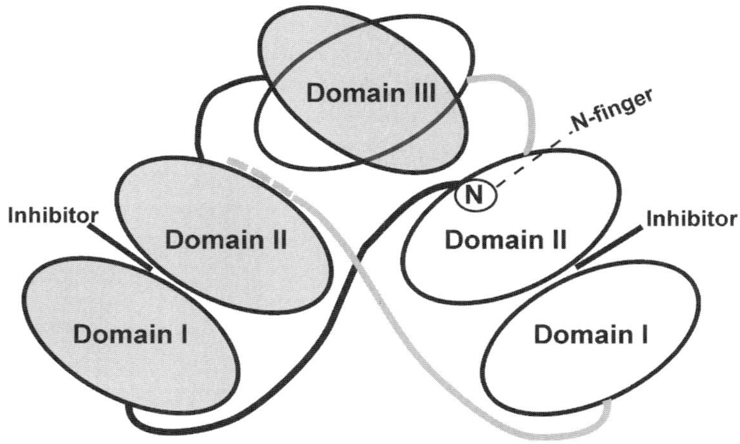

Figure 7. Schematic drawing of the SARS-CoV M^{pro} dimer as seen in the crystal structure at pH 6.0. Note the important role of the "N-finger".

Glu166 becoming more mobile and partly filling the S1 pocket, thereby decreasing the activity of the enzyme. This is presumably due to the deprotonation of His172 at the high pH value. The pK value of histidine residues involved in salt bridges has been shown to be around 8.0 to 8.5, fully consistent with our interpretation of the phenomenon. Thus, we propose that the low-pH and high-pH flanks of the bell-shaped pH-activity curve (Fig. 5) are determined by the protonation and deprotonation of His163 and His172, respectively. In this respect, our interpretation differs from that of Lai and coworkers who proposed that deactivation of the enzyme at high pH is due to deprotonation of the active-site cysteine [26]. In our opinion, the latter would only play a role at even higher pH values of >9.

The different protonation states of His163 and His172 and their influence on the conformation of the substrate-binding site were further explored by molecular-dynamics calculations over 10 ns each (Tan et al., in preparation). The results are in full agreement with the interpretation of the crystal structures put forward here. Furthermore, molecular dynamics calculations have the advantage that they can simulate states of the system under investigation that are not easily accessible to experiment. A dynamics run at pH 5.0, with His163 protonated in both monomers of the dimer, revealed a tendency of the two S1 pockets to collapse, with Glu166 switching between the protonated His163 and His172 residues over the time of the simulation.

It is important to note that none of the conformational differences seen between monomers "A" and "B" of the SARS-CoV M^{pro} when crystallized at pH 6.0 is due to crystal packing artefacts. Symmetry-related contacts between dimers mainly involve domain III of both molecules; the only residues in domains I and II to display strong crystal contacts are His A134, Asn B53, Asp B56, Ile B59, Arg B60, His B134. Furthermore, the fact that the conformation of monomer B flips back to the normal, active one within the same crystal lattice after equilibration of the crystals at higher pH values, proves that crystal packing does not play a role here.

The amino terminus of the SARS-CoV M^{pro} plays an important role in our structural model, by interacting with essential residues of the substrate-binding site of the other monomer in the dimer. Like a finger, the N-terminus docks into its specific binding site (Fig. 7) and flicks on the enzymatic activity of the other monomer. Hydrogen bonding from the "N-finger" to the main chain of Phe140 helps shape the oxyanion loop, and ion-pair formation with Glu166 prevents the latter from blocking the S1 specificity pocket. If a free N-terminus is not available at position 1 of the M^{pro}, such as in the maltose-binding protein (MBP) fusion protein or in the presence of an N-terminal histidine tag, the enzymatic activity should be reduced and this has indeed been observed, at least with the MBP fusion protein [13]. In order to further demonstrate the importance of the N terminus, we deleted residues 1 to 5 in the TGEV M^{pro} and indeed found the enzyme to be almost totally inactive [13]. This observation also solves the mystery of the importance of the "extra" helical domain III of the main proteinase. Its task is to provide defined interaction points for the N-terminal segment and thereby locating the tip of the N-finger to its specific interaction site with Phe140 and Glu166 of the other monomer. Accordingly, deletion of domain III also results in an inactive enzyme [13]. The enzyme is dimeric because of the essential role played by the N-finger, but the N-terminal segment is not essential for dimerization, as shown recently by Shi et al. [24] and also indicated by steered molecular dynamics calculations of a SARS-CoV M^{pro} dimer devoid of the N-terminal residues (Tan et al., personal communication).

A transition between a catalytically competent and an incompetent conformation of the oxyanion-binding site has also been seen in the crystal structure of equine arterivirus main proteinase (nsp4), where the loop structurally equivalent to the M^{pro} 139–143 loop undergoes a peptide flip, resulting in misorientation of the amide corresponding to Gly143 [30]. Also, we have little doubt that the same pH-induced conformational changes that we observed in the SARS-CoV M^{pro} does exist in all other coronavirus main proteinases. We simply failed to detect it earlier because we had crystallized the M^{pro}s of TGEV and HCoV 229E at pH >8.0, i.e. with both monomers adopting an active conformation [13, 18].

In conclusion, SARS-CoV M^{pro} appears to possess a pH-triggered activation switch, which may regulate proteolytic activity in different cellular compartments. Such a pH switch would provide the virus with a mechanism to synchronize the polyprotein processing with the microenvironment. Further mutagenesis and biochemical studies on the details of the switch are clearly desirable.

Self-activation of the main proteinases

The M^{pro} is part of the viral polyprotein itself and has to be activated by autocleavage from this inactive precursor before it can cleave the polyprotein at other cleavage sites. So far, it has been completely unclear how this autoactivation might occur but the crystallographic work on SARS-CoV M^{pro} now provides a clue. The pH-dependent conformational changes seen in the X-ray structures [19] could well correlate with the structural arrangements occurring during self-activation of the enzyme.

Moreover, a comparison with the transition between chymotrypsin and its proenzyme, chymotrypsinogen, reveals a remarkable similarity in the mechanisms used. In mature chymotrypsin, the charged amino terminus, created after cleavage of the proenzyme at the Arg15-Ile16 bond, forms an ion pair with Asp194, a residue involved in forming the wall of the S1 specificity pocket. In chymotrypsinogen, on the other hand, the N-terminal extension of the polypeptide chain by 15 residues causes disruption of this ion pair [31]. The Asp194 side chain changes conformation and so does, along with it, Gly193, whose amide forms part of the oxyanion hole. As a consequence, interaction of Gly193, which corresponds to Gly143 of SARS-CoV M^{pro}, with the tetrahedral intermediate is no longer possible. In SARS-CoV and other coronaviruses, the polyprotein upstream to the N-terminal autocleavage site of the M^{pro} corresponds to the propeptide in chymotrypsinogen. The role of Asp194 of the latter is taken by Glu166 in SARS-CoV M^{pro} and its proenzyme, and the oxyanion-binding region changes in a similar way. The major difference between the two enzymes is that the event is *intra*molecular in chymotrypsin but *inter*molecular in SARS-CoV M^{pro}.

It is a matter of debate whether the autocleavage of the M^{pro}s from the polyprotein precursors occur in *cis* or in *trans*. In the case of mouse hepatitis (corona)virus (MHV) M^{pro}, autocleavage has exclusively been observed in *trans* [28]. On the other hand, it has been shown for several picornavirus 3C proteinases, e.g. hepatitis A virus $3C^{pro}$ [32], that the first step of autocleavage of the enzyme, i.e. processing at the N-terminal cleavage site, occurs in *cis*, followed by other cleavage reactions in *trans*. Molecular modeling studies based on the TGEV M^{pro} crystal structure suggested that N-terminal precursor cleavage in cis should be possible, because by introducing a bend around residues 11 to 13, the extended N-terminal chain can be quite easily folded back into the active site of its own molecule, even though the distance between the amino terminus (A1) and CysA145 $S\gamma$ is about 34 Å [13]. On the other hand, bringing the N terminus from the position seen in the crystal structure into the catalytic site of the other molecule in the dimer proves quite difficult, even though the distance is only about 11 Å. Thus, the fact that the M^{pro}s are dimers does not necessarily support cleavage in *trans*. The SARS-CoV M^{pro} structure rather suggests a different role for the dimerization, the mutual activation of the subunits by transition from the proenzyme conformation to that of the active enzyme, triggered by binding of N-fingers to the activation switch. Clearly, asymmetric dimers consisting of one molecule in the mature conformation and one in the proenzyme conformation, as seen in the SARS-CoV M^{pro} crystal structure at pH 6.0, would be important intermediates in this process. Polyprotein processing in SARS-CoV-infected cells could thus be initiated by the occasional dimerization of two membrane-anchored M^{pro} domains within polyproteins and mutual activation through the N-finger tips, or by the rare event of cis-autocleavage of a single M^{pro} domain which then binds to another one within polyprotein, again activating it through the N-finger. The results are highly active M^{pro} dimers which can then cleave other substrates in *trans*. Such a mechanism could lead to self-acceleration of M^{pro} autoprocessing, after a slow onset triggered by a rare initial event. This mechanism is consistent with the fact that in cells infected with HCoV 229E or MHV, long-lived cleavage intermediates are usually not observed, but polyprotein is processed with increasing speed, once the first cleavage has occurred [28, 33].

Complex of the SARS-CoV M^{pro} with a chloromethyl ketone inhibitor

After dissecting the details of conformational dynamics of the SARS-CoV main proteinase, we are now finally in the position to competently discuss the interactions of the enzyme with substrate. To visualize these, the substrate-analoguous hexapeptidyl CMK inhibitor, Cbz-Val-Asn-Ser-Thr-Leu-Gln-CMK, was soaked into the crystals of the SARS-CoV enzyme grown at pH 6.0, and the structure of the complex was determined at 2.5 Å resolution [19]. We expected to see one of two possible cases, i.e. either i) the inhibitor would only bind to the protomer in the active conformation (monomer “A”), or ii) it would bind to the inactive protomer (monomer “B”) as well, thereby imposing the active conformation onto the latter by an induced-fit mechanism. Quite unexpectedly, neither assumption turned out to be true. Instead, whereas the inhibitor does bind to both subunits and covalent bonds are being formed between the Sγ of Cys145 and the methylene group of the CMK, the inhibitor exhibits two different modes of binding, each of which is unusual and unexpected (Fig. 3B, C). Protomer “B” remains in the inactive conformation, and the inhibitor does not open the occluded S1 pocket to allow the P1 Gln to enter the specificity site (Fig. 3C). Instead, the P1 Gln points out of the substrate-binding cleft and towards bulk solvent. On the other hand, P2 Leu and P4 Ser bind to the appropriate specificity pockets that have been observed in the structure of TGEV M^{pro} [13], whereas P3 Thr is oriented toward bulk solvent. This result can be interpreted as resulting from the high chemical reactivity of the CMK moiety with obvious concurrent inability of the inhibitor to overcome the protonation of HisB163 at the bottom of the S1 pocket at pH 6.0.

Binding of the CMK inhibitor to protomer A, which exhibits the active conformation, is even less conventional (Fig. 3B). The P1 glutamine resides in the S1 pocket and its side-chain carbonyl accepts a 2.8-Å hydrogen bond from the Nε2 atom of HisA163, whereas its side-chain amide nitrogen donates a 2.8-Å hydrogen bond to the carboxylate of GluA166, ensuring the specificity for glutamine in the S1 subsite. However, the P2 residue fails to penetrate the S2 subsite and becomes partially solvent-accessible. This non-canonical binding results in a frameshift in subsite interaction: P3 Thr occupies the S2 pocket instead and P5 Asn binds at the S4 subsite. We note that the P2 residue specificity of SARS-CoV M^{pro} is less stringent than that of other CoV M^{pro}s, which, with few exceptions, are restricted to leucine [28]. The unexpected binding mode of the substrate-like inhibitor may well be a consequence of the more relaxed specificity requirements of the SARS-CoV M^{pro}, compared to other coronaviral main proteinases. However, before further conclusions are made, it has to be excluded that the binding mode observed is due to an artefact, perhaps because the sequence of the peptidyl CMK inhibitor had been derived from the TGEV M^{pro} and not the SARS-CoV M^{pro} N-terminal autocleavage site. Therefore, we are presently determining the crystal structures of the complexes of SARS-CoV M^{pro} with other inhibitors, both peptidic and non-peptidic.

Structure-based design of anti-SARS inhibitors

When the genome sequence of the SARS coronavirus was published on the internet on April 13, 2003 [16], we immediately located the segment in orf1a coding for the main proteinase and aligned the amino acid sequence of the enzyme with the M^{pro}s of other coronaviruses. Next, we constructed a homology model of the SARS-CoV M^{pro}, based on this alignment and our crystal structures of the TGEV and HCoV 229E main proteinases [18]. This theoretical model revealed that the substrate-binding site of the SARS-CoV enzyme is very similar to those of the two other viral enzymes. At that time, less than one month after the discovery of the new SARS virus and at the peak of the epidemic in China, this structural model was the best we could get, and it proved in fact very useful (see below). Of course, a theoretical homology model will always be inferior to an experimental crystal structure, but in the absence of the latter, it can provide a reasonably good basis for structure-assisted drug discovery [34, 35]. When we had determined the crystal structure of the SARS-CoV M^{pro} another 10 weeks later [19], the overall r.m.s. deviation for all Cα atoms of the protein between theoretical model and experimental structure was found to be as high as 3.8 Å. However, this unreasonably high value is only caused by large deviations of the last four residues at the flexible C-terminus, which deviate by more than 12 Å, and by slight differences of the mutual orientation of the three domains. If the models for the individual domains are compared with the crystal structure, and only this is a fair comparison in view of the large flexibility of the enzyme, the r.m.s. deviation is down to little more than 1 Å.

Whatever the view taken on this issue, the homology model served primarily one purpose, and that was to facilitate the design of anti-SARS inhibitors directed at the main proteinase. With the template of the peptidyl CMK inhibitor – as bound to the TGEV M^{pro} – at hand, we compared its binding mode to those seen for all other inhibitors of cysteine proteinases that occupy the N-terminal half of the substrate binding site (subsites Sn-S1), as long as atomic coordinates were available in the Protein Data Bank (PDB). We found that AG7088, a compound carrying a vinylogous ethyl ester instead of a CMK group and designed to block human rhinovirus (HRV) 3C proteinase [36], interacted in much the same way with its target enzyme than did our CMK inhibitor (Fig. 8) [18].

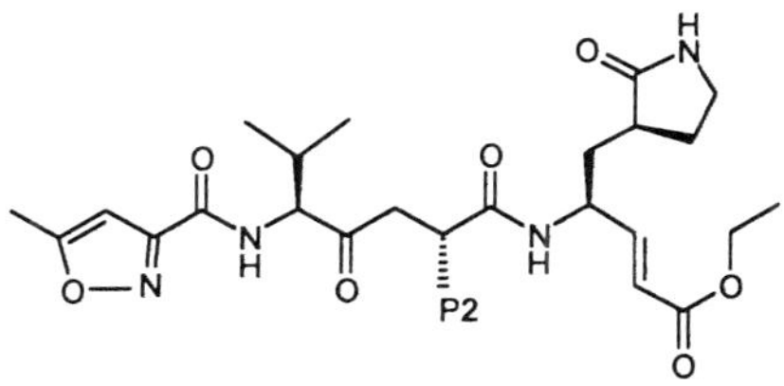

P2 = *p*-fluoro-benzyl: AG7088 (CAS number: 223537-30-2, Pfizer Inc.)

As mentioned before, the picornavirus 3C proteinases ($3C^{pro}$) have a chymotrypsin-related structure, reminiscent of domains I and II of the coronavirus M^{pro}, although several of the secondary-structure elements are arranged differently, making structural alignment difficult with sequence identities < 10%. Also, they completely lack a counterpart to domain III of coronavirus M^{pro}s. Nevertheless, the substrate specificity of picornavirus $3C^{pro}$s [32, 37] for the P1', P1 and P4 sites is similar to that of the coronavirus M^{pro}s (hence the original designation "3C-like" for the latter; see Tab. 1). Only parts of the two structures, TGEV M^{pro} in complex with the CMK inhibitor and HRV-2 in complex with AG7088, can be spatially superimposed (Fig. 8; r.m.s. deviation of 2.10 Å for 134 pairs of Cα positions out of the ~180 residues in domains I and II). Both inhibitors, the hexapeptidyl CMK and AG7088, bind to their respective target proteinases through formation of an antiparallel β-sheet with strand eII. However, completely different segments of the polypeptide chain interact with the substrate analogues on the opposite site: residues 188 to 191 of the loop connecting domains II and III in M^{pro}, as opposed to the short β-strand 126 to 128 in HRV $3C^{pro}$. As a result, the architectures of the S2 subsites are entirely different between the two enzymes; hence, the different specificities for the P2 residues of the substrates (Leu *versus* Phe). The inhibitor

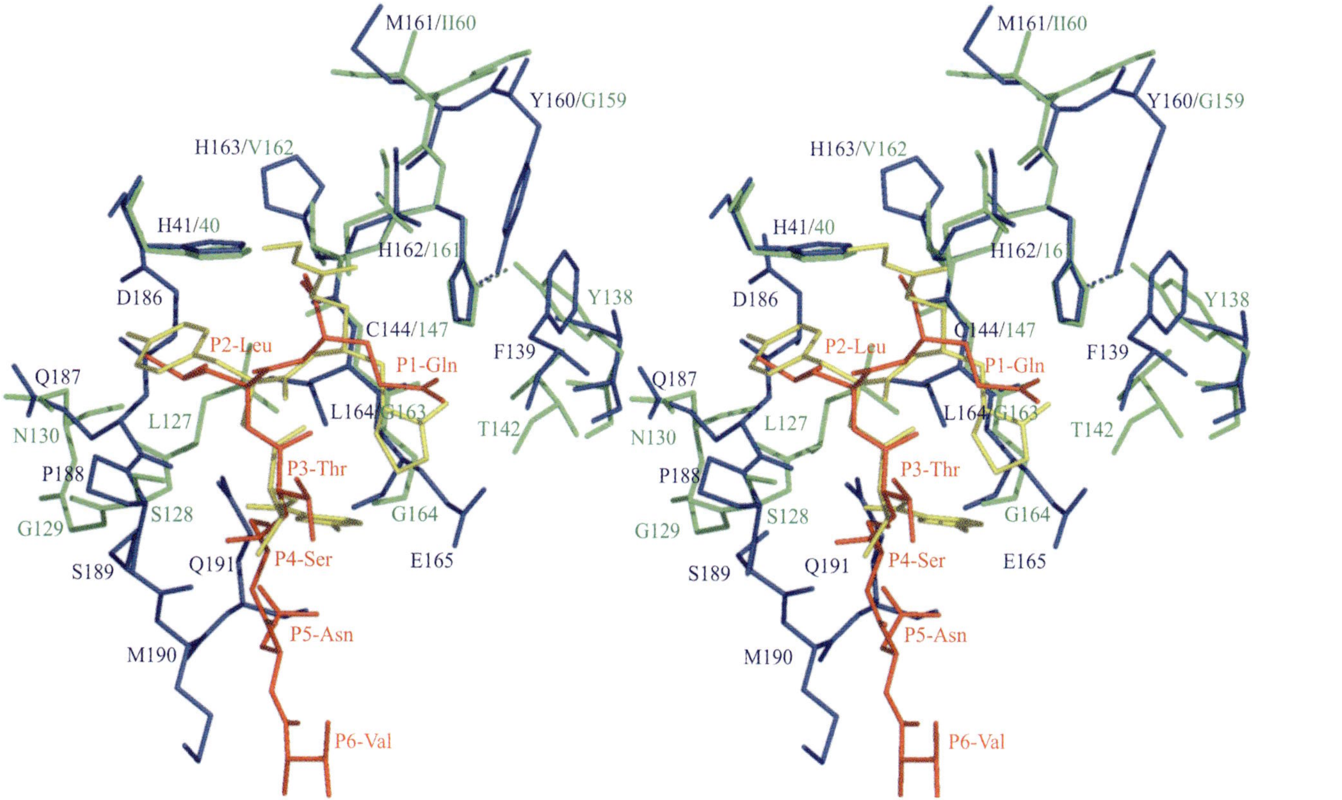

Figure 8. Superimposed structures of TGEV M^{pro} (blue) in complex with CMK inhibitor (red) and HRV-2 (green) in complex with AG7088 (yellow). Only the substrate-binding sites are shown. Stereo illustration. From [18], with permission of the American Association for the Advancement of Science (AAAS).

AG7088 has a *p*-fluorophenylalanine side chain (*p*-fluorobenzyl) in this position. Based on molecular modeling, we proposed that this side chain might be too long to fit into the S2 pocket of coronavirus M^{pro}, but an unmodified benzyl group would probably fit, as evidenced by Phe occurring in the P2 position of the C-terminal autocleavage site of the SARS coronavirus enzyme (see Tab. 1). Apart from this difference, the superimposition of the two complexes (Fig. 8) suggested that the side chains of AG7088 binding to subsites S1 (lactone derivative of glutamine) and S4 (5-methyl-isoxazole-3-carbonyl) can be easily accommodated by the coronavirus M^{pro}. Thus, we proposed that AG7088 could serve as a starting point for modifications which should quickly lead to an efficient and bioavailable inhibitor for coronavirus main proteinases. In fact, such modifications have been applied (work mostly unpublished so far; a published proposal for modification is found in [38]) and we will see a number of good inhibitors designed on this basis appear in the literature in the next few months.

Another possible approach to inhibiting the SARS-CoV main proteinase could make use of the insight into the importance of the N-finger in activating the enzyme. One could screen for competitve inhibitors that prevent M^{pro} dimerization through binding to the N-finger docking site, but without activating the Glu166/Phe140 switch. Such an approach would open a second front in addition to active site-directed inhibitors, in the urgent search for substances efficiently blocking the SARS coronavirus.

Several groups have proposed to use HIV-1 proteinase inhibitors as starting points for designing inhibitors directed at the SARS-CoV M^{pro}. However, many of these studies remained at the modelling level and failed to prove the usefulness of the HIV-1 proteinase inhibitors experimentally [39, 40]. Some of the reports did not even seem to acknowledge the fact that the enzymatic mechanisms of HIV-1 proteinase, an aspartic proteinase, and SARS-CoV main proteinase, a cysteine proteinase, are very different. One of the few studies reporting a clinical usefulness of the application of HIV-1 proteinase inhibitors was published by Peiris et al. [41]. According to their results, a combination of the HIV-1 proteinase inhibitor kaletra and ribavirin was more effective than ribavirin alone, which, however, was basically inactive, as shown later [42]. Based on the present structural knowledge, it is not obvious how HIV-1 proteinase inhibitors should block SARS-CoV.

In conclusion, prospects for discovering and developing inhibitors of the SARS-CoV main proteinase are good, given the structural knowledge that is available for the target today. It should also be emphasized that the crystal structures of the various M^{pro}s allow very efficient virtual screening [43] for existing organic compounds that might bind and inhibit the target. This approach is currently yielding promising inhibitors, which also exhibit anti-SARS activity on virus-infected Vero cells (Jiang, personal communication).

Conclusions

The three-dimensional structures presented here for coronavirus main proteinases provide a solid basis for the design of anti-coronaviral drugs. The binding modes of peptidic inhibitors and substrates have been revealed by the crystal structure of TGEV M^{pro} in complex with a hexapeptidyl chloromethyl ketone, and, within limitations, of the complex with the SARS-CoV M^{pro} and the same inhibitor. The structure of the SARS-CoV enzyme was determined at three different pH values and revealed a pH-dependent activation switch for the M^{pro}. The pH-activity profile of the main proteinase was shown to be governed by the protonation and deprotonation of two histidine residues in the substrate-binding site. The conformational changes observed also suggested a mechanism for the self-activation of the M^{pro} by autocleavage from the viral polyprotein. On the basis of structural comparisons between the TGEV M^{pro} in complex with a hexapeptidyl CMK inhibitor and the HRV 3C proteinase in complex with the vinylogous ethyl ester AG7088, it has been proposed that whereas the latter would not be a good inhibitor of the SARS-CoV M^{pro}, it should be a good starting point for designing such inhibitors. Such design studies are being performed at the moment and will start to yield potent anti-SARS compounds in the next few months and years.

Acknowledgements

The work described here was, in part, supported by grants from the "Deutsche Forschungsgemeinschaft", the "Sino-German Center for the Promotion of Science", the "Sino-European Project on SARS Diagnostics and Antivirals" (SEPSDA) of the European Commission, the Chinese Ministry of Science and Technology, and the "Fonds der Chemischen Industrie".

References

1 Drosten C, Günther S, Preiser W, van der Werf S, Brodt HR, Becker S, Rabenau H, Panning M, Kolesnikova L, Fouchier RAM et al (2003) Identification of a novel coronavirus in patients with severe acute respiratory syndrome. *N Engl J Med* 348: 1967–1976

2 Ksiazek TG, Erdman D, Goldsmith CS, Zaki SR, Peret T, Emery S, Tong S, Urbani C, Comer JA, Lim W et al (2003) A novel coronavirus associated with severe acute respiratory syndrome. *N Engl J Med* 348: 1953–1966

3 Cavanagh D (1997) *Nidovirales*: a new order comprising *Coronaviridae* and *Arteriviridae*. *Arch Virol* 142: 629–633

4 Cowley JA, Dimmock CM, Spann KM, Walker PJ (2000) Gill-associated virus

of *Penaeus monodon* prawns: an invertebrate virus with ORF1a and ORF1b genes related to arteri- and coronaviruses. *J Gen Virol* 81: 1473–1484
5 den Boon JA, Snijder EJ, Chirnside ED, de Vries AA, Horzinek MC, Spaan WJ (1991) Equine arteritis virus is not a togavirus but belongs to the coronavirus-like superfamily. *J Virol* 65: 2910–2920
6 Enjuanes L, van der Zeijst BAM (1995) Molecular basis of transmissible gastroenteritis virus epidemiology. In: SG Siddell (ed): *The Coronaviridae*. Plenum Press, New York, NY, 337–376
7 Saif LJ, Wesley R (1999) Transmissible gastroenteritis virus. In Straw BES, Allaire WL, Mengeling WL, Taylor DJ (eds): *Diseases of Swine*, 8th edn. Iowa State University Press, Ames, Iowa, 295–325
8 Myint SH (1995) Human coronavirus infections. In: Siddell SG (ed): *The Coronavirdae*. Plenum Press, New York, 389–401
9 Lee N, Hui D, Wu A, Chan P, Cameron P, Joynt GM, Ahuja A, Yung MY, Leung CB, To KF et al (2003) A major outbreak of severe acute respiratory syndrome in Hong Kong. *N Engl J Med* 348: 1986–1994
10 Herold J, Raabe T, Schelle-Prinz B, Siddell SG (1993) Nucleotide sequence of the human coronavirus 229E RNA polymerase locus. *Virology* 195: 680–691
11 Thiel V, Herold J, Schelle B, Siddell SG (2001) Viral replicase gene products suffice for coronavirus discontinuous transcription. *J Virol* 75: 6676–6681
12 Ziebuhr J, Herold J, Siddell SG (1995) Characterization of a human coronavirus (strain 229E) 3C-like proteinase activity. *J Virol* 69: 4331–4338
13 Anand K, Palm J, Mesters J, Siddell SG, Ziebuhr J, Hilgenfeld R (2002) Structure of coronavirus main proteinase reveals combination of a chymotrypsin fold with an extra α-helical domain. *EMBO J* 21: 3213–3224
14 Ziebuhr J, Snijder EJ, Gorbalenya AE (2000) Virus-encoded proteinases and proteolytic processing in the *Nidovirales*. *J Gen Virol* 81: 853–879
15 Hegyi A, Ziebuhr J (2002) Conservation of substrate specificities among coronavirus main proteases. *J Gen Virol* 83: 595–599
16 Marra M, Jones SJ, Astell CR, Holt RA, Brooks-Wilson A, Butterfield YS, Khattra J, Asano JK, Barber SA, Chan SY et al (2003) The genome sequence of the SARS-associated coronavirus. *Science* 300: 1399–1404
17 Rota PA, Oberste MS, Monroe SS, Nix WA, Campagnoli R, Icenogle JP, Penaranda S, Bankamp B, Maher K, Chen MH et al (2003) Characterization of a novel coronavirus associated with severe acute respiratory syndrome. *Science* 300: 1394–1399
18 Anand K, Ziebuhr J, Wadhwani P, Mesters J, Hilgenfeld R (2003) Coronavirus main proteinase ($3CL^{pro}$) structure: basis for design of anti-SARS drugs. *Science* 300: 1763–1767
19 Yang H, Yang M, Ding Y, Liu Y, Lou Z, Zhou Z, Sun L, Mo L, Ye S, Pang H et al (2003) The crystal structures of severe acute respiratory syndrome virus main protease and its complex with an inhibitor. *Proc Natl Acad Sci USA* 100: 13190–13195
20 Tsukada H, Blow DM (1985) Structure of a-chymotrypsin refined at 1.68 Å resolution. *J Mol Biol* 184: 703–711

21 Allaire M, Chernaia MM, Malcolm BA, James MN (1994) Picornaviral 3C cysteine proteinases have a fold similar to chymotrypsin-like serine proteinases. *Nature* 369: 72–76

22 Bergmann EM, Mosimann SC, Chernaia MM, Malcolm BA, James MN (1997) The refined crystal structure of the 3C gene product from hepatitis A virus: specific proteinase activity and RNA recognition. *J Virol* 71: 2436–2448

23 Fan K, Wei P, Feng Q, Chen S, Huang C, Ma L, Lai B, Pei J, Liu Y, Chen J, Lai L (2004) Biosynthesis, purification, and substrate specificity of severe acute respiratory syndrome coronavirus 3C-like proteinase. *J Biol Chem* 279: 1637–1642

24 Shi J, Wei Z, Song J (2004) Dissection study on the severe acute respiratory syndrome virus 3C-like protease reveals the critical role of the extra domain in dimerization of the enzyme. *J Biol Chem* 279: 24765–24773

25 Polgár, L (1974) Mercaptide-imidazolium ion-pair: the reactive nucleophile in papain catalysis. *FEBS Lett* 47: 15–18

26 Huang C, Wei P, Fan K, Liu Y, Lai L (2004) 3C-like proteinase from SARS coronavirus catalyzes substrate hydrolysis by a general-base mechanism. *Biochemistry* 43: 4568–4574.

27 Hegyi A, Friebe A, Gorbalenya AE, Ziebuhr J (2002) Mutational analysis of the active centre of coronavirus 3C-like proteases. *J Gen Virol* 83: 581–593

28 Ziebuhr J, Snijder EJ, Gorbalenya AE (2000) Virus-encoded proteinases and proteolytic processing in the *Nidovirales*. *J Gen Virol* 81: 853–879

29 Heisen B (2004) Expression, Reinigung und Aktivitätsbestimmung der Hauptproteinase des SARS-Coronavirus. Bachelor Thesis, University of Lübeck, 2004

30 Barrette-Ng IH, Ng KK, Mark BL, Van Aken D, Cherney MM, Garen C, Kolodenko Y, Gorbalenya AE, Snijder EJ, James MN (2002) Structure of arterivirus nsp4. The smallest chymotrypsin-like proteinase with an alpha/beta C-terminal extension and alternate conformations of the oxyanion hole. *J Biol Chem* 277: 39960–39966

31 Bode W, Schwager P, Huber R (1978) The transition of bovine trypsinogen to a trypsin-like state upon strong ligand binding. The refined crystal structures of the bovine trypsinogen-pancreatic trypsin inhibitor complex and of its ternary complex with Ile-Val at 1.9 A resolution. *J Mol Biol* 118: 99–112

32 Ryan MD, Flint M (1997) Virus-encoded proteinases of the picornavirus supergroup. *J Gen Virol* 78: 699–723

33 Ziebuhr J, Heusipp G, Siddell SG (1997) Biosynthesis, purification, and characterization of the human coronavirus 229E 3C-like proteinase. *J Virol* 71: 3992–3997

34 Hillisch A, Pineda F, Hilgenfeld R (2004) The use of homology models in the drug discovery process. *Drug Discov Today* 9: 659–669

35 Hillisch A, Hilgenfeld R (eds) *Modern Methods of Drug Discovery*. Birkhäuser, Basel, 2002.

36 Matthews DA, Dragovitch PS, Webber SE, Fuhrman SA, Patick AK, Zalman LS, Hendrickson TF, Love RA, Prins TJ, Marakovits JT (1999) Structure-assist-

ed design of mechanism-based irreversible inhibitors of human rhinovirus 3C protease with potent antiviral activity against multiple rhinovirus serotypes. *Proc Natl Acad Sci USA* 96: 11000–11007
37 Kräusslich HG, Wimmer E (1988) Viral proteinases. *Annu Rev Biochem* 57: 701–754
38 Chou K, Wei D, Zhong W (2003) Binding mechanism of coronavirus main proteinase with ligands and its implication to drug design against SARS. *Biochem Biophys Res Commun* 308: 148–151
39 Jenwitheesuk E, Samudrala R (2003) Identifying inhibitors of the SARS coronavirus proteinase. *BMC Lett* 13: 3989–3992
40 Zhang XW, Yap YL (2004) Old drugs as lead compounds for a new disease? Binding analysis of SARS coronavirus main proteinase with HIV, psychotic, and parasite drugs. *Bioorg Med Chem* 12: 2517–2521
41 Peiris JSM, Chu CM, Cheng VCC, Chan KS, Hung IFN, Poon LLM, Law KI, Tang BSF, Hon TYW, Chan CS et al (2003) Clinical progression and viral load in a community outbreak of coronavirus-associated SARS pneumonia: a prospective study. *Lancet* 361: 1767–1762
42 Cyranoski D (2003) Critics slam treatment for SARS as ineffective and perhaps dangerous. *Nature* 423: 4
43 Shen J, Xu X, Cheng F, Liu H, Luo X, Shen J, Chen K, Zhao W, Shen X, Jiang H (2003) Virtual screening on natural products for discovering active compounds and target information. *Curr Med Chem* 10: 1241–1253

Coronaviruses with Special Emphasis on First Insights Concerning SARS
ed. by A. Schmidt, M.H. Wolff and O. Weber

Environmental survival and microbicide inactivation of coronaviruses

Manfred H. Wolff,[1] Syed A. Sattar,[2] Olusola Adegbunrin[2] and Jason Tetro[2]

[1] *Faculty of Bioscience, Institute of Microbiology and Virology, Stockumer Str. 10, D-58453 Witten, Germany*
[2] *Centre for Research on Environmental Microbiology (CREM), Faculty of Medicine, University of Ottawa, Ottawa, Ontario, Canada K1H 8M5*

Introduction

Since their first isolation from chickens in 1937 [1], coronaviruses have proven to be significant pathogens of many types of wild as well as economically important domesticated animals. Though coronaviruses were first identified as human respiratory pathogens in 1965 [2], only recently, with their established link with the severe acute respiratory syndrome (SARS), has there been a sudden upsurge of interest in this group of viruses.

Taxonomically, these enveloped, positive-sense RNA viruses [1] belong in the genus *Coronavirus* of the family *Coronaviridae* in the order *Nidovirales* [3]. To date, the genus contains some 14 members. Birds and mammals are the known hosts with a wide variety of species affected. In mammals, coronaviruses have been isolated from pigs, cattle, mice, rats, dogs, horses, cats, and humans [1], and in birds mainly from chickens [4] and turkeys [5].

Coronaviruses 229E and OC43 are recognized respiratory pathogens of humans. The causative agent of SARS (SARS-CoV), which has now been fully characterized [6], awaits its formal inclusion in the genus. Genomic studies show SARS-CoV to be unique as it contains elements of both mammalian and avian ancestry [7] and the effect of this recombination has been disastrous for humans. In the first recorded outbreak in 2003, the virus caused 8,461 clinical cases and 804 recorded deaths globally [8]. Fortunately, and in spite of its seemingly high mutation rates [9], the spread of the virus was effectively controlled, mainly through general public health measures and basic infection control practices. Nevertheless, the SARS incident has had a significant impact on human health and the global economy [10] and thus highlighted the need to better understand the modes and vehicles for its spread and proper means to interrupt its environmental transmission.

Pathogenesis and shedding of infectious virus

Depending on the type of coronavirus and the animal host species, virus shedding can occur from the respiratory and/or gastrointestinal tract [11] and the two main portals of virus entry into susceptible animals are the nose and the mouth [12]. In humans, coronaviruses normally cause the common cold, SARS being a notable exception because it causes severe pneumonia as well as acute gastroenteritis. The risk of environmental contamination with the SARS-CoV is thus much higher. The evidence available thus far from outbreak investigations is strongly suggestive of droplet transmission [13] and to a much limited degree by aerosols [14]. It is not known if the SARS-CoV can also be acquired through the mouth or the conjunctivae, nor do we know if inhaled virus deposited in the throat can be directly translocated to the gut.

In SARS, massive spiking of the immunological response leads to hypoxia and eventual respiratory distress syndrome [15]. Infection of the gastrointestinal tract causes acute diarrhea and may also result in peritonitis and necrotizing colitis [16]. The simultaneous involvement of the respiratory as well as the gastrointestinal tracts in SARS [11] is highly reminiscent of coronavirus infections in cattle [17] and other animals.

Based on the pig model, the infectious period for coronaviruses is approximately 6 days post-infection [12, 18] with a peak at day 4 post-infection. This holds true for bovine [17, 19] and human infections [20, 21] as well. In pigs, virus release from the nose peaks on the fourth day of infection with yields of $>5.5 \log_{10}$ $TCID_{50}$/g of nasal discharge, with the air around such animals containing nearly 2 $\log_{10}$ of infectious virus/m^3 [12]. Similarly, infectious virus has been detected in the nasal discharge and feces of SARS patients [11].

Environmental survival and spread of coronaviruses

In general, a given pathogen must remain viable outside the host to allow for environmental spread, and the combined effect of many biotic and abiotic factors determines how long such viability can be retained. While environmental survival of coronaviruses has been studied to some degree under experimental conditions [22, 23] including SARS (Tab. 1), we know much less about the types and relative significance of vehicles in the in-nature spread of coronaviruses, in particular those that can infect humans. For example, infectious virus has been recovered from both droplets and air in the vicinity of pigs experimentally infected with the porcine respiratory coronavirus [12], but the potential, if any, of droplets and aerosols in the spread of the virus to susceptible animals in the vicinity is unknown.

The following is a summary of the available information on the environmental survival and spread of coronaviruses.

Table 1. Environmental survival of SARS-CoV (modified from [20]

Environment	Number of hours virus infectivity remained detectable
Fluid	
Cell culture fluid at 4°C	>120
Cell culture fluid at room temperature	60
Autoclaved water	72
Serum	72
Sputum	96
Feces	96
Urine	<6
Non-porous environmental surface	
Glass	60
Mosaic	60
Metal	72
Plastic	60
Porous materials	
Cloth	72
Filter paper	72
Autoclaved soil (Beijing, China)	<6

Air

The effect of relative humidity (RH) and air temperature has been studied on the airborne survival of experimentally aerosolized human coronavirus 229E [22]. As is true for enveloped viruses in general, 229E survived better at 30-50% RH than at 80% RH when the air temperature was about 20°C. Under these conditions, the half-lives of the virus at 30%, 50% and 80% RH were 27, 67 and 3 hours, respectively. Lowering the air temperature to 6°C increased the half-lives of the virus at 30% and 50% RH to 34 and 103 hours, respectively. But the lower air temperature produced the most dramatic effect on virus survival at 80% RH and changed its half-life from 3 to over 86 hours.

The available epidemiological evidence strongly suggests that SARS spreads through droplets [13] and such spread is much easier to control than that through aerosols. However, the pattern of spread of SARS-CoV in at least two instances is highly suggestive of airborne spread.

A cluster of 329 SARS cases was recorded in one apartment complex in Hong Kong with the majority of them occurring on several floors in one wing [24]. This pattern of spread is highly suggestive of virus dissemination by air, and the aerosolization of the virus was speculated to have occurred from malfunctioning sewers in the building [24]. Rodent pests in the building have been hypothesized as possible amplifiers and disseminators of the virus [25]; the virus, most likely acquired from infected residents, may have multiplied in the rodents, being released in their excreta and then possibly becoming airborne. While hantaviruses, for example, can infect humans from aerosolized rodent excreta [26], the role of air in the transmission of SARS-CoV in this outbreak remains speculative at this stage. However, a more detailed analysis of the outbreak of SARS at that apartment complex suggests that the virus released by the patients themselves may have spread through air [27].

Limited airborne spread of SARS may have occurred on board commercial aircraft. In one such instance, a symptomatic index case infected at least 22 of 120 (18.3%) passengers and crew during a three-hour flight [14]. Some of those infected were seated over 2 m (90 inches) away from the index case, a distance much longer than the 0.9 m (36 inches) generally believed to be the limit for droplet transmission. In such retrospective investigations it is virtually impossible to rule out the role of other possible means of virus spread. Also, the inside of an aircraft combines features which may be more conducive to airborne spread of pathogens.

A recent report from Canada suggests that oxygen delivery masks with open vents could promote the dispersal of respiratory pathogens such as SARS-CoV through their enhanced release in mists of exhaled pulmonary gases [28]. The exhaled moist air ejected from such oxygen masks is believed to carry pathogen-laden droplets over longer distances and possibly contribute to an increased risk of spread of respiratory infections in nosocomial settings. Additional investigations are needed to first prove that viruses such SARS-CoV can retain their infectivity better in the warm, moisture-laden air exhaled from oxygen masks. The findings on the influence of RH and air temperature on the airborne survival of coronavirus 229E would tend to suggest otherwise [22].

Sewage and biosolids

SARS-CoV can survive for up to 96 hours in body fluids such as sputum, feces and serum, but is less stable in urine [20]. The fecal excretion of SARS-CoV generated much concern on the safety of handling and spreading municipal solids on lands [29]. There are no reports of the recovery of infectious SARS-CoV from raw sewage or sludge and if the behavior of other enveloped viruses such as HIV is an indication, it would be highly unlikely that the virus can survive in such wastes long enough to pose any risks to human health. In view of this, it is even less likely that the virus would survive the conventional methods of sewage and biosolids treatment. Therefore, any suggestion of health risk from handling of municipal wastes or their proper disposal would be difficult to justify [29].

Skin

Since safety and ethical considerations would not permit the experimental contamination of the hands of human subjects with SARS-CoV, we have used 229E as a surrogate to study the potential of coronaviruses to survive on hands. Preliminary findings from such experiments indicate that nearly 45% of infectious virus remains viable on the hands of adult subjects after 1 hour. This is in contrast to other enveloped respiratory viruses (e.g. parainfluenzavirus) which become essentially undetectable in about 10 minutes on human skin [30].

Food and water

We are not aware of any published information on the survival of coronaviruses in food. Recent studies have shown SARS-CoV to survive in water to a very limited degree [20]. There is no evidence to suggest the spread of coronaviruses through food or water.

Environmental surfaces

SARS-CoV [20] and 229E and OC43 [23] can retain their infectivity for several hours on porous and non-porous environmental surfaces. While such survival is better than that of other enveloped human pathogens [30], there is no evidence to suggest that environmental surfaces play any direct or indirect role in the spread of coronaviruses.

Activity of microbicides against coronaviruses

Because of their enveloped nature coronaviruses are more susceptible to microbicides than non-enveloped viruses. In a comparative study, an animal parvovirus (non-enveloped) required 20- to 500-fold higher concentrations of the tested microbicides than were needed to inactivate an animal coronavirus [31].

Even before the advent of SARS considerable evaluation of the activity of microbicides against this virus group had been carried out. The following is a summary of this information.

Virucidal activity of several microbicides was tested against the mouse hepatitis virus (MHV) and the canine coronavirus (CCV), Kilham rat virus and canine parvovirus [32]. Both coronaviruses were readily inactivated by ethanol, isopropanol, benzalkonium chloride, iodophor, sodium hypochlorite, sodium chlorite, cresol soap and formaldehyde whereas the two parvoviruses proved to be considerably more resistant.

The relative resistance of 229E to microbicides was compared to that of coxsackievirus B3, adenovirus type 5, and parainfluenzavirus type 3 using the second tier of a quantitative carrier test (QCT-2) [33]. Stainless steel disks were used as carriers and each one received 10 μl of the test virus, suspended in either faeces or mucin and the inoculum allowed to dry for 1 h under ambient conditions. After 1 min exposure to 20 μl of the disinfectant, the virus from the disks was immediately eluted and plaque assayed. The efficacy criterion of a $\geq 3 \log_{10}$ reduction in virus infectivity was used. As expected, the coronavirus proved to be generally less resistant to microbicides than the two non-enveloped viruses.

In a more recent study, Wood and Payne [34] used a suspension test to assess the activity of chloroxylenol, benzalkonium chloride and cetrimide/chlorhexidine against three types of enveloped viruses (herpesvirus type 1, HIV-1 and a human coronavirus). The coronavirus was found to be generally more resistant than the other two enveloped viruses tested. While this observation is of interest, the findings have limited practical significance because the testing was based on a suspension test which presents the test microbicide with a weaker challenge than a carrier test protocol. A summary of all findings can be found in Table 2.

Alcohols

Most alcohols used in disinfection are ethanol and isopropyl alcohol, both usually at a concentration of 70% [32, 34]. Without soil load, the transmissible gastroenteritis virus (TGEV) was reduced 4.5 $\log_{10}$ by ethanol in the suspension test over 5 minutes [35]. Similarly, using QCT-2 and organic load, ethanol reduced 229E [33] by at least 3 log10 over the course of 5 minutes.

Chlorine and other halides

In tests using varying concentrations of sodium hypochlorite, 1000 ppm was effective against TGEV [34], bovine coronavirus [31] and 229E [33] irrespective of test conditions. Chloramine T ($C_7H_7SO_2NNaCl$) had similar results against bovine coronavirus and 229E. Povidone-iodine at a concentration of 1% reduced 229E by $>3 \log_{10}$ with the QCT-2 test.

Aldehydes

Formaldehyde at 4% is used as an overall disinfecting and sterilizing solution albeit its use as a general disinfectant is not recommended. It is effective against TGEV, reducing it over 5 $\log_{10}$ in under 5 minutes in suspension. At 2%, glutaraldehyde can inactivate 229E over 3 $\log_{10}$ [33] in the QCT-2 test.

Table 2. Effect of microbicides on coronaviruses

Active ingredient(s)	Virus	Test condition	Time	≥3 Log_{10} reduction	Refs.
		Ethanol			
70%	229E	QCT-2 + SL	5 min	Yes	[32]
70%	TGEV	Suspension	5 min	Yes	[34]
		Chlorine			
Sodium hypochlorite (100 ppm)	229E	QCT-2 + SL	5 min	No	[32]
Sodium hypochlorite (1000 ppm)	229E	QCT-2 + SL	5 min	Yes	[32]
Sodium hypochlorite (1500 ppm)	TGEV	Suspension	5 min	Yes	[34]
Chloramine T (1500 ppm)	229E	QCT-2 + SL	5 min		[32]
		Iodine			
1%	229E	QCT-2 + SL	5 min	Yes	[32]
1%	TGEV	Suspension	5 min	Yes	[34]
0.5%	Bovine	Suspension + SL	60 min	Yes	[30]
		Formaldehyde			
0.3%	Bovine	Suspension + SL	60 min	Yes	[30]
		Glutaraldehyde			
2%	229E	QCT-2 + SL	5 min		[32]
2%	TGEV	Suspension	5 min	Yes	[34]
		Quaternary ammonium compounds – benzalkonium chloride			
100 ppm	TGEV	Suspension	5 min	Yes	[34]
		Chlorhexidene gluconate			
80 ppm	229E	QCT-2 + SL	5 min	No	[32]
80 ppm + 70% ethanol	229E	QCT-2 + SL	5 min	Yes	[32]
		Phenolics			
O-phenylphenol (200 ppm)	229E	QCT-2 + SL	5 min	No	[32]
O-phenylphenol + sodium lauryl sulfate (0.6%)	229E	QCT-2 + SL	5 min	Yes	[32]
O-phenylphenol + 70% ethanol	229E	QCT-2 + SL	5 min	Yes	[32]
O-phenylphenol + 5% isopropyl alcohol	TGEV	QCT-2 + SL	5 min	Yes	[34]

SL, soil load; QCT-2, quantitative carrier test – Tier 2; TGEV, transmissible gastroenteritis virus

Quaternary ammonium compounds

A quaternary ammonium disinfectant requires the presence of an ammonium ion and at least one of its hydrogen atoms substituted by an organic radical. As a result, the list of quaternary ammonium compounds is rather extensive. This type of disinfectant is usually cationic and affects a

Table 3. Data on stability and resistance of SARS-CoV compiled by members of WHO laboratory network (modified from [35])

Substrate	Initial viral count log_{10} PFU	Condition	Survival time		Method of testing viability
Government Virus Unit, Dept. of Health, Hong Kong, SAR China					
Virus spiked in baby stool	1.00E+03	pH 6–7	3 hr		Virus isolation in cell culture
Virus spiked in normal stool	7.50E+03	pH 8	6 hr		Virus isolation in cell culture
Virus in diarrheal stool	7.50E+03	pH 9	4 days		Virus isolation in cell culture
Queen Mary Hospital, The University of Hong Kong, Hong Kong, SAR China					
Stool	1.00E+03	Room temperature	at least 2 days		Virus isolation in cell culture
Urine	1.00E+03	Room temperature	at least 24 hr		Virus isolation in cell culture
Virus culture medium + 1% bovine serum	1.00E+03	On plastic surface in room temperature	at least 2 days		Virus isolation in cell culture
Virus culture medium + 1% bovine serum	1.00E+04	30–37°C	at least 1hr		Virus isolation in cell culture
Virus culture medium + 1% fetal calf	1.00E+04	56°C	degradation of serum titre over time (10 000 infectious virus units in 15 min)		Virus isolation in cell culture
Virus in acetone, 10% formaldehyde and paraformaldehyde, 10% clorox, 75%ethanol, 2% phenol	1.00E+06	Room temperature	less than 5 min		Virus isolation in cell culture
National Institute of infectious Diseases, Tokyo, Japan					
Virus culture + 2% bovine serum	1.00E+06	minus 80°C	at least 4 days		Virus isolation and RT-PCR
Virus culture + 2% fetal calf serum	1.00E+06	4°C	at least 4 days		Virus isolation and RT-PCR
Virus culture + 2% fetal calf serum	1.00E+06	37°C	less than 4 days		Virus isolation and RT-PCR
Virus culture + 2% fetal calf serum	1.00E+05	56°C	less than 30 min		
University of Marburg, Germany					
Virus culture	1.00E+06	4°C	at least 21 days		Virus isolation
Virus culture	1.00E+06	minus 80°C	at least 21 days		Virus isolation
Chinese University, Hong Kong					
Virus in phosphate buffered saline (PBS)	9.00E+04	Room temperature on	PBS	Stool	Virus isolation in cell culture
Virus in sterilized		Plastered wall	24h	36 h	
		Plastic surface	36h	72 h	
		Formica surface	36h	36 h	
		Stainless steel	36h	72 h	
		Wood	12h	24 h	
		Cotton cloth	12h	24 h	
		Pig skin	?24h	?24 h	
		Glass slide	72h	96 h	
		Paper file cover	24h	36 h	

cell by adhering to its negatively charged membrane and disrupting the ionic potential of the cell. In the case of viruses, this adherence can disrupt the envelope, rendering the virus noninfectious. The quaternary ammonium compounds are best represented by chlorhexidine gluconate, which is widely used in health care institutions and in consumer disinfectants and antiseptics. In both suspension and QCT-2 tests, chlorhexidine gluconate faired well against TGEV [35] and 229E [33, 34]. Concentrations ranging from 500 to 15,000 ppm were effective in reducing the virus by at least 3 $\log_{10}$.

Phenolics

The phenolic compounds have a long history as their ancestry dates back to the use of coal tar soaps, whose active ingredients were creosol-based. Although some disinfectants continue to use the same historical active ingredient, creosol, most have developed over time to become more active against various microbes. For example, *o*-phenylphenol at 200 ppm is highly ineffective against most viruses, including 229E in the QCT-2 test [33]. However, the addition of either a detergent, such as sodium lauryl sulphate, or ethanol, proves highly effective against the virus over 3 $\log_{10}$ reduction is seen after 5 minutes. In the same way, many phenolic compounds rely on the helper effect of other chemicals to work effectively.

Survival and inactivation of the SARS coronavirus

The World Health Organization Laboratory Network has summarized the available data on SARS-CoV survival and inactivation [36], which are redrawn for this chapter as Table 3. Tables 4 and 5 summarize more recent studies on the inactivation of 229E by environmental surface disinfectants and antiseptics, respectively.

Concluding remarks

Despite the enhanced awareness of the potential of coronaviruses as animal and human pathogens, our understanding of their environmental survival and the exact means of their spread remains weak. Such information would be essential to design and implement more rational approaches to prevention and control of outbreaks of coronaviral infections. This is particularly relevant for the recently discovered SARS-CoV. However, the limited data available indicate that coronaviruses as a group are more stable in the environment that other enveloped viruses.

Table 4. Activity of microbicides against coronavirus 229E (Sattar et al., unpublished data)

Microbicide	Dilution tested (ppm)	Contact time (min)	Log_{10} reduction
Accelerated H_2O_2	Undiluted (5000)	3	4.0
Spray (26 g ethanol +	Undiluted	3	4.4
11.5 g 2-propanol +		1	4.4
0.054 g polyhexanide/100 g)			
Ethanol	75% (v/v)	5	4.0
Potassium monopersulfate	1% (w/v) solution	0.5	2.3
23.0% + sodium dichloro-s-	in water	1	4.1
triazinetrione 5.0%			
5.25% sodium hypochlorite	1:50 (1000)	3	4.0
(bleach)			
5.25% sodium hypochlorite	2 ml 5% acid	0.5	2.2
+ 5% acetic acid (vinegar)	+ 8 ml water (5000)		
Spray (ethanol 79.646%	Undiluted	3	3.3
+ a quat.)		10	3.1
4.8% chloroxylenol	1:40 (1200)	10	4.1
A mixture of two quat. ammoniums	1:128 (660)	10	4.0
A mixture of two phenolics	1:256 (820)	10	4.1

The second tier of the quantitative carrier test (QCT-2) with stainless steel disks was used. Ten μl of the virus suspension with a soil load was dried on each carrier and the inoculum exposed to 50 μl of the test microbicide at 23±2°C.

Table 5. Activity of an ethanol-based hand rub against coronavirus 229E (Sattar et al., unpublished data)

Treatment	Mean ± SD	% Reduction
Baseline	$1.32 \times 10^4 \pm 0.4$	–
Hard water (200 PPM $CaCO_3$)	$3.02 \times 10^3 \pm 2.0$	77.0
75% (v/v) ethanol	0	>99.99
Ethanol (60%) containing gel	0	>99.99

The fingerpad method (ASTM 1838) was used. Ten μl of virus in soil load was placed on each fingerpad & dried. The dried inoculum was exposed to 1 ml of control or test solution for 30 seconds. The fingerpads were eluted & eluates plaque assayed.

References

1 Holmes KV, Lai MMC (1996) Coronaviridae: The viruses and their replication. In: Fields BN, Knipe DM, Howley PM (eds): *Virology*. Vol. 1. 3rd ed. Philadelphia: Lippincott-Raven, 1075–1093

2 Kapikian AZ (1975) The coronaviruses. *Dev Biol Stand* 28: 42–64

3 International Committee on Taxonomy of Viruses. ICTV Index to Virus Classification and Nomenclature. http://www.ncbi.nlm.nih.gov/ICTVdb/Ictv/index.htm.

4 Grattan DA (1968) Infectious bronchitis in laying fowls. *Vet Rec* 83: 157

5 King DJ (1975) Comments on the etiology and immunity of transmissible (coronaviral) enteritis of turkeys (bluecomb). *Am J Vet Res* 36: 555–556

6 Rota PA, Oberste MS, Monroe SS, Nix WA, Campagnoli R, Icenogle JP, Penaranda S, Bankamp B, Maher K, Chen MH et al (2003) Characterization of a novel coronavirus associated with severe acute respiratory syndrome. *Science* 300: 1394–1399

7 Stavrinides J, Guttman DS (2004) Mosaic evolution of the severe acute respiratory syndrome coronavirus. *J Virol* 78: 76–82

8 World Health Organization. Severe acute respiratory syndrome (SARS) Report by the Secretariat. Nov. 23, 2003 EB113/33. http: //www.who.int/gb/EB_WHA/PDF/EB113/eeb11333.pdf 8422 and 908

9 Brown EG, Tetro JA (2003) Comparative analysis of the SARS coronavirus genome: a good start to a long journey. *Lancet* 361: 1756–1757

10 Chandler C (2003) SARS attacks, China shudders. *Fortune* 147: 32

11 Leung WK, To KF, Chan PK, Chan HL, Wu AK, Lee N, Yuen KY, Sung JJ (2003) Enteric involvement of severe acute respiratory syndrome-associated coronavirus infection. *Gastroenterology* 125: 1011–1017

12 Bourgueil E, Hutet E, Cariolet R, Vannier P (1992) Experimental infection of pigs with the porcine respiratory coronavirus (PRCV): measure of viral excretion. *Vet Microbiol* 31: 11–18

13 Inouye S (2003) SARS transmission: language and droplet production. *Lancet* 362: 170

14 Olsen SJ, Chang HL, Cheung TY, Tang AF, Fisk TL, Ooi SP, Kuo HW, Jiang DD, Chen KT, Lando J et al (2003) Transmission of the severe acute respiratory syndrome on aircraft. *N Engl J Med* 349: 2416–2422

15 Wong GW, Fok TF (2004) Severe acute respiratory syndrome (sars) in children. *Pediatr Pulmonol* 37 (S26): 69–71

16 Kennedy M, Citino S, McNabb AH, Moffatt AS, Gertz K, Kania S (2002) Detection of feline coronavirus in captive *Felidae* in the USA. *J Vet Diagn Invest* 14: 520–522

17 Hasoksuz M, Hoet AE, Loerch SC, Wittum TE, Nielsen PR, Saif LJ (2002) Detection of respiratory and enteric shedding of bovine coronaviruses in cattle in an Ohio feedlot. *J Vet Diagn Invest* 14: 308–313

18 Van Reeth K, Nauwynck H, Pensaert M (1996) Dual infections of feeder pigs with porcine reproductive and respiratory syndrome virus followed by porcine respiratory coronavirus or swine influenza virus: a clinical and virological study.*Vet Microbiol* 48: 325–335

19 Hoet AE, Smiley J, Thomas C, Nielsen PR, Wittum TE, Saif LJ (2003) Association of enteric shedding of bovine torovirus (Breda virus) and other enteropathogens with diarrhea in veal calves. *Am J Vet Res* 64: 485–490

20 Duan SM, Zhao XS, Wen RF, Huang JJ, Pi GH, Zhang SX, Han J, Bi SL, Ruan L, Dong XP; SARS Research Team (2003) Stability of SARS coronavirus in human specimens and environment and its sensitivity to heating and UV irradiation. *Biomed Environ Sci* 16: 246–255

21 Cho KO, Hoet AE, Loerch SC, Wittum TE, Saif LJ (2001) Evaluation of con-

current shedding of bovine coronavirus via the respiratory tract and enteric route in feedlot cattle. *Am J Vet Res* 62: 1436–1441

22 Ijaz MK, Brunner AH, Sattar SA, Nair RC, Johnson-Lussenburg CM (1985) Survival characteristics of airborne human coronavirus 229E. *J Gen Virol* 66: 2743–2748

23 Sizun J, Yu MW, Talbot PJ (2000) Survival of human coronaviruses 229E and OC43 in suspension and after drying onsurfaces: a possible source ofhospital-acquired infections. *J Hosp Infect* 46: 55–60

24 Ng SK (2004) The mystery of Amoy Gardens. In: Loh C. and Civic Exchange (eds): *At the Epicentre: Hong Kong and the SARS Outbreak*. Hong Kong: Hong Kong University Press, 117–138

25 Ng SK (2003) Possible role of an animal vector in the SARS outbreak at Amoy Gardens. *Lancet* 362: 570–572

26 Peters CJ, Khan AS (2002) Hantavirus pulmonary syndrome: the new American hemorrhagic fever. *Clin Infect Dis* 34: 1224–1231

27 Yu ITS, Li Y, Wong TW, Tam W, Chan AT, Lee JH, Leung DY, Ho T (2004) Evidence of airborne transmission of the severe acute respiratory syndrome virus. *N Eng J Med* 350: 1731–1739

28 Somogyi R, Vesely AE, Azami T, Preiss D, Fisher J, Correia J, Fowler RA (2004) Dispersal of respiratory droplets with open vs closed oxygen delivery masks: implications for the transmission of severe acute respiratory syndrome. *Chest* 125: 1155–1157

29 Environmental Science & Engineering Magazine. Biosolids not affected by SARS virus. *Environ Sci Eng* June, 2003, http: //www.esemag.com/0603/sars.html

30 Sattar SA, Springthorpe VS (1996) Transmission of viral infections through animate and inanimate surfaces and infection control through chemical disinfection. In: C Hurst (ed): *Modeling Disease Transmission and Its Prevention by Disinfection.* Cambridge University Press, Cambridge, UK, 224–257

31 Maris P (1990) Virucidal efficacy of eight disinfectants against pneumovirus, coronavirus and parvovirus. *Ann Rech Vet* 21: 275–279

32 Saknimit M, Inatsuki I, Sugiyama Y, Yagami K (1988) Virucidal efficacy of physico-chemical treatments against coronaviruses and parvoviruses of laboratory animals. *Jikken Dobutsu* 37: 341–345

33 Sattar SA, Springthorpe VS, Karim Y, Loro P (1989) Chemical disinfection of non-porous inanimate surfaces experimentally contaminated with four human pathogenic viruses. *Epidemiol Infect* 102: 493–505

34 Wood A, Payne D (1998) The action of three antiseptics/disinfectants against enveloped and non-enveloped viruses. *J Hosp Infect* 38: 283–295

35 Brown TT Jr (1981) Laboratory evaluation of selected disinfectants as virucidal agents against porcine parvovirus, pseudorabies virus, and transmissible gastroenteritis virus. *Am J Vet Res* 42: 1033–1036

36 World Health Organization. First data on stability and resistance of SARS coronavirus compiled by members of WHO laboratory network. http: //www.who.int/csr/sars/survival_2003_05_04/en/

Coronaviruses with Special Emphasis on First Insights Concerning SARS
ed. by A. Schmidt, M.H. Wolff and O. Weber

Disease management strategies in SARS

Andrea Ammon

Department for Infectious Disease Epidemiology, Robert Koch-Institut, Seestraße 10, 13353 Berlin, Germany

Introduction

Disease management as understood here does not mean therapy or diagnostics; here the focus will be on the public health management.

When the first SARS cases became known, decisions about the management of these cases, but also regarding the management of their contact persons had to be based on very limited evidence. Although an unprecedented cooperation of scientists around the world led to a rapid accumulation of knowledge about key features of the disease and finally the detection of the virus, the first weeks were characterized by uncertainty and fears. Strategies for managing the disease were necessary on each level of the health systems where patients occurred, i.e. the private practices that saw the patients often before they were transferred to a hospital, and the hospitals. In particular the public health service had to develop strategies for the containment of further spread in the absence of an effective vaccine and a therapeutic option.

In the following chapter, the currently available information about management strategies for SARS in the various areas of health systems will be summarized.

General considerations

For the development of an effective management strategy, several epidemiological features of a disease have to be known, e.g. length of the incubation period, period of infectiousness, the stability of the pathogen in the environment, mode(s) of transmission, risk factors for transmission. Length of incubation period for example has implications for recommendations on isolation of cases and their contact persons. The following section describes the facts known so far [1]. The reader should keep in mind that during the first weeks of the SARS outbreak none of these observations were known to the decision makers.

Incubation period

The incubation period of an infectious disease includes the time from infection to the onset of first symptoms. Usually, an average time is given as well as the range from minimal to maximum number of days. Estimation of the incubation period of SARS was based on cases where a single defined contact to a SARS patient has been observed. Table 1 shows the observations compiled by WHO within the epidemiology working group [1]. Median incubation period was 4–5 days, mean 4–6 days. The minimum time reported was 1 day and the maximum were 14 days. The time which all recommendations were based on had a maximum of 10 days. Therefore, these outlier observations exceeding the 10 days raised concern.

Donnelly et al. commented on their data that they were based on a small number of cases resulting in a high variance and which also may be subjected to reporting bias [2]. The group's consensus and one of the recommendations for further research was to investigate these outliers in more detail before extending the incubation period beyond 10 days.

Period of infectiousness

For the assessment of how long patients should be isolated and at which times exposure to patients may have posed a risk for their contact persons, the period of infectiousness has to be known. Particular anxiety was caused by some patients who infected a high number of persons (so-called "super spreading events").

The infection by sub-clinically ill patients or transmission in prodromal phase has not been reported so far.

Data so far available are based on small numbers of observations, but they offer an orientation. In general, the estimation of the infectious period can be derived from several observations. At which point in the clinical course can virus be detected in which clinical materials? Ideally, consecutive samples of various clinical materials should be taken.

Transmission seems to be greatest from severely ill patients, usually in the second week of their illness [1]. Data from Singapore show that few secondary cases arise when SARS patients are isolated within 5 days of onset of illness [1]. Using RT-PCR, Peiris et al. [3] detected SARS-associated coronavirus RNA in nasopharyngeal aspirates in 24 of 75 patients with a mean of 3.2 days after onset of illness, in 68% this test was positive at day 14. Twenty of the initially positive patients were followed up in 3-day intervals, and their samples were quantitatively investigated. At days 5, 10 and 15 they found mean geometric viral loads of 2.3×10^5, 1.9×10^7, and 9.8×10^4 copies per ml respectively, indicating a peak of viral load around day 10. These data support the epidemiological observations. Single reports of transmission from patients in their early phase of disease seem to contra-

Table 1: Summary of SARS incubation period estimates [1]

Country	Min.	Mean	Median	Max.	Basis
Canada	2	4.8	4.2	10	42 cases
China	1	4	4	12	70 cases; 5 cases > 10 days
Hong Kong	–	6.4	–	16.7	57 cases; 95% of cases ≤ 14.2 days [2]
China, Taiwan				10–14	Household transmission studies
Singapore	1	5.3	5	10	46 cases
Viet Nam	5	6–7	–	10	Health care associated exposure
WHO Euro	5	7.2	7	10	5 cases

dict these observations. Current guidelines from WHO on the clinical management and discharge of SARS patients are based on a 10-day interval since defervescence and a normal chest X-ray [4], since there are no reports of transmission beyond 10 days of fever resolution (Clinical management document, WHO [5]). Most countries follow these guidelines. Hong Kong, however, discharges patients only 19 days after the end of fever and normal chest X-ray [1].

Stability of SARS coronavirus

SARS-CoV is stable in faeces and urine at room temperature for at least 1-2 days. In stool from patients with diarrhoea it may be stable up to 4 days. The virus has been isolated from stool on various surfaces such as stainless steel and plastic up to 72 hours. It is susceptible to commonly used disinfectants and fixatives (Clinical management document, WHO [5]) [6].

Modes of and risk factors for transmission

It is now understood that SARS emerged in Guangdong in November 2002. More than one third of the first cases with onset dates before February 1, 2003, occurred in food handlers [7], indicating a primary source in wildlife. Despite many efforts and testing of a variety of animals, e.g. palm civets, racoon dogs, rats, hares, beaver, so far the reservoir has not been found [8–11]. It is unclear whether the animals harbouring the virus are the source or just a vehicle from the primary reservoir to humans.

The basic reproduction number R_0, which is the average number of secondary cases generated by one infected person in a susceptible population, has been estimated to be around 3 [12, 13] which is compatible with moderate transmissibility like the spread by direct contact or larger droplets that travel only a few meters. However aerosolizing procedures during health care – which may include bronchoscopy, intubation, suction, and nebulised aerosol therapy – or as shown in the Amoy Gardens outbreak, may amplify transmission *via* aerosols also for a longer distance [14, 15].

The primary mode of transmission seems to be direct mucous membrane contact with infectious respiratory droplets or by exposure to fomites [16, 17]. Cases have occurred primarily among persons with close contact to SARS patients during health care or in households [1]. Transmission occurred also during flights when infected persons were on board during the symptomatic phase of their illness [18, 19]. The risk of transmission during flights is difficult to assess, since either active surveillance was not thoroughly done [19] or the flight crew and/or passengers also had other possible exposures.

However, there was evidence [20, 21] that in the case of the unique outbreak of Amoy Gardens, starting from an index patient with extremely high SARS-CoV concentrations in his faeces and urine, the virus was spread via airborne virus-laden aerosols generated in the vertical soil stack of the apartment building due to improperly functioning of the drainage system.

Tsang et al. [15] describe a so-called super-spreading event in Hong Kong: Nine contact persons of an index patient fell ill, some after short contact times (three times for 10 minutes in the ICU) and one after indirect contact while wearing a surgical mask. The Hotel "M" in Hong Kong played a pivotal role in the international spread of SARS. An infected physician spent one night in February 2003 in this hotel and became the index case for four national and international clusters and cases in two countries without further secondary spread. Although sharing the same floor in that night was a risk factor in a retrospective cohort study, the specific mode of transmission within the hotel still remains unclear [22]. It is unclear whether viral factors, environmental factors, host factors or their combination were important for the occurrence of these events ([23].

Strategy for management

The management should essentially aim at two goals: the early detection of cases and the limitation of further spread. For the early detection it is important to alert health care workers (HCW) to potential cases of SARS. Thus, updated information on clinical symptoms and training in hygiene measures should be continuously given to all HCW [23]. To assure that criteria for defining cases are similarly used in all affected countries, case definitions are necessary. A systematic approach for the management of clinical cases as well as their contact persons should be pursued. While during the outbreak phase in 2003 these approaches sometimes had to be decided upon very limited evidence, meanwhile several studies have been published which tried to assess the effectiveness of control measures (see below).

Although some of them are based on small numbers of study subjects, they provide some guidance.

Involved in the implementation of these goals are the public health service and HCW in a broad sense both in private practices and hospitals.

Early detection of cases

Surveillance

Risk assessment on country level

For assessing the risk of the occurrence of SARS, three categories of risk zones (see Box 1) have been proposed by WHO [24]. The categorization should be done according to the experience during the epidemic in 2002–2003 and the postepidemic phase. Different levels of activities are recommended in the different risk zones. For areas at risk of emerging SARS-CoV-like viruses from wildlife or other animal reservoirs it is recommended to implement the SARS alert, conduct enhanced surveillance in populations at risk and to carry out special studies for SARS-CoV infections in animals and human populations. For areas at a higher risk of SARS-CoV emergence or introduction the implementation of the SARS alert and enhanced surveillance is recommended, while areas at low risk should implement the SARS alert.

Enhanced surveillance and special studies should be done in populations at risk and could include, depending on the area and the risk assessment [24]:

- Surveillance for pneumonia in settings such as nursing homes, rehabilitation units, community health care centres and in private practice.
- Surveillance of persons discharged from hospital with a diagnosis of unspecified atypical pneumonia during and following an outbreak of SARS.
- Surveillance for absenteeism among HCW caring for patients with SARS and laboratory staff working with SARS-CoV.
- Laboratory-based surveillance of SARS-CoV infection.
- Surveillance for requests for laboratory testing for SARS-CoV.
- Surveillance for unexplained deaths following an acute respiratory illness.
- Serological and clinical surveillance of high risk populations (HCW, animal handlers, laboratory staff working with SARS-CoV, etc).
- Community-based serological surveys to monitor changes in the seroprevalence of SARS-CoV infection.
- Sero-surveys among wildlife populations.

Case definition – SARS alert

During the outbreak phase of SARS (March through July 2003), the case definition for SARS provided by WHO for global surveillance was based

Box 1: Risk categories for the emergence of SARS [24]

Emergence of SARS-CoV-like viruses from wildlife or other animal reservoirs
Countries/areas identified as source(s) of the epidemic in 2002-2003 in southern China or areas with an increased likelihood of animal to human transmission of SARS-CoV-like viruses from wildlife or other animal reservoirs.

Areas at higher risk of SARS-CoV emergence or introduction
Countries/areas at potentially higher risk of SARS-CoV-emergence or introduction due to the presence of laboratories in which SARS-CoV and/or SARS-CoV-like viruses are being studied or in which clinical specimens infected with SARS-CoV are being processed or stored.

OR

Countries/areas with entry of large numbers of persons from areas in which wildlife or other animal reservoirs of SARS-CoV-like viruses are found.

Low risk of SARS-CoV emergence or introduction
Countries/areas that never reported cases or reported only imported cases during the 2002–2003 epidemic, and that do not conduct research using live SARS-CoV-like viruses or store clinical samples from SARS cases.

on the clinical picture of a respiratory disease. Important elements to increase specificity were the criteria of a stay in affected areas and having had contact to a SARS patient [25]. Experience with this case definition in Hong Kong and Singapore showed that the specificity of the case definition was 96% in both studies, and the sensitivity was 26 and 27.8%, respectively, indicating that many patients my have atypical presentation of symptoms and a careful examination and observation period is required for persons with an exposure suspicious of SARS ([26, 27]).

For the post-outbreak period the definition of a "SARS alert" ([24], see box 2) was created: According to the observation that many HCW were affected, the SARS alert is based on the detection of clusters of HCW. The recently occurring infections in laboratory workers resulted in a revision to also include persons in the SARS alert who are working in laboratories where SARS-CoV is handled [24]. The observations of atypical clinical presentations mentioned above were included now into the current description of the clinical picture [24]. Beside the symptoms mentioned for the clinical picture it is now clearly stated that no individual symptom or cluster of symptoms has proven to be specific, even fever may be absent on initial measurement.

Particularly the non-specific disease signs and symptoms, the long mean incubation period of 6.4 days, the long time between onset of symptoms and hospital admission from 3 to 5 days, and a lack of a reliable diagnostic test in the early phase of illness can lead to potential transmission to frontline HCW and the community [2, 16].

Box 2: Definition of the SARS alert [24]

1. An individual with clinical evidence of SARS *AND* with one or more of the following epidemiological risk factors for SARS-CoV infection in the 10 days before the onset of symptoms:

- Employed in an occupation associated with an increased risk of SARS-CoV exposure (e.g. staff in a laboratory working with live SARS-CoV/SARS-CoV-like viruses or storing clinical specimens infected with SARS-CoV; persons with exposure to wildlife or other animals considered a reservoir of SARS-CoV, their excretions or secretions, etc.).
- Close contact (having cared for, lived with, or had direct contact with the respiratory secretions or body fluids) of a person under investigation for SARS.
- History of travel to, or residence in, an area experiencing an outbreak of SARS.

OR

2. Two or more health care workers with clinical evidence of SARS in the same health care unit and with onset of illness in the same 10-day period.

OR

3. Three or more persons (health care workers and/or patients and/or visitors) with clinical evidence of SARS with onset of illness in the same 10-day period and epidemiologically linked to a health-care facility.

Once a SARS alert has been raised, the public health management includes immediate isolation of patients and the implementation of transmission-based precautions (see below); the rapid establishment of a diagnosis; the tracing and quarantine of contact persons. Laboratory confirmed cases have to be reported to WHO.

Transit site surveillance

In affected areas, fever checks of persons leaving or entering affected areas were suggested to prevent international spread. These measures were particularly recommended for airports and ports and were accompanied by recommendations for the management of possible cases on international flights, disinfection of aircrafts after carrying suspect cases and surveillance of persons who have been in contact with suspect cases while undertaking international travel [28]. For the post-outbreak period these measures are of course abandoned.

Limitation of further spread

Management of contact persons

For the assessment of risk of certain exposures of contact persons, it was attempted to categorize this risk according to the closeness and intensity of the contacts resulting in different levels of protection but also in different levels of control measures for contact persons. Exposures supposed to confer a higher risk were close contacts with a SARS patients while applying no or inadequate protective measures, including direct contact with respiratory secretions, close/intimate contact with a SARS patient, examining or caring for a SARS patient, living in the same household with a SARS patient or staying within the same room.

Exposures involving the aforementioned situations during which appropriate protective measure were applied presumably conferred a lower risk.

Contact persons should be traced and placed under quarantine, mostly at home or in designated sites [29] until SARS is ruled out in the index patient or the maximum incubation period of 10 days since the last contact with the index patient has elapsed. Quarantine means the separation or movement restriction of persons who are supposed to have been exposed but are not (yet) ill. Quarantined persons are required to monitor their temperature twice a day which should be controlled daily by public health authorities. If persons under quarantine develop fever, they should immediately be brought to hospital and be treated in isolation units.

Strategies for the prevention of transmission in health care settings

In particular in the absence of evidence of SARS transmission in the world, the main challenge is to be sufficiently alert but not to overload the system with unnecessary differential diagnoses and false alarms.

Risk assessment in the health care setting

The risk assessment within the health care setting should be carried out for the different groups within such a facility (type of facility; isolation unit or general ward, HCW: depending on years of experience and training, visitors, the current management strategies) (Clinical management document, WHO [5]).

Experience showed that infections occurred in areas of assumed lower risk due to patients with atypical symptoms who were not suspected to have SARS at initial examination [30]. Thus, this approach should be cautiously viewed in particular for the clinical management.

Risk assessment of the individual patient (differential diagnosis)

Most important is the assessment of patients with symptoms compatible with SARS. A number of flow charts and clinical decision rules have been reported to standardize the decision making process (examples [31–33]) which were used during the SARS outbreak. So far no agreed upon process for risk assessment of patients in the post-outbreak period has been published although WHO is trying to put together a consensus approach. Despite laboratory tests being available, there is still a lack for a rapid, reliable and early test. Thus, the risk assessment has to be based mainly on clinical grounds and epidemiological information (Clinical management document, WHO [5]). The indication for a SARS-CoV test should take into account that in low risk areas false positive test results are more likely. Thus the test should be considered only in the context with clinical and epidemiological evidence that SARS-CoV might be the causative agent. The challenge is to have sufficient sensitivity to screen suspected SARS cases out of the group of atypical pneumonia without raising false alarms too often. This is important to reduce the risk of activating unnecessarily response teams in hospitals and public health service.

Standard precautions

There is no doubt that the application of standard precautions will reduce the nosocomial transmission of infections in general. Standard precautions include hand hygiene after each patient contact or contact with infectious materials, wearing gloves for contact with body fluids, non-intact skin, routine cleaning and disinfection of frequently touched surfaces, safe handling and disposal of needles and other sharp instruments (Clinical management document, WHO [5]).

Risk reduction strategies

Since the main transmission pathways are droplets, aerosols or direct/indirect contact with patients, clinical material or indirect *via* contaminated surfaces, precautions should be established to reduce or better, to avoid these contacts.

When a patient is admitted to a health care setting (i.e. private practice or hospital), and there is evidence from the clinical picture and the epidemiological information that SARS could be suspected, the patient should be given a surgical mask and be seated and examined in a separate room. The HCW should also be protected with a surgical mask, possibly with a N95 mask which corresponds to FFP2 masks in Europe [34]. Use of these masks depends on the medical procedures to be performed. If the patient has to be admitted to the hospital – either because the suspicion is corroborated or for further evaluation –, he/she should be placed there in an isolation room with own bathroom facilities and if possible an anteroom. In case of several cases, cohort isolation would be a possibility.

Personal protective equipment of staff caring for these patients should consist of N 95 masks, with even higher protection depending on the kind of medical procedures to be performed, gloves, goggles and gown when entering the room. All equipment has to be disposed safely before leaving the room and hands should be disinfected after removing the gloves. All surfaces have to be cleaned and disinfected daily with proven virucidal disinfectants.

Certain aerosol generating procedures should be carried out only if absolutely necessary and in these circumstances, additional precautions should be employed, i.e. use of N100 or FFP3 masks. If possible these procedures should be carried out by the most experienced staff trained in the use of appropriate protective measures including respiratory protection. Among these high risk procedures are: resuscitation, bronchoscopy, endotracheal intubation, airway suctioning, diagnostic sputum induction, aerosolized medications such as nebulizers) (Clinical management document, WHO [5]).

Access to the isolation unit should be restricted to essential staff only and they should not care for other patients if possible. The number of visitors should also be limited as much as possible [35].

Effectiveness of measures

Quarantine

This measure got new appreciation during the SARS outbreak due to a lack of vaccine and therapeutic options [36]. However, the effectiveness was difficult to assess, first because only a few of the quarantined persons developed suspect or probable SARS and secondly, because a series of control measures were applied in addition to quarantine which made the evaluation of the relative contribution of each of the measures difficult [37]. In Taiwan, less than 0.5% of the >130,000 persons under quarantine developed suspect or probable SARS [38], whereas in Beijing the attack rate among quarantined persons varied widely from 0.4% in work or school contacts to 15.4% among spouses. There was also a strong dependence of the attack rate among household members according to age, ranging from 5.0% for persons <30 years to 27.6% in 60- to 69-year old persons [29].

Precautions against droplets

Seto et al. showed that all infected staff members of five Hong Kong hospitals omitted at least one of the recommended measures (mask, gloves, gowns, hand-washing); masks being the most important single measure [39].

Reasons for nosocomial outbreaks

As mentioned above, omission of at least one of the recommended personal protective measures was the most frequent cause of staff members getting infected. In addition, atypical clinical presentation of SARS patients was another factor that contributed to the spread of SARS among health care staff and close contacts of patients. In a hospital in Singapore atypical clinical presentation of an index patient led to 51 infections (24 HCW, 15 other patients, 12 family members) [40]. Similarly, Ho et al. described an outbreak among hospital workers in Hong Kong which resulted from exposure of staff to patients with unsuspected SARS in low-risk general wards [30].

Transit site surveillance
Pang et al. report the results of this measure from the Beijing area [29]. Fever checks using infrared thermometers were instituted at the Beijing airport, major train stations and all 71 roads connecting Beijing to other areas. A total of almost 14 million people were screened at these sites between late April through end of June 2003, identifying 12 probable SARS cases. The costs of these measures were not reported.

Lessons learnt for future management

Strengthening of public health infrastructure
The SARS epidemic has helped to sensitize health authorities world wide to strengthen the public health infrastructure which is necessary for combating rapidly spreading infections [41].

Contact tracing and quarantine
"Old fashioned" public health concepts like contact tracing, quarantine for exposed persons and isolation of cases should be revisited and instituted early in the outbreak

Infection control measures
SARS has emphasised the need for strict infection control measures on a routine basis. Therefore, these infection control measures have to be simple, but effective.

Patients suspected with SARS should be isolated, obviously those with probable SARS.

Continuous training and communication
Training and education for health professionals at all levels should be continuously offered. Communication efforts for health care professionals, policymakers and the public have to be enhanced [42]. The purpose of informing and warning the public is to increase the risk perception which may lead to an earlier reporting of symptoms as well as improvements in personal hygiene [2].

Global cooperation
Another important lesson is the necessity of global cooperation in the containment of infectious diseases. SARS gave an impressive example that diseases which seem to be happening in one part of the world can spread within no time over the world. The rapid exchange of information between public health institutions world wide, coordinated by WHO, was pivotal in being able to contain the outbreak within months.

References

1 WHO (2003) Consensus document on the epidemiology of SARS. *Wkly Epidemiol Rec* 78: 373–375

2 Donnelly CA, Ghani AC, Leung GM, Hedley AJ, Fraser C, Riley S, Abu-Raddad LJ, Ho LM, Thach TQ, Chau P et al (2003) Epidemiological determinants of spread of causal agent of severe acute respiratory syndrome in Hong Kong. *Lancet* 361: 1761–1766

3 Peiris JSM, Yuen KY, Osterhaus ADME, Stöhr K (2003) Clinical progression and viral load in a community outbreak of coronavirus-associated SARS pneumonia: a prospective study. *Lancet* 361: 1767–1772

4 http://www.who.int/csr/sars/discharge/en/, accessed 31/5/2004

5 http://www.who.int/csr/resources/publications/SARSNEWGUIDANCE/en/, accessed 28/12/2004

6 http://www.who.int/csr/sars/survival_2003_05_04/en/index.html, accessed 28/12/2004

7 Breiman RF, Evans MR, Preiser W, Maguire J, Schnur A, Li A, Bekedam H, MacKenzie JS (2003) Role of China in the quest to define and control severe acute respiratory syndrome. *Emerg Infect Dis* 9: 1037–1041

8 CDC (2003) Prevalence of IgG antibody to SARS-associated coronavirus in animal traders – Guangdong province, China, 2003. *MMWR* 52: 986–987

9 Guan Y, Zheng BJ, He YQ, Liu XL, Zhuang ZX, Cheung CL, Luo SW, Li PH, Zhang LJ, Guan YJ et al (2003) Isolation and characterization of viruses related to the SARS Coronavirus from animals in Southern China. *Sciencexpress*: 1–8

10 Enserink M (2003) Clues to the animal origin of SARS. Science 300: 1351

11 Ng SKC (2003) Possible role of an animal vector in the SARS outbreak at Amoy Gardens. *Lancet* 362: 570–572

12 Lipsitch M, Cohen T, Cooper B, Robins JM, Ma S, James L, Gopalakrishna G, Chew SK, Tan CC, Samore MH et al (2003) Transmission dynamics and control of severe acute respiratory syndrome. *Science* 300: 1966–1970

13 Riley S, Fraser C, Donnelly CA, Ghani AC, Abu-Raddad LJ, Hedley AJ, Leung GM, Ho LM, Lam TH, Thach TQ et al (2003) Transmission dynamics of the etiological agent of SARS in Hong Kong: impact of public health interventions. *Science* 300: 1961–1966

14 Dwosh HA, Hong HHL, Austgarden D, Herman S, Schabas RE (2003) Identification and containment of an ourbreak of SARS in a community hospital. *Journal of the Canadian Medical Association (CMAJ)* 168: 1415–1420

15 Tsang KW, Ho PL, Ooi GC, Yee WKS, Wang T, Chang-Yeung M, Lam WK, Seto WH, Yam LYC, Cheung TM et al (2003) A cluster of cases of severe acute respiratory syndrome in Hong Kong. *N Engl J Med* 348: 1977–1985

16 Abdullah ASM, Tomlinson B, Cockram CS, Thomas GN (2003) Lessons from the severe acute respiratory syndrome outbreak in Hong Kong. *Emerg Infect Dis* 9: 1042–1045

17 Tomlinson B, Cockram C (2003) SARS: experience at Prince of Wales Hospital, Hong Kong. *Lancet* 361: 1486–1487

18 Olsen SJ, Chang HL, Cheung TYY, Tang AFY, Fisk TL, Ooi SPL, Kuo HW, Jiang DDS, Chen KT, Lando J et al (2004) Transmission of the severe acute respiratory syndrome on aircraft. *N Engl J Med* 349: 2416–2422
19 Wilder-Smith A, Paton NI, Goh KT (2003) Low risk of transmission of severe acute respiratory syndrome on airplanes: the Singapore experience. *Trop Med Int Health* 8: 1035–1037
20 Yu ITS, Li Y, Wong TW, Tam W, Chan AT, Lee JHW, Leung DYC, Ho T (2004) Evidence of airborne transmission of the severe acute respiratory syndrome virus. *N Engl J Med* 350: 1731–1739
21 WHO (2003) Inadequate plumbing systems probably contributed to SARS transmission. *Wkly Epidemiol Rec* 78: 371–372
22 Radun D, Niedrig M, Ammon A, Stark K (2003) Retrospective cohort study among German guests of the Hotel "M", Hong Kong, identified an early SARS case. *Euro Surveill* 8: 228–230
23 Lee N, Sung JJY (2003) Nosocomial transmission of SARS. *Current Infect Dis Rep* 5: 473–476
24 http://www.who.int/csr/resources/publications/en/WHO_CDS_CSR_ARO_2004_1.pdf, accessed 28/12/2004
25 http://www.who.int/csr/sars/casedefinition/en/print.html, accessed 31/5/2004
26 Tambyah PA, Singh KS, Habib AG (2003) SARS: understanding the coronavirus. *BMJ* 327: 620
27 Rainer TH, Cameron PA, Smit D, Ong KL, Hung ANW, Nin DCP, Ahuja AT, Si LCY, Sung JJY (2003) Evaluation of WHO criteria for identifying patients with severe acute respiratory syndrome out of hospital: prospective observational study. *BMJ* 326: 1354–1358
28 WHO (2003) WHO recommended measures for persons undertaking international travel form areas affected by severe acute respiratory syndrome (SARS). *Wkly Epidemiol Rec* 78: 97–110
29 Pang Y, Zhu Z, Xu F, Guo J, Gong X, Liu D, Liu Z, Chin DP, Feikin DR (2003) Evaluation of control measures implemented in the severe acute respiratory syndrome outbreak in Beijing, 2003. *JAMA* 290: 3215–3221
30 Ho AS, Sung JJY, Chan-Yeung M (2003) An outbreak of severe acute respiratory syndrome among hospital workers in a community hospital in Hong Kong. *Ann Int Med* 139: 546–567
31 Ho, W (2003) Guideline on management of severe acute respiratory syndrome (SARS). *Lancet*, online publication
32 Wang TL, Jang TN, Huang CH, Kao SJ, Lin CM, Lee FN, Liu CY, Chong CF, Lin CM, Dorji H et al (2004) Establishing a clinical decision rule of severe acute respiratory syndrome at the emergency department. *Ann Emerg Med* 43: 17–22
33 Chen SY, Su CP, Ma MHM, Chiang WC, Hsu CY, Ko PCI, Tsai KC, Yen Z, Shih FY, Chen SC et al (2004) Predictive model of diagnosing probable cases of severe acute respiratory syndrome in febrile patients with exposure risk. *Ann Emerg Med* 43: 1–5
34 Puro VN, Magnavita N, Ippolito G (2003) SARS and masks. *J Hosp Infect* 56: 73–74

35 Wenzel RP, Edmond MB (2003) Managing SARS amidst uncertainty. *N Engl J Med* 348: 1947–1948
36 Diamond B (2003) SARS spreads new outlook on quarantine models. *Nat Med* 9: 1441
37 CDC (2003) Efficiency of quarantine during an epidemic of severe acute respiratory syndrome – Beijing, China, 2003. *MMWR* 52: 1037–1040
38 CDC (2003) Use of quarantine to prevent transmission of severe acute respiratory syndrome – Taiwan, 2003. *MMWR* 52: 680–683
39 Seto WH, Tsang D, Yung RWH, Ching TY, Ng TK, Ho M, Ho LM, Peiris JSM (2003) Effectiveness of precautions against droplets and contact in prevention of nosocomial transmission of severe acute respiratory syndrome. *Lancet* 361: 1519–1520
40 Chow KY, Lee CE, Ling ML, Heng DMK, Yap SG (2004) Outbreak of severe acute respiratory syndrome in a tertiary hospital in Singapore, linked to an index patient with atypical presentation: epidemiological study. *BMJ* 328: 195–199
41 Emanuel EJ (2003) The lessons of SARS. *Ann Int Med* 139: 589–591
42 Hughes J (2003) The SARS response – building and assessing an evidence-based approach to future global microbial threats. *JAMA* 290: 3251–3253

Index